Pain in Shoulder and Arm

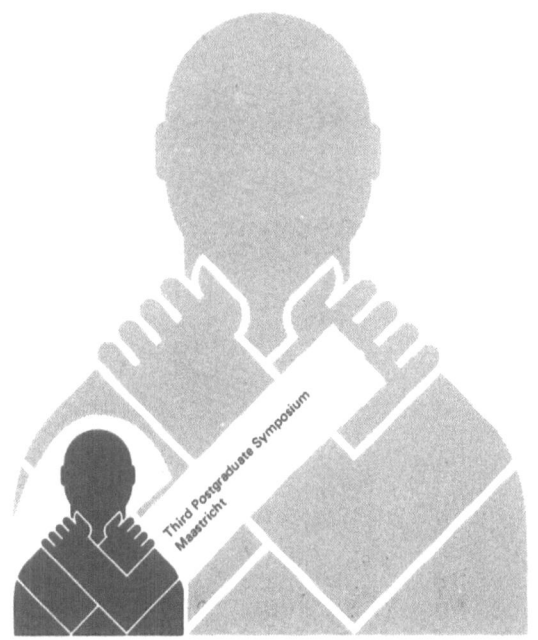

DEVELOPMENTS IN SURGERY

Volume 1

Pain in Shoulder and Arm

An Integrated View

edited by

J.M. GREEP M.D. *(Maastricht)*
H.A.J. LEMMENS M.D. *(Maastricht)*
D.B. ROOS M.D. *(Denver)*
H.C. URSCHEL M.D. *(Dallas)*

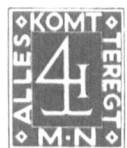

1979
MARTINUS NIJHOFF PUBLISHERS
THE HAGUE/BOSTON/LONDON

The distribution of this book is handled by the following team of publishers

for the United States and Canada

Kluwer Boston, Inc.
160 Old Derby Street
Hingham, MA 02043
USA

for all other countries

Kluwer Academic Publishers Group
Distribution Center
P.O. Box 322
3300 AH Dordrecht
The Netherlands

———————————

Library of Congress Cataloging in Publication Data   CIP

Main entry under title:

Pain in shoulder and arm.

(Developments in surgery; 1)
1. Shoulder-Diseases. 2. Arm-Diseases. 3. Pain. 4. Thoracic outlet syndrome.
I. Greep, J.M. II. Lemmens, H.A.J. III. Roos, D.B. IV. Urschel, H.C.
IV. Series. [DNLM:1. Shoulder-hand syndrome-Congresses. W1 DE998S
v. 1/WE810 P144 1978]
RC939.P34   617'.572'072   79-16449

ISBN-13: 978-94-009-9305-1   e-ISBN-13: 978-94-009-9303-7
DOI: 10.1007/978-94-009-9303-7

———————————

Preface

The "shoulder-hand syndrome" or pain in the shoulder or arm is an extremely vital subject for the multi-disciplinary approach and usually requires more than one speciality for complete evaluation. The proceedings of this symposium – organized by the department of general surgery of the University of Limburg – cover the field thoroughly with contributions from outstanding specialists from all over the world. Rheumatological, neurosurgical, orthopedic, and traumatological aspects are covered. Vascular surgeons considering both venous and arterial problems entwine with thoracic surgeons to review the thoracic outlet problem. Establishing a diagnosis in this multi-disciplinary field is extremely important and encompasses a combination of disciplines including neurology, orthopedics, surgery, and physical medicine. Likewise, the role of each contributing factor must be assessed when multiple sources were responsible for pain. In addition to adequate diagnosis, it is important to institute the appropriate therapy and to establish the proper priority and timing of such therapies. The follow-up techniques particularly regarding thoracic outlet syndrome are extremely important to provide an objective basis for evaluation.

Although many advances have been made in the field of objective diagnosis and therapy, there still is a great deal of overlap and confusion which has to be clarified.

Professor Greep and his organizing committee have done a wonderful job in composing a program covering all aspects of this field. They are to be congratulated on bringing us a "timely current status" report on pain in the shoulder and arm.

HAROLD C. URSCHEL M.D.

Acknowledgement

After the successful conference on Pain in Shoulder and Arm, held in Maastricht in 1977, we felt the necessity to present a selection of the discussed topics in book form. The selection is a result of editorial policy; the topics have been selected to cover a wide range from neurophysiology to orthopedics and general surgery. We hope that these chapters will serve the purpose of promoting an objective view of all aspects of the field of Pain in Shoulder and Arm with as goal a better care for our patients' problems.

The editors would like to thank A.R. Smith M.D., the department of medical illustrations and the secretaries of the department of surgery in Maastricht for their great help in preparing this book and last but not least all the authors for their contributions.

Maastricht, July, 1979.   J.M. Greep M.D.

Table of contents

List of contributors

D.J. Bakker M.D., Wilhelminagasthuis, The Netherlands.

M. Beaujean M.D., Institut de Chirurgie, Hôpital de Bavière, 66, Boulevard de la Constitution, 4020-Liège, Belgium

J.P. Caillens M.D., 17 Avenue de Palavas, Montpellier, France

H. Claessens M.D., University Hospital, Department of Physical medicine and Orthopedic surgery, De Pintelaan 135, B-9000 Gent, Belgium

J. Cyriax M.D. M.R.C.P., Former Orthopaedic Physician, St. Thomas Hospital, London, England

H. Denck M.D., Surgical Department, Vienna City Hospital-Lainz, Wolkersbergenstrasse 1, Austria

R. van Dongen M.D., Wilhelminagasthuis, Amsterdam, The Netherlands

J. Drewes M.D., Chirurgische Universitätsklinik 19, 4 Düsseldorf, Moorenstrasse 5, The Federal Republic of Germany

J.H. Dunant F.A.C.S., St. Jakobs Strasse 40, CH-4052 Basel, Switzerland

R.W. Gilliatt M.D., Institute of Neurology, National Hospital London, Queen Square, London WC1N 3BG, England

J.M. Greep M.D., University of Limburg, Department of Surgery, Maastricht, The Netherlands.

P. Hirschfeld M.D., Zentral Krankenhaus, Städtische Krankenanstalt, Bremen-2800, Federal Republic of Germany

B. Janevski M.D., Department of Radiology, St. Annadal Hospital, University of Limburg, Maastricht, The Netherlands

L. Kinzl M.D., University Hospital Ulm, D-79 Ulm, Federal Republic of Germany

J. van der Korst M.D., Center for Rheumatic Diseases, Slotervaartziekenhuis, The Netherlands

H.A.J. Lemmens M.D., Surgical Department, University of Limburg, Maastricht, The Netherlands

K.A.E. Meijers M.D., Department of Rheumatology,Leiden University Hospital, Leiden, The Netherlands

A. McBeath M.D., Division of Orthopedic Surgery, University of Wisconsin, Medical School, 1300 University Avenue, Madison, Wisconsin 53706, U.S.A.

G. Padberg M.D., Department of Neurology, St. Annadal Hospital, Maastricht, The Netherlands

E. Parry M.D., Broadgreen Hospital, Thomas Drive, Liverpool – 14, England

D.B. Roos M.D., P.C., University of Colorado, School of Medicine, Department of Surgery, Franklin Building Suite 7000, 2045 Franklin Street, Denver, Colorado 80205, U.S.A.

F. Spaans M.D., Department of Neurophysiology, De Wever-Ziekenhuis, Heerlen, The Netherlands.

A.R. Smith M.D., University of Limburg, Department of Surgery, Maastricht, The Netherlands.

H. Urschel M.D., Baylor University, Department of Thoracic and Cardio-Vascular Surgery, 1201 Barnett Tower, 3600 Gaston Avenue, Dallas, Texas 75246, U.S.A.

Part I
Investigation and diagnosis

1. Examination of the shoulder and treatment of shoulder pain

JAMES CYRIAX M.D.*

EXAMINATION OF THE SHOULDER

The only way to reach a diagnosis in the conditions commonly affecting the shoulder is by clinical examination. Accurate diagnosis is most rewarding, since equally accurate treatment is often immediately successful. Though lesions of bone show up radiologically, in the majority of shoulder lesions the X-ray appearances are negative or even misleading. A frequent error is to X-ray the neck and shoulder to find spondylosis on the former, and no abnormality at the shoulder joint. The symptomless stiffness at the cervical joints is then treated and the shoulder lesion left untouched owing to undue reliance on X-ray appearances. Beware of labels that do not name the tissue at fault: e.g. frozen shoulder, rotator cuff syndrome, periarthritis.

LOCATION OF PAIN

Where the pain is felt provides little help. With one exception, all tissues at the shoulder are derived in whole or in part from the fifth cervical segment. Hence, whatever the lesion a pain occupying some part of the fifth cervical dermatome is created, i.e. along the front of the arm to the radial side of the forearm. The exception is the acromio-clavicular joint, which is developed within the fourth cervical segment; pain originating there is felt at the point of the shoulder and cannot radiate to the arm.

Acromio-clavicular joint	C4
Shoulder capsule	C5
Sub-deltoid bursa	C5
Supraspinatus	C5
Infraspinatus	C5 (6)
Subscapularis	C5–6
Biceps tendon	C5–6

*Former Orthopaedic Physician, St. Thomas's Hospital, London.

J.M. Greep, H.A.J. Lemmens, D.B. Roos and H.C. Urschel (eds.).
Pain in shoulder and arm: an integrated view, 3–7. All rights reserved.
Copyright © 1979 by Martinus Nijhoff Publishers, The Hague/Boston/London.

PRELIMINARY EXAMINATION

Before examining the shoulder in detail, it is important to be sure that it is the shoulder whence symptoms originate. The routine examination of the entire length of the cervical segments is therefore carried out first from neck to fingers.

The six active neck movements are performed and, if some of them cause scapular pain, a cervical disc protrusion has to be considered. Painless limitation and radiographic evidence of osteophytosis is ignored. Then, resisted cervical rotation tests the muscles supplied by the first and second cervical roots. Scapular elevation and approximation are tested next. They assess the muscles supplied by the third and fourth cervical roots. Limited active and passive elevation indicates contracture of the costo-coracoid fascia such as occurs with apical pulmonary neoplasm. If maintained elevation brings on paraesthesia in the hands, compression of the lower trunk of the brachial plexus against a cervical or a first rib is suggested. A tight thoracic outlet also leads to disappearance of the pulse on scapular approximation.

Table 1. Cervical roots tested by resisted movements.

Cervical root	Resisted movements
C5	resisted abduction at shoulder and flexion at the elbow.
C6	resisted flexion at the elbow and radial extension at the wrist.
C7	resisted adduction at the shoulder, extension at the elbow and flexion at the wrist.
C8	resisted ulnar deviation at the wrist, adduction and extension of thumb.
T1	weakness of the small muscles of the hand. This suggests a cervical rib or a Pancoast tumour.

SHOULDER EXAMINATION

If this preliminary examination reveals no abnormality, the shoulder is examined in detail by means of twelve movements. These are:

1. *Active elevation*
   Abduction range: 90°
   Scapular rotation: 60°
   Adduction of the humerus with the acromion and coracoid processes now pointing upwards: 30° The patient states if any pain is provoked.

2. *Passive elevation*

   The doctor raises the arm as high as possible and then notes: a) range, b) end-feel, c) if it hurts. d) if so, where. In shoulder-joint lesions, the range of passive elevation should correspond to the range of active abduction, minus 60° scapular rotation.

3. *Painful area*

   The patient is asked to raise his arm up and to describe when pain starts and then stops. Pain may be felt as the arm passes the horizontal, ceasing above that level. If so, the tender tissue lies in a pinchable position, i.e., between one or other humeral tuberosity and acromion.

4. *Passive scapulo-humeral abduction*

   The doctor fixes the lower angle of the scapula with the thumb of one hand and raises the arm passively with the other until he feels the scapula start to rotate. This angle indicates the range of abduction at the shoulder-joint.

5. *Passive lateral rotation*

   The forearm is held in the saggital plane, the elbow flexed to a right angle. From this position, passive lateral rotation is carried out. Range and end-feel are noted. The normal range is 90°

6. *Passive medial rotation*

   From the same starting position the humerus is rotated medially. Again the normal range is 90°.

   There follow six resisted movements to test the function of the muscles.

7. *Resisted abduction*

   Deltoid and supraspinatus.

8. *Resisted lateral rotation*

   Infraspinatus and teres minor.

9. *Resisted medial rotation*

   Subscapularis. Latissimus dorsi, pectoralis major, teres major.

10. *Resisted adduction*

    Latissimus dorsi, pectoralis major, teres major.

11. *Resisted flexion of elbow*

    Biceps: long head

12. *Resisted extension of elbow*
   Triceps

INTERPRETATION

Four categories of lesion emerge:
1. Limited range: Capsular pattern
This means that abduction is so much limited, lateral rotation more and medial less in degree. Limited movement in the capsular pattern indicates arthritis, even if the radiographic appearance is normal. This may be traumatic, rheumatoid, monoarticular, osteo-arthrosis, chondrocalcinosis or palindromic.
2. Limited range: Non-capsular pattern
The common cause is acute subdeltoid bursitis.
3. Full passive range: One resisted movement hurts
This indicates tendinitis.
   Now accessory tests show which part of the tendon. Tendinitis cannot give rise to limited passive movement. Which movement is painful indicates which tendon is affected.

   Resisted abduction: Supraspinatus
   Resisted lateral rotation: Infraspinatus
   Resisted medial rotation: Subscapularis

   It should be remembered that a painful arc should be given second place in interpretation. If say, supraspinatus tendinitis is present. The arc indicates which part of that tendon. But the converse is not justified; for a painful arc occurs also with infraspinatus and subscapular tendinitis or localised bursitis. If a painful arc exists but no resisted movement hurts, localized subdeltoid bursitis is present.
4. Weakness: Tendon rupture or neuritis is the likely cause.
Rupture of the supraspinatus tendon leads to paralysis of active abduction and to a painful arc on passive abduction. Long thoracic neuritis prevents the serratus anterior from rotating the scapula actively. Hence voluntary elevation is 60° limited but passive full and painless. Supra-scapular neuritis leads to three week's scapular aching with painless weakness of the two spinatus muscles. In spinal accessory neuritis, active elevation is only 5° limited, but this is full and painless passively. An axillary palsy leads to no active limitation, but to marked wasting of the deltoid.

None of these diagnoses – arthritis, bursitis, tendinitis or neuritis – can be reached other than clinically.

TREATMENT

Treatment at the shoulder is extremely simple and immediately effective. Arthritis responds to intra-articular steroid injections. After the first, the pain is greatly relieved, but several more must be given at increasing intervals to keep the joint comfortable. Osteoarthrosis requires gradual stretching.

Acute bursitis responds to steroid infiltration; chronic bursitis responds equally well to local anaesthesia.

Tendinitis gets well with one or two steroid infiltrations. Massage to the tendon is also effective but takes longer to succeed.

All in all, the shoulder is extremely responsive to treatment. The only difficulty is a really accurate diagnosis.

2. Arthrography of the shoulder: technique, results, indications

J.P. CAILLENS M.D.*

ABSTRACT

Technique and results of shoulder arthrography as well as its indications are discussed on the basis of experience with more than 400 cases of shoulders with pain, limitation of motion, or instability. Opaque contrast medium was used by preference.

The results in simple painful shoulder, acute painful shoulder, frozen shoulder and rupture of the short rotator muscles are discussed. The images obtained in paralytic shoulder, rheumatoid shoulder, fractures and dislocations of the shoulder are described.

Four indications are presented: 1) diagnostic, in atrophy of the shoulder, blockage and instability; 2) preoperative, in rupture of the rotator cuff, chronic tendinitis and recurrent dislocation; 3) therapeutic, for intraarticular dilatation in frozen shoulder; and 4) medicolegal, in the etiologic assessment of shoulder atrophy.

Shoulder arthrography was first performed in 1933 by Oberholzer. This author, who had a wide experience in knee arthrography, used gaseous injections. Since then many investigators have reported their experiences with this diagnostic procedure in medical and surgical lesions of the shoulder.

Our own experience is based on more than 400 examinations in which we have most often used opaque contrast material.

TECHNIQUE

Contrast media

Radiopaque substances, which were developed in 1929, were first iodides, soon thereafter diiodides and, since 1952, triiodinated derivatives (radioselectan 60, contrix 28). Insufflations of air have been used, but capsulosynovial leakage is often observed and makes this technique less reliable.

Injection equipment

We use needles with stylets, 6 cm long and 2 mm in diameter, and three

*Rheumatology Clinic of the Medical Center, Montpellier, France.

J.M. Greep, H.A.J. Lemmens, D.B. Roos and H.C. Urschel (eds.).
Pain in shoulder and arm: an integrated view, 9–23. All rights reserved.
Copyright © 1979 by Martinus Nijhoff Publishers, The Hague/Boston/London.

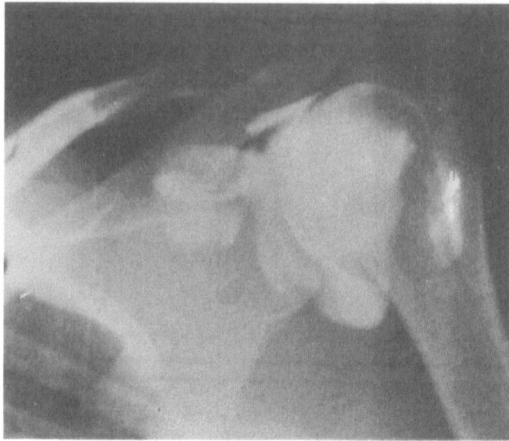

Figure 1. Normal opaque arthrography. Frontal view.

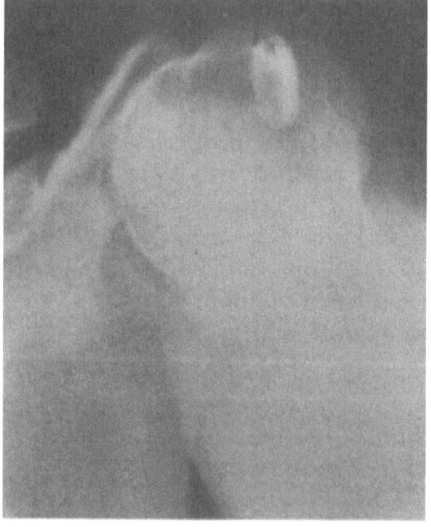

Figure 2. Normal opaque arthrography. View of bicipital groove.

syringes as follows: one of 20 ml for the contrast medium, one of 10 ml for an analgesic, and one of 21 ml for a cortisone derivative.

Radiologic equipment

We use a conventional roentgenologic installation. The puncture of the joint is done with an image intensifier under control on a television screen.

Arthrocentesis

The patient is positioned on his back and turned to his side so that his body forms a 30-degree dihedral angle with the examining table. This position opens the articular interspace to be examined. The point of injection corresponds to a dimple located 1 cm medial to the anterior part of the acromioclavicular joint, and this dimple can readily be deepened by the tip of a finger (Verpyck). Directing the needle inferiorly and anteriorly in relation to the patient, the examiner extends the analgesia of the soft tissues as he advances. Keeping the needle in the glenohumeral interstice, he readily injects a few milliliters of the analgesic. A reflux at the mouth of the needle is a sign of successful injection. Then the contrast medium is injected into the joint under control on the television screen. Successive films taken after each injection of 2 ml make progressive monitoring of the filling of the joint space possible.

Radiographic technique

The radiologic examination is essentially based on four arthrograms: three frontal views, with the humerus in the neutral position, in external rotation and internal rotation, and one lateral view. Additional views are sometimes necessary: view of the bicipital groove, the patient standing with weight-bearing arm, then with the arm in abduction against resistance; tomograms may be added, to be taken in the frontal and sagittal planes, and a 16-mm movie may be made with a camera joined with an image intensifier. Intraarticular pressures can be measured with an electronic manometer during and after the injection of the radiopaque material.

RESULTS

Normal opaque arthrography

The injected dye spreads medially over the head of the humerus as far as the anatomical neck, outlining the upper part of the articular cartilage by a fine border whose thickness diminishes from laterally to medially. The lower part of the joint space is marked by a large, rounded pouch which extends medially into the subscapular recess and laterally along the anatomical neck of the humerus. Medially, the subscapular recess of the joint space extends to the middle portion of the glenohumeral space below the coracoid process. Laterally, the tendon of the long head of the biceps with its sheath is visible like a rail of 3 or 4 cm in length.

In external rotation, the medial recess is obliterated because the serous

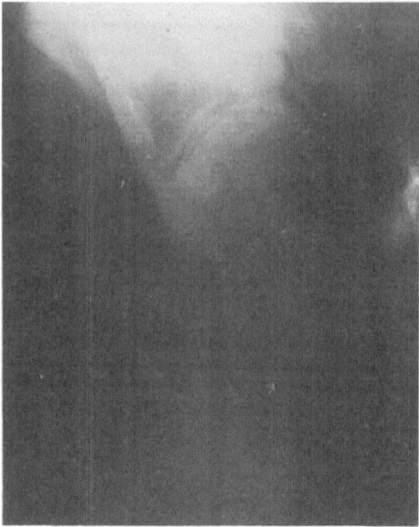

Figure 3. Normal shoulder arthrography. Lateral view. Note the prearticular translucent triangle outlining the anterior portion of the glenoid lip.

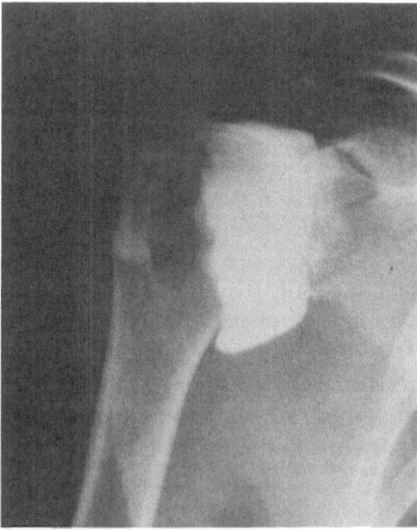

Figure 4. Periarticular calcification. Normal aspect of joint space.

bursa is compressed by the subscapularis muscle. In internal rotation, this recess is readily visualized. In the lateral view the anterior and posterior portions of the glenoid lip are seen as radiolucent triangles and the subscapular recess is in contact with the articular cavity.

Opaque arthrograms of normal shoulders never show an infiltration – even not a partial one – of the subacromial or subdeltoid bursa. While we habitually inject 12 to 14 ml of the dye, the joint space can admit up to 35 ml.

Painful and restricted shoulders

Simple painful shoulder This condition corresponds to the type of capsule described by Cyriax; there is no joint restriction. Opaque arthrography is of value: in a total of 16 cases of simple painful shoulder it revealed 8 rotator cuff tears.

Periarticular calcification. Acute painful shoulder In a certain number of cases of shoulders with periarticular calcium deposits arthrography could show the practically constant absence of any associated rupture of the short rotator muscles. In the acutely painful shoulder the limitation is of antalgic nature, and the arthrogram is normal.

Frozen shoulder There are various causes of restriction in the mobility of the shoulder. The most typical, if not the most frequent, is a contracture of the joint capsule. It is readily demonstrated by arthrography. The picture is characteristic: there is global reduction of the extent of the contrast medium, the axillary recess and the subscapularis bursa are obliterated, and the dye is less expanded over the humeral head. In most cases the biceps sheath is visible but poorly injected. During the filling of the joint space there is resistance to the injection, the increase in the intraarticular pressure being proportional to the quantity of injected material and to the degree of capsular contracture. We classify the contractures as very severe, severe, and moderate. In the very severe type the lower and medial recesses are not visualized. In the severe contractures of the capsule there is definite obliteration of the axillary recess and the subscapularis bursa. The interpretation of moderate contractures of the capsule is more difficult. The findings on the film must be evaluated in relation to the resistance upon injection or to the intraarticular pressure. In these cases, periarticular calcific deposits are as frequent as in painful shoulders in general, while signs of associated rupture of the rotator cuff are less often found. A high degree of intraarticular pressure often causes rupture of the subscapularis bursa and of the tendon sheath of the biceps.

The injection of radiopaque material into the shoulder joint results in its

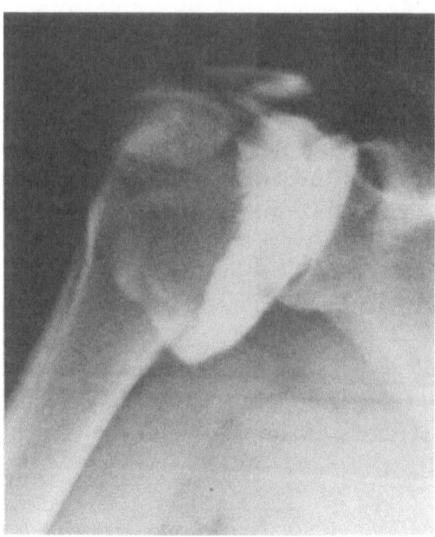

Figure 5. Slight injection of subdeltoid bursa. Small rupture of the rotator cuff.

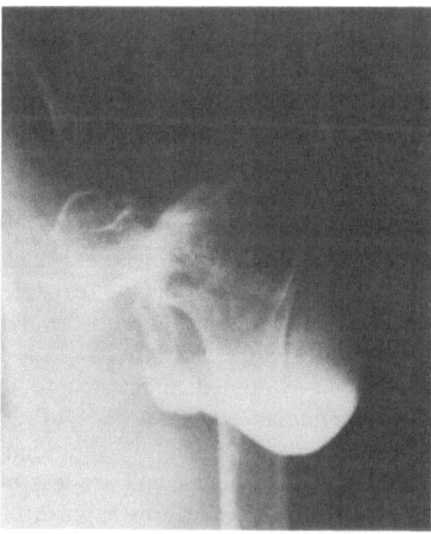

Figure 6. Rupture of long standing. Image of capsule-bursa.

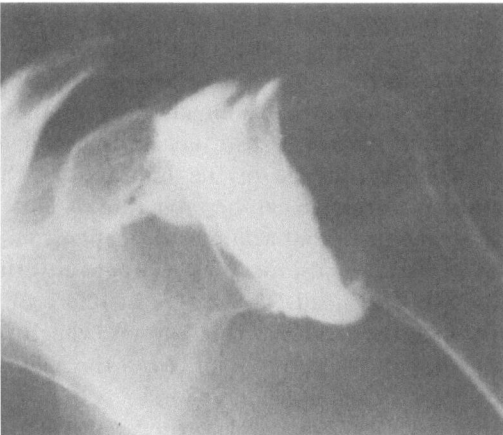

Figure 7. Frank capsular contracture. Retracted axillary recess and subscapularis bursa.

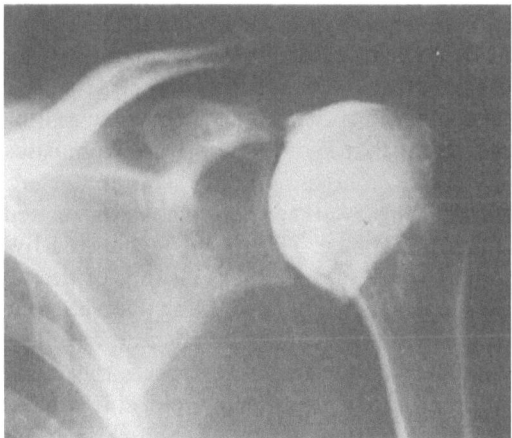

Figure 8. Severe capsular contracture. Note the disappearance of the axillary recess and of the subscapularis bursa. The biceps sheath is not injected.

dilatation, hence in a notable improvement of its mobility. This observation led Andrén and Lundberg in 1965 to raise shoulder arthrography to the rank of a therapeutic procedure. In cases of painful shoulders with limited motions opaque arthrography sometimes helps to differentiate between antalgic blockage, mechanic blockage, and blockage due to a lesion of soft tissues, such as bursitis or tenosynovitis of the long head of the biceps.

Rupture of the rotator cuff The flow of a more or less considerable amount of radiopaque liquid into the subdeltoid bursa is a fundamental arthrographic sign of rupture or avulsion of the rotator cuff tendons. The object of controversy by anatomists, later declared as a lesion by surgeons, such rupture became better known and understood thanks to arthrography. While the joint space is filling, the examiner observes the leakage of the liquid and can most often locate the tear, generally found medially to the upper facet of the greater tubercle of the humerus at the level of the supraspinatus tendon. The leakage can be moderate or large. The injection of the bursa is always complete but volume and expansion may vary. The subdeltoid bursa filled with liquid looks like a cupule covering the top and lateral aspect of the humeral head. The degree of filling of the subdeltoid bursa is proportional to the degree of the rupture which may vary from small to large. At the upper part of the joint cavity the leakage of the liquid may produce the image of a button hole or a niche in the shape of a burning flake and indicating an incomplete rupture.

An irregular and abundant filling as well as an early spreading of the dye reveal an important tear which is always observed in rotator cuff ruptures of long standing.

The axillary and subscapular recesses are usually normal. However, they may be contractured, thus revealing the combination of a rupture and a retraction of the capsule. Calcific deposits are found less often together with ruptures. There is a correlation between arthrographic and plain roentgenographic signs to the extent that it often limits the diagnostic indications for arthrography. Among the roentgenographic signs is Leclerc's sign, i.e. the elevation of the humeral head, either spontaneous or elicited by abduction of the humerus against resistance. The sign is recognized by the narrowing of the humeroacromial space and by the widening of the lower portion of the scapulohumeral space according to Welfling. De Sèze and his coworkers have shown that the elevation of the humeral head is followed by signs of humeroacromial and scapulohumeral arthrosis, the result – at times asymptomatic – of rotator cuff rupture. An old cuff rupture (Serre), often bilateral and symmetric, is marked by such arthrosis which has often reached an advanced stage. We deal here with a precise etiology of scapulohumeral arthrosis as opposed to osteoarthritis of the shoulder, which is in general not associated with degenerative involvement of the rotator cuff.

In the etiology of the painful shoulder the long head of the biceps plays a particular role. The frequency of its involvement in the rupture of the rotator cuff has been observed by many authors. Lesions of the biceps can be demonstrated by arthrography, but the interpretation of the signs is not always easy. Anomalies in the filling of the tendon sheath, features of rupture of the short rotator muscles, and capsular retractions in the anterior type of painful shoulder have been reported. In dislocation or subluxation of the long head of the biceps arthrography affords often very conclusive results.

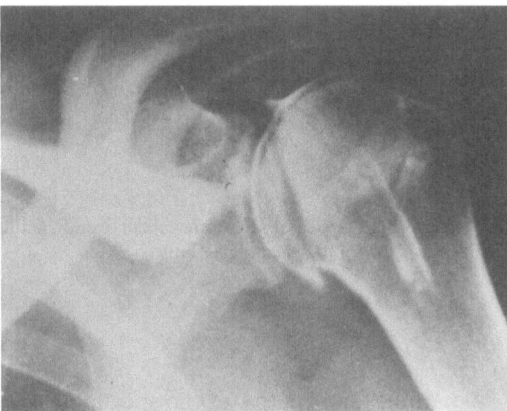

Figure 9. Arthrographic image of severe capsular contracture with medial leakage of contrast medium due to high pressure.

The rheumatoid shoulder

Little information is available on arthrography of the rheumatoid shoulder except for that by Ennevaara who in 1967 published an extensive study on 200 arthrographies.

Localized or diffuse synovitis Filling defects appear as rounded patches, fairly well defined and of varied sizes, and revealing the presence of synovial pannus. the joint capsule appears "moth-eaten" and its outline is poorly defined. This aspect may be localized in the zone of attachment of the capsule to the humerus, or there may be diffuse synovitis.

Biceps sheath anomalies Ennevaara recognizes the following features: poor and uneven filling, non-filling, signs of adhesion between the tendon and its sheath, "ampulla" sheath, and tear of the sheath.

Capsular contracture Images of capsular retraction have been observed by all authors. Their frequencies range from 16 to 37%.

Lesions of the rotator cuff Tears of the rotator cuff occur often. The most frequent type is complete perforation which occurs in between 19 and 54% of the cases, depending upon the statistics. The finding of a tear in a cuff raises the question of its relationship with rheumatoid involvement. In the opinion of many authors ruptures are independent of rheumatoid arthritis, whereas Ennevaara ascribes an etiological role to this disease.

Involvement of the shoulder joint is part of the clinical picture in rhizomelic joint disease of the elderly. Images of capsular retraction as well as of cuff rupture may be found and arthrograms are nonspecific.

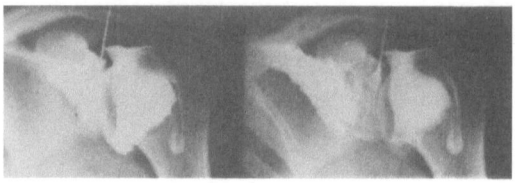

Figure 10*A*. Dilated join space in moderate capsular contracture.
B. Tear at the level of the subscapularis bursa.

The paralytic shoulder

Flaccid paralysis A painful neuropathy of the shoulder is at times difficult to distinguish from a syndrome of periarthritis, particularly if in the latter there is loss of abduction. Indeed, the loss of power of the shoulder may be of neurologic origin or may be due to a rupture of the rotator cuff. Theoretically (de Sèze), a cuff rupture which results in pseudoparalysis of the abductor muscles with conservation of the deltoid and without atrophy or reflex sensory changes is in all points different from paralyses which are associated with a global deficit including atrophy of the muscles, sensory and often reflex changes. Moreover, differences between the two syndromes are found by conventional roentgenography, arthrography and electro-diagnostic procedures. However, in practice the differentiation between rupture and paralysis is not always that simple: the circumstances of onset are often similar and the traumatism in particular is apparently inconsequential. A dislocation of the shoulder may initiate either condition. The sequence of events may cloud the clinical picture of rupture and atrophy may develop.

With a radiographic examination of the shoulder an assessment can be made of possible traumatic lesions of bones and joints. X-rays can discover indirect trophic signs of rupture frequently observed after the age of 50, presenting the problem of differentiating it from a neurologic lesion. Similarly, a complete rupture may be discovered in a patient with a neurologic lesion of traumatic origin.

However, opaque arthrography remains of great diagnostic value. Normal findings will support the neurologic etiology of the disturbance.

The hemiplegic shoulder Shoulder pain is the most frequent complication of hemiplegia and is often quite disabling. In patients with hemiplegia of various etiologies we have found normal arthrograms in one-fourth of the cases, all others having capsular contractures, often quite pronounced. This great frequency is not astonishing. Indeed, hemiplegia is a well-known cause of the syndrome of periarthritis. The retraction of the capsule is a manifestation of painful reflex dystrophy which occurs early or late in the condition.

Sequelae of obstetric paralysis Opaque arthrographies were taken of the shoulder joints of 13 children (9 boys, 4 girls) between 6 and 16 years of age (average age 9 years) with obstetric paralysis. The arthrograms of 10 shoulders were frankly pathologic. In each case the image was asymmetric as compared with the contralateral arthrogram. There was definite diminution of the axillary recess and the subscapularis bursa, presenting the typical picture of capsular contracture. The contracture was severe in 4 cases, moderate in 6. It was associated with flattening of the humeral head, well seen in the lateral projection, and clinically with limitation in abduction and external rotation. Contracture of the capsule is frequently present among the late sequelae of obstetrical paralysis. We have no doubt that it is characterized by its arthrographic image and by the phenomenon of reflux due to the high intraarticular pressure. These findings are related to a frequently observed limitation of passive motions of the glenohumeral joint. This fact is of practical significance for the treatment of the shoulder with birth palsy. It illustrates the importance of passive mobilization in all directions. The therapeutic plan that we use is that of the frozen shoulder due to capsular contracture.

Dislocations and fractures of the shoulder

Acute dislocation Opaque arthrography reveals a capsular leakage at the level of the lower recess. Acute dislocation being a frequent cause of cuff rupture, arthrography enabled Reeves to differentiate capsular rupture from capsular detachment. The latter requires a longer immobilization of the shoulder, whereas in the former the shoulder may be mobilized as early as one week after the accident.

Recurrent anterior dislocation Frontal arthrograms are characterized by an expansion of the articular limits and contours. The capacity of the joint is always increased and amounts sometimes to over 40 ml. In the lateral projection a recurrent dislocation is characterized by the disappearance of the radiolucent triangular area which corresponds to the anterior portion of the glenoid lip. The great frequency of cuff lesions in traumatic dislocations in people over the age of 50 should be underlined, as well as its rarity in recurrent dislocations.

Posterior dislocation The rare occurrence of posterior dislocation and the difficulty to diagnose it have often been mentioned. Arthrography reveals

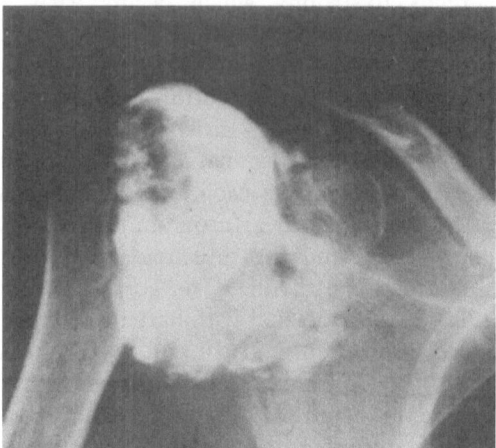

Figure 11. Diffuse synovitis in rheumatoid arthritis. Tomentose aspect of synovial membrane and uneven capsular attachments.

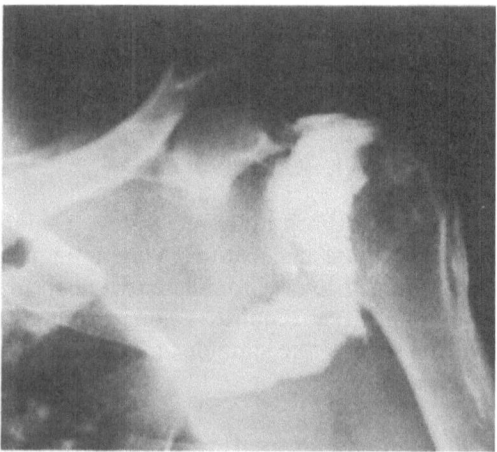

Figure 12. Sequelae of anteromedial dislocation. Note the considerable leakage of dye at the level of the lower recess.

the disappearance of the image of the posterior glenoid lip and a large posterior pouch.

Recurrent posterior dislocation   In most cases of this condition the clinical diagnosis is obvious. Radiographic assessment substantiates the posterior displacement of the humeral head past the glenoid cavity. At times there is aplasia of the glenoid cavity. Opaque arthrography reveals hyperlaxity of the joint, the presence of a large posterior pouch, and the absence or poor visualization of a radiolucent triangle posteriorly.

Fractures Fractures of the greater tubercle of the humerus, whose displacement is often missed for lack of an axillary view, are often responsible for severe capsular retraction consecutive to prolonged immobilization. An associated rupture of the rotator cuff may be detected.

Fractures of the surgical neck are first accompanied by pseudoparalysis of the shoulder and inferior subluxation of the humeral head. Secondarily, following a period of often too long immobilization, pronounced retraction of the capsule ensues.

INDICATIONS

The indications for shoulder arthrography are limited according to many authors. Indeed, the clinical assessment of shoulder lesions is at present well established. Indirect radiologic signs of tendinous involvement lead to recognize the condition of the rotator cuff. The medical treatment, rehabilitation procedures, and the clinical course of the syndrome under the effects of these therapies suffice in most cases to confirm the part played by the capsule in a blockage or that of a tendon in a functional deficiency.

There are at present four types of indications.

Diagnostic

In the presence of atrophy of the shoulder area there are immediate diagnostic problems in which arthrography is a diagnostic adjuvant of great – even irreplaceable – value. A normal arthrogram speaks in favor of the neurologic origin of the atrophy. Evidence of a rupture combined with a neurologic deficiency must be noted and only arthrography can substantiate the degree of the lesion.

Limitation of motions and blockage are frequent indications. The role played by the contracture of the capsule in the stiff and painful shoulder can initially be assessed only by arthrography. This procedure can also help to evaluate the condition of the cuff and of the bicipital sheath.

An unstable shoulder, often observed in young patients, should lead the examiner to look for an anterior or posterior subluxation, a glenoid lip syndrome, and a dislocation or subluxation of the long head of the biceps. Intraarticular foreign bodies can be demonstrated and their position localized by this examination.

Preoperative

In the preoperative evaluation rupture of the cuff, chronic tendinitis or recurrent dislocation arthrography is indispensable. Indeed, numerous authors believe in particular that a shoulder with atrophy should not be operated upon without prior arthrographic examination.

Therapeutic

Our personal experience, although of short duration, fully confirms Lundberg's conclusion of the double value of arthrography: it gives us a record of the degree of capsular contracture and it shortens the duration of treatment of the frozen shoulder.

Medicolegal

In the medicolegal evaluation of an atrophy, in order to assess the role played by the rupture of the short rotators due to a traumatism, on the one hand, and that by a degenerative process, on the other, arthrography of both shoulders is indicated.

CONCLUSION

Shoulder arthrography is a simple procedure which can give valuable information. Two main types of images can be recognized: 1. images of addition (leakage) in ruptures of the rotator cuff or of the synovial capsule, and 2. images of subtraction (filling defects) in capsular contractures. The value of arthrography is to be underlined in the diagnosis of atrophy of the shoulder, scapulohumeral blockage, instability, and intraarticular foreign body. Arthrography is part of the preoperative evaluation of a cuff rupture, a tendinitis, and a recurrent dislocation. The intraarticular dilatation affords an indisputable improvement in the mobility of the joint and is particularly indicated in cases where manipulations under general anesthesia are not feasible. Finally, arthrography is of medicolegal value, particularly in cases of atrophy of the shoulder.

Arthrography brought a large share to the knowledge of scapulohumeral pathology. It contributed very much to the understanding of the painful and stiff shoulder. In certain fields of medicine as well as in orthopedic surgery the recognition of its value is likely to increase.

REFERENCES

1. L. Andren, B.J. Lundberg. Treatment of rigid shoulders by joint distention during arthrography Acta orthop. scand. 36: 36–45, 1965.
2. J-P. Caillens. L'arthrographie de l'epaule. Paris, Masson Edit. 1 vol, 148, 1974.
3. J-P. Caillens, Y. Jarrousse. Place de la dilatation intra-articulaire au cours de l'arthrographie opaque dans le traitement des rétractions capsulaires serrées. In Actualités en Rééducation Fonctionnelle et Réadaptation, 2ème série, Paris, Masson Edit. 116–118, 1977.
4. H. Serre, L. Simon, M. Vialla, J-P. Caillens. Mesure des pressions intra-articulaires au cours de l'arthrographie de l'épaule. Rev. Rhum. 31: 377–383, 1964.
5. S. de Sèze, H. Ryckewaert, H. Caroit, A. Hubault, G. Poinsard, J.C. Renier, J. Welfling. Les ruptures traumatiques de la coiffe des rotateurs. Revue du Rheum. XVII, 11:443–453, 1960.

3. Angiography of the upper extremity

B. JANEVSKI M.D.*

ABSTRACT

Angiographic technique for the investigation of the arteries of the upper extremity is described, this includes modifications of the methods for percutaneous catheterization as well as the use of vasodilators for peripheral hand angiograms. The conclusions are based on the author's own experience in 730 selective studies of the arteries of the upper extremities.

A brief review of the angiographic findings in the different vascular conditions affecting the shoulder and arm is included, with examples from the author's own series. In addition, an attempt is made to differentiate thromboangiitis obliterans from arteriosclerosis obliterans based on roentgenographic findings.

During the past 20 years the angiographic investigation of the upper extremity has been in full motion. New techniques of examination have been developed. Various types of procedures have been performed under increasingly satisfactory technical conditions. Better and less toxic contrast media have become available.

The engineering achievement at the present time has certainly made possible greater progress in vascular radiology, than in other branches of medicine. Angiography is now generally considered to be the most important special radiological procedure for the diagnosis of vascular abnormalities of the upper extremity. Selective vasodilatation, high-volume injections of contrast media and subtraction technique, have improved the diagnostic value of angiography and led to better understanding and more precise therapy for a varity of vascular morbid conditions, particularly of the hand and the thoracic outlet region.

EXAMINATION TECHNIQUE

There are different techniques used for subclavian and brachial angiography at the present time:

*Department of Radiology, St Annadal Hospital, University of Limburg, Maastricht, The Netherlands.

J.M. Greep, H.A.J. Lemmens, D.B. Roos and H.C. Urschel (eds.).
Pain in shoulder and arm: an integrated view, 25–48. All rights reserved.
Copyright © 1979 by Martinus Nijhoff Publishers, The Hague/Boston/London.

- catheterization transfemoral technique (Seldinger)
- brachial cut-down technique
- percutaneous brachial artery puncture
- retrograde axillary puncture with antegrade positioning
- of the catheter (Hawkins and Hudson)

It is up to the radiologist to decide what kind of technique to use in each individual case.

In the majority of cases subclavian and brachial angiography are performed by passing the catheter percutaneously via the femoral artery by the Seldinger technique. In a very small number of cases, usually older patients with tortuous arteriosclerotic arteries or stenosis and occlusion of the femoral and iliac vessels, surgical exposure of the brachial artery is needed. In our department, in such cases the brachial cut-down technique is the method of choice.

For catheterization of the right and the left subclavian arteries, the congenital variations in the origin of the aortic arch vessels must be kept in mind.

Since most subclavian artery stenoses occur at, or distal to the first rib, and in maximal abduction of the arm the subclavian compression appears at the same place, the catheter has to be left just proximal to the first rib, but beyond the origin of the vertebral artery and thyrocervical trunk (Figures 1A and 1B). Because of the important neurotoxicity of the contrast media, the cathetertip in subclavian arteriography has to be placed distal to the origin of the vertebral artery and thyrocervical trunk, otherwise a large volume of contrast material reaches the brain and the cervical spinal cord. For the same reason only water-soluble methylglucamine salts of contrast media are used. (Methylglucamine Metrizoate = Isopaque cerebral or Meglumine Ioxitalamate = Telebrix 30.)

Radiographs are first taken of the upper chest and shoulder in a neutral position; with the upperarm along the thoracic wall. Sixteen cubic centimeters of Telebrix 30 meglumine or Isopaque cerebral with an injection rate of 8 ml per second, are injected over a period of four seconds. The injection is made by an automatic pressure injector. The roentgenograms in this study, six in total, are made by a serial film-changer, with a frequency of two exposures per second, for the first four films, and one exposure per second for the next two seconds.

In patients with thoracic outlet compression syndrome, a second series of radiographs has to be taken with the upper arm in a provocative position. The patient is asked sequentially to abduct the arm, turn and extend the head and take a deep breath until one or all of these manoeuvers result in damping or obliteration of the radial pulse. Sometimes other manoeuvers have to be used, for the same purpose (the simple hyperabduction manoeuver; Adson test; modified Adson test and the Allen test). The total

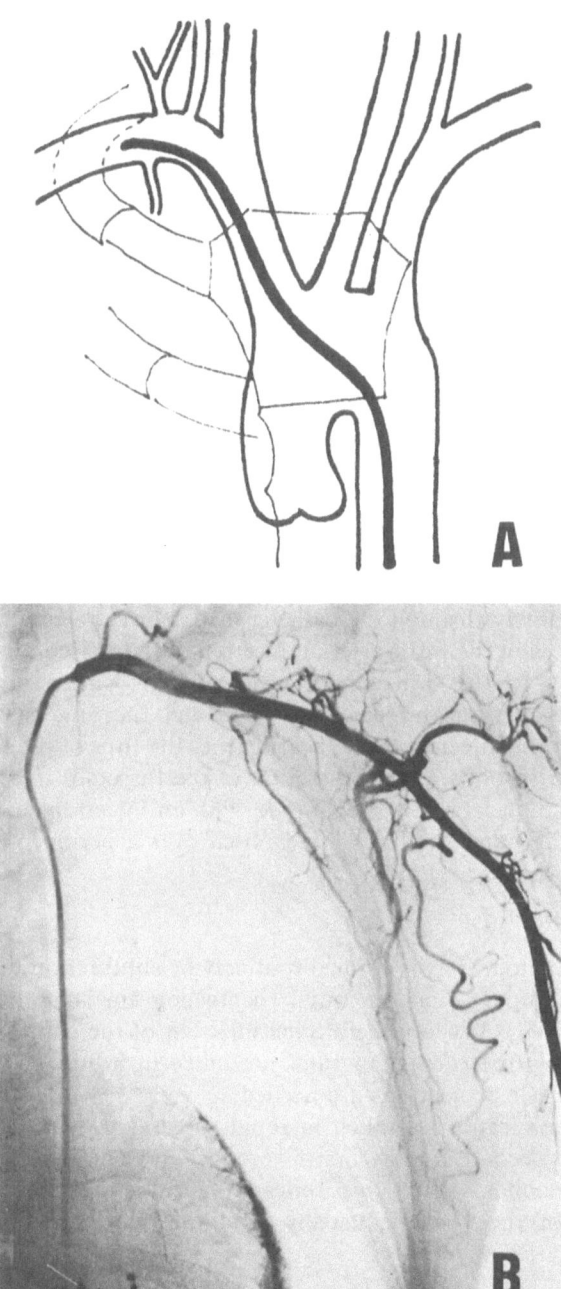

Figure 1*A*. Correct position of the catheter in right subclavian arteriography.
B. Left subclavian arteriogram in neutral position. Note the optimal filling of the left shoulder and upper arm arteries, but no opacification of the left vertebral artery.

volume of contrast material and the frequency of the exposures are exactly the same as in the previous study.

Where a severe compression or complete obstruction of the subclavian artery exists, the total volume of contrast medium should be diminished. Otherwise, because of the obstruction, a large volume of contrast goes to the cerebral vessels (Figures 2A and 2B). In brachial angiography the catheter has to be advanced as deep as possible, usually in the distal part of the brachial artery, 5 to 10 cm up to the antecubital fossa (Figure 3). This position of the catheter is possible, only if a normal anatomy of the brachial artery exists, namely if the bifurcation of the brachial artery in radial and ulnar artery is below the elbow joint. In case of high bifurcation the cathetertip has to be left proximal to the bifurcation, otherwise the possibility exists of super-selective injection in one of the forearm arteries. These arteriograms we called territorial arteriograms (Figures 4A and 4B).

For a good visualization of the digital arteries, a vasodilator has to be injected intraarterially, prior to contrast injection. For this purpose we use 20 mg tolazoline hydrochloride (Priscol) diluted with normal physiologic saline up to 20 ml for one site angiography. The vasodilator has to be injected very slowly through the catheter, usually over a period of 100–120 seconds. Following the intra-arterial injection of the Priscol a characteristic local reddening of the skin can be observed. The patient usually feels a slight warmth over the forearm, the palm and the fingers. The contrast medium should be injected, as the heat reaches the tops of the fingers, which is about 10–15 seconds after completion of the Priscolin injection. A total volume of 18 ml Telebrix 30 meglumine, with an injection rate of 5 ml per second is injected and the films are exposed over a period of 8 seconds.

Roentgenography

The brachial angiography is studied routinely by subtraction technique. The program is set up so that an initial roentgenogram is obtained for sub-traction purposes 0.3 second before the injection of the contrast material is begun. Normally the roentgenograms are taken in frontal (AP) projection, occasionally other projections are needed.

The roentgenograms are taken in rapid succession, with a frequency of three films per second, for the first 3 seconds, and one film per second for the next 5 seconds. With this series of roentgenograms an optimum angiography of the hand is usually obtained, with good filling of the arteries, capillaries and veins.

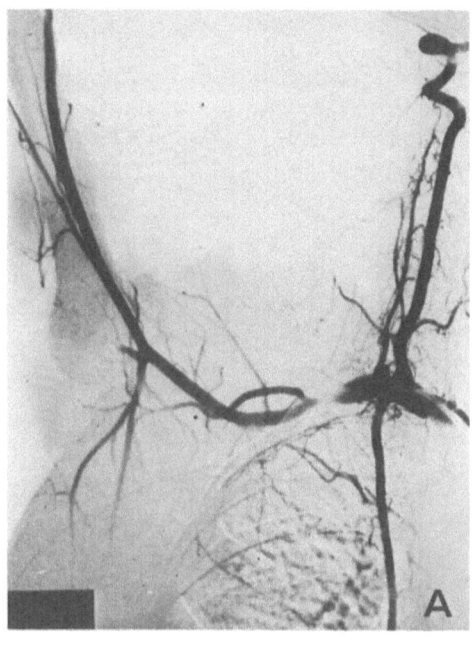

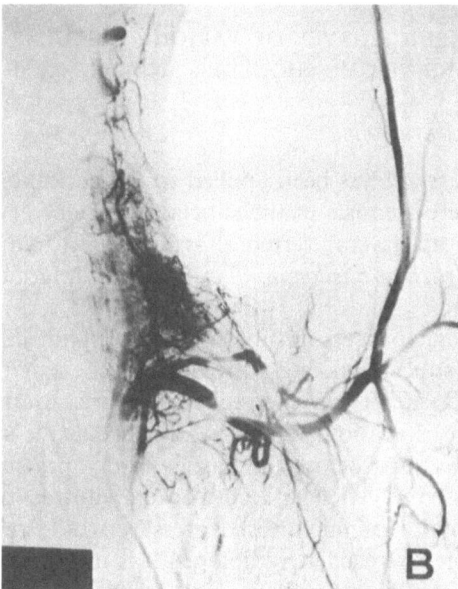

Figure 2*A* and *B*. Right and left subclavian arteriograms in hyperabduction. Severe costo-clavicular compression of the subclavian arteries, a large volume of contrast goes to the vertebral artery and thyrocervical trunk, due to the compression.

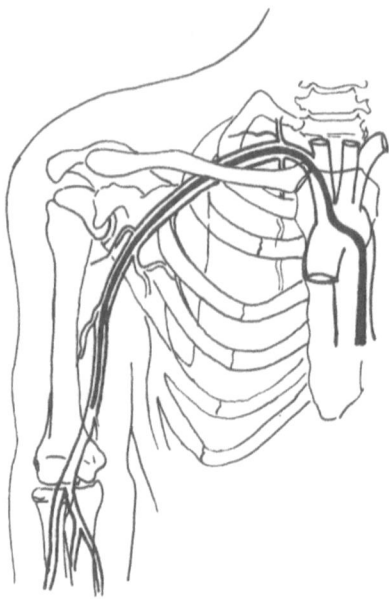

Figure 3. Final position of the catheter in right brachial angiography.

A BRIEF ANGIOGRAPHIC SURVEY OF VARIOUS VASCULAR MORBID CONDITIONS OF THE SHOULDER AND THE ARM

The subclavian steal syndrome

The term *subclavian steal* has been applied to the condition whereby either obstruction, or severe stenosis of the subclavian artery at its origin causes reversal flow in the ipsilateral vertebral artery, often followed by cerebral arterial ischemia. *Brachial-basilar insufficiency* is an alternative term for the same syndrome.

The basic pathologic process in subclavian steal syndrome is an occlusion or a stenosis of the subclavian artery proximal to the origin of the vertebral artery. Occlusive disease at this site reduces the pressure in the subclavian artery distal to the obstruction. When the pressure at the subclavian end of the vertebral artery drops below the basilar artery pressure, the vertebral artery flow is reversed. Reivich and co-workers showed that a subclavian pressure 10% less than systemic arterial pressure would reverse flow in the vertebral artery. For the vascular radiologist it is important to know that a 50% reduction in the lumen of the subclavian or inominate artery is necessary to produce the critical pressure gradient of 10%.

Patients with subclavian steal syndrome may be asymptomatic; however, cerebral symptoms or complaints referable to the arm are more frequent.

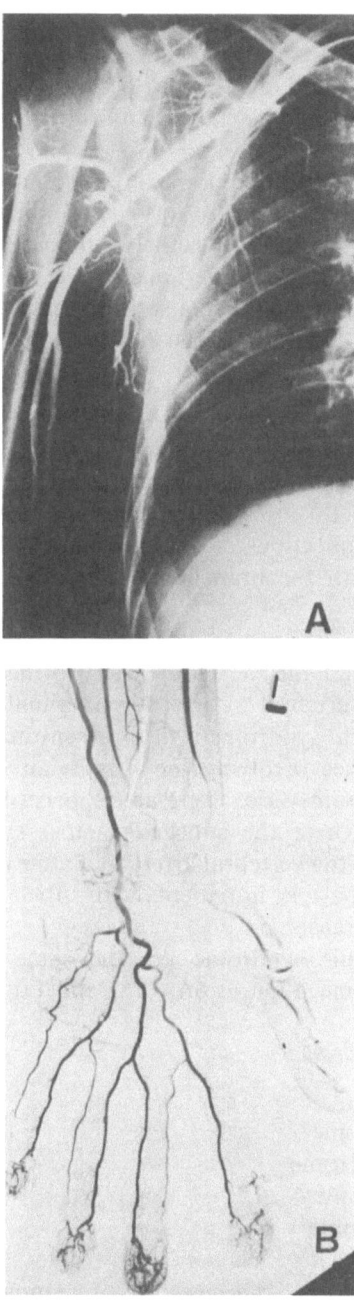

Figure 4*A*. High bifurcation of the brachial artery.
B. Territorial arteriography of the ulnar artery.

Intermittent or constant pain of the affected extremity, precipitated initially by increased activity of the arm, paresthesia and weakness. Basilar artery insufficiency is characterized by vertigo, occipital headache, ataxia, inco-ordination, loss of equilibrium, syncope and transitory attacks of bilateral blurred vision.

The most suitable angiographic procedure to demonstrate the retrograde vertebral flow in subclavian steal is aortic arch aortography. Injection of contrast material with pressure injector in the ascending aorta permits visualization of prograde flow in the nonstenotic vessels immediately after injection, and the late films will demonstrate reverse flow down the vertebral artery and into the subclavian artery (Figures 5A and 5B).

Thyrocervical steal syndrome

This syndrome has previously been reported as a variant of the subclavian steal syndrome. It means filling of the subclavian artery distally from the stenosis by reversal flow through the branches of the thyrocervical trunk, as a result of anatomic connections of the muscular branches of the vertebral and carotid arteries with the branches to the thyrocervical trunk in the neck.

The *thyrocervical steal* is present in patients with total occlusion of the subclavian artery beyond the vertebral artery orifice, namely subclavian stenosis distal to the vertebral artery, but proximal to the thyrocervical trunk. Thyrocervical steal syndrome is also present in patients with arteriosclerotic occlusive disease involving the subclavian artery as well as the vertebral artery on the same side. There are reports of this syndrome in the literature in patients where the subclavian steal syndrome was treated surgically by ligation of the vertebral artery and after operative damage and ligation of the vertebral artery in patients with subclavian steal undergoing neck surgery for other reasons.

The symptoms in this syndrome are the same as in patients with subclavian steal syndrome (Figures 6A, B, C and D).

The thoracic outlet syndrome

Cervical rib syndrome
Scalenus anticus syndrome
Costo – clavicular syndrome
Hyperabduction syndrome
Pectoralis minor syndrome

The term, *thoracic outlet syndrome* was recommended by Rob and Standeven in 1958. It is a general term for a number of neurovascular syndromes which have in common compression of the brachial plexus,

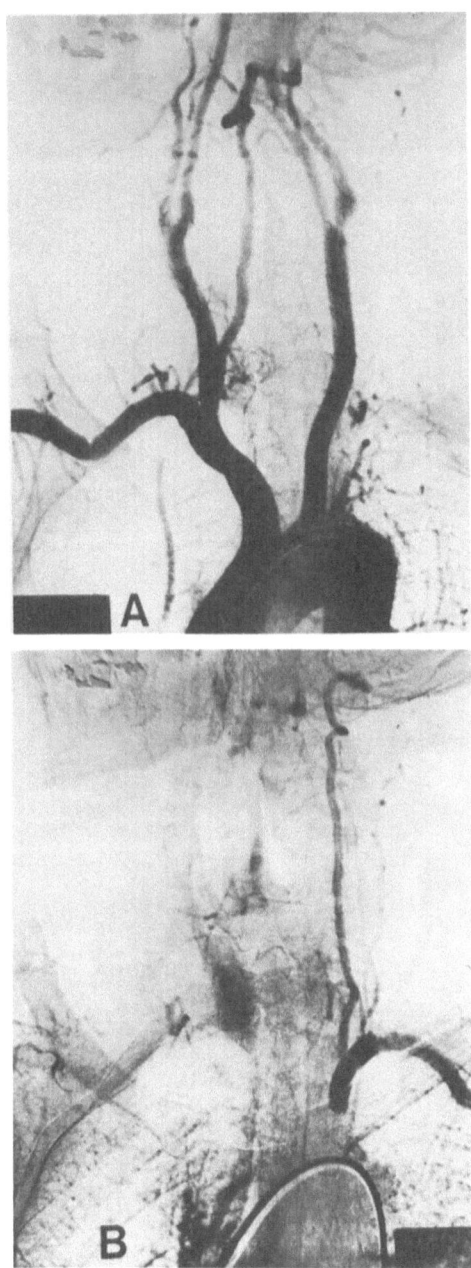

Aortic arch aortography.

Figure 5A. Simultaneous opacification of the right subclavian artery and carotid arteries. There is no opacification of the left subclavian artery.

B. Late and retrograde opacification of the left subclavian artery from the left vertebral artery. There is an occlusion of the proximal intrathoracic portion of the subclavian artery.

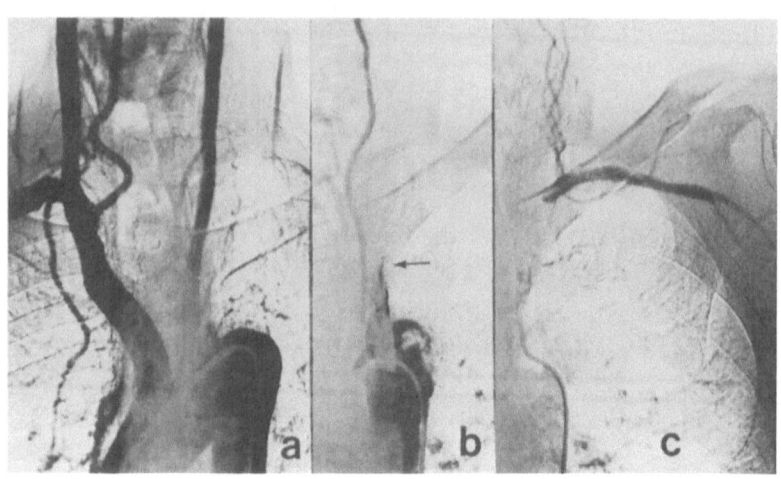

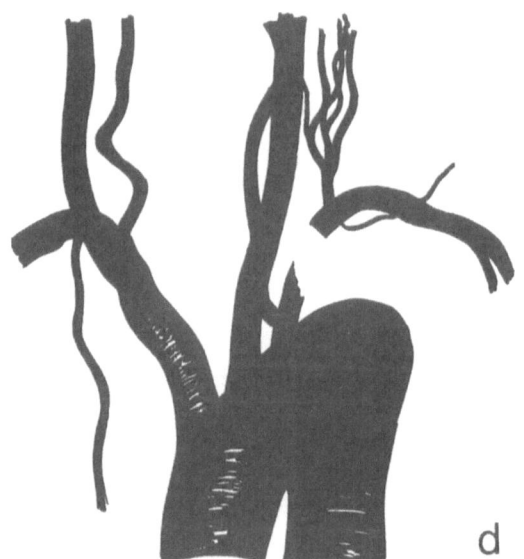

Figure 6A. Aortic arch injection demonstrates filling of both carotids and both vertebral arteries. No filling of the left subclavian artery.

    B. Selective injection in the orifice of the left subclavian artery demonstrate a normal filling of the left vertebral artery. There is a total obliteration of the left subclavian artery (arrow) just beyond the vertebral take off.

Figure 6C. Later film in sequence, demonstrates filling of the left subclavian artery, by retrograde flow through ascending cervical branches of the left thyrocervical trunk.

    D. Schematic diagram of angiographic findings in the reported case.

subclavian artery or vein at the superior aperture of the thorax. The scalenus anticus syndrome; Costo-clavicular syndrome; Cervical rib syndrome and hyperabduction syndrome were first grouped under the term *thoracic outlet compression.*

The pathophysiology of the thoracic outlet syndrome rests upon the fact that as the brachial plexus and the subclavian artery and vein leave the neck and chest on their way to the upper extremity, they travel through a common tunnel. The roof of this tunnel consists of the clavicle and the floor of the first rib. When these bony structures, or their membranous ligaments contract toward each other, the brachial plexus, the subclavian vein and the subclavian artery are compressed. The degree of the compression force and its location will determine what symptoms are produced. It should be noted that any of the three structures (vein, artery and nerve) may be compressed by these bony-ligamentous structures selectively or in combination. Therefore, this syndrome can produce vascular symptoms, neurologic symptoms or a combination of both. The neurologic symptoms are, early in this condition more frequent than the vascular.

Neural symptomes include tingling, numbness or pain in the arm, hand shoulder and neck, especially following abduction of the arm.

Routine X-ray studies should include chest, cervical spine and shoulder. The chest X-ray for example, may reveal a superior sulcus (Pancous) tumor invading the brachial plexus, mimicking outlet compression. Cervical ribs, an elongated C7 transverse process, bifid first ribs, exostosis of the first rib, or malformed ribs, clavicular deformity such as a tumor or callus due to fracture, can also be seen on the chest and spine X-ray. Presence of these abnormalities helps to confirm the diagnosis, but they are not definitely diagnostic.

The thoracic outlet syndrome is fairly common in adults. The pre-operative diagnosis of the exact location and a etiology of the arterial lesion is important to the surgeon attempting correction of the causes for this syndrome.

Patients with thoracic outlet compression syndrome can be divided into two groups: a) Patients with *static* arterial compression and permanent vascular changes, and b) those who have only *dynamic*, inconstant arterial compression and no permanent vascular changes (Figure 7A and 7B). The patients with static arterial compression are generally subjects with congenital bony abnormalities of the first rib or clavicle. In those patients the most important complications of the thoracic outlet syndrome may usually be found, namely stenosis of the subclavian artery with post-stenotic dilatation (aneurysm), total occlusion of the subclavian artery or vein, and in the digital arteries at the ipsilateral site, and distal arterial occlusions (thromboembolisms) (Figures 8, 9, and 10A, B).

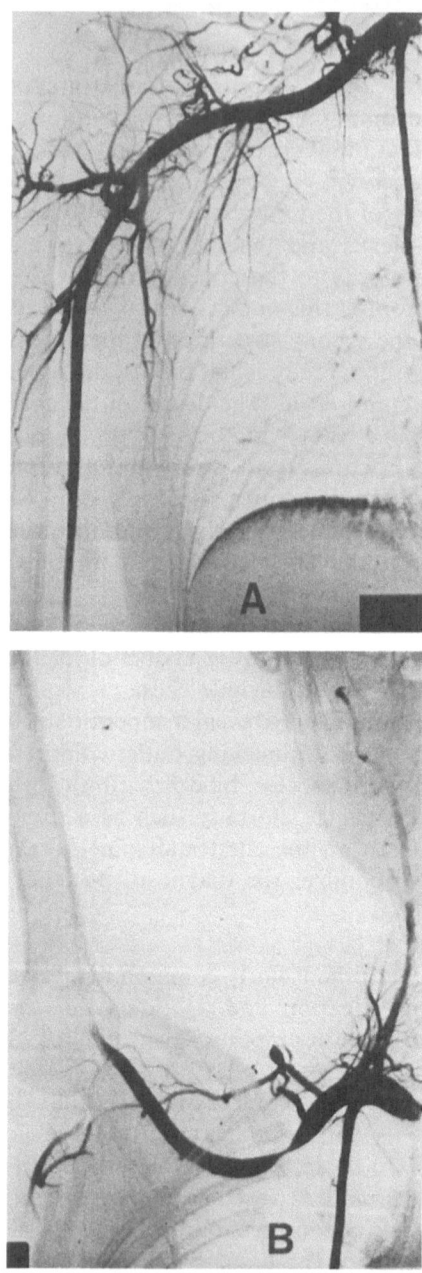

Dynamic, inconstant arterial compression

Figure 7*A*. Normal right subclavian arteriogram performed in neutral position of the arm.
B. Severe costo-clavicular compression of the subclavian artery during hyperabduction-external rotation test.

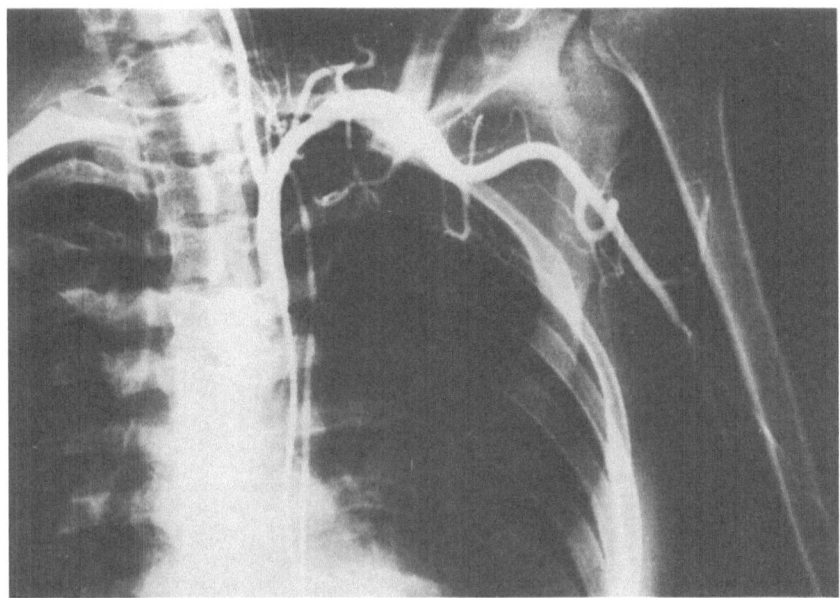

Figure 8. An arteriogram of the left subclavian artery in neutral position demonstrates post-stenotic dilatation (fusiform aneurysm) caused by static compression from a rudimentary cervical rib.

The vascular complaints in these patients are generally always present. The symptoms may be divided into arterial and venous. Intermittent compression of the subclavian artery produces; numbness, coldness, weakness and blanching. Venous symptoms range from oedema and stiffness of the fingers to venous engorgement in certain elevated positions. The periferal arterial thromboembolism causes ischemic symptoms in the hand.

The hypothenar hammer syndrome

This post-traumatic digital ischemia is a clinical entity, characterized by varying degree of digital ischemia from traumatic occlusion of the ulnar artery. The main cause of the ulnar artery injury is repetitive blunt trauma to the palm. The syndrome is often found in individuals subjected to occupational trauma, mechanics, lathe-operators, metal workers and others.

The ulnar artery bifurcates into superficial and deep palmar branches in a groove (Guyon's tunnel) bounded medially by the pisiform bone and hook of the hamate, and dorsally by the transverse carpal ligament. For its proximal 2 cm it is vulnerable to injury, lying superficially in the palm, covered only by skin, subcutaneous tissues, and the palmaris brevis muscle.

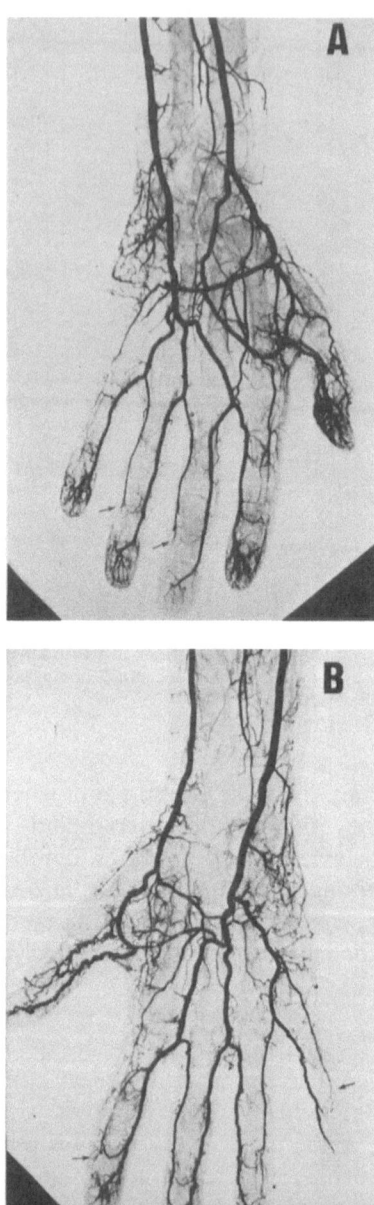

Figure 9*A*. Hand arteriograms in two patients with static arterial compression at the thoracic outlet.
B. Both arteriograms demonstrate post embolic occlusions of the proper digital arteries (arrows).

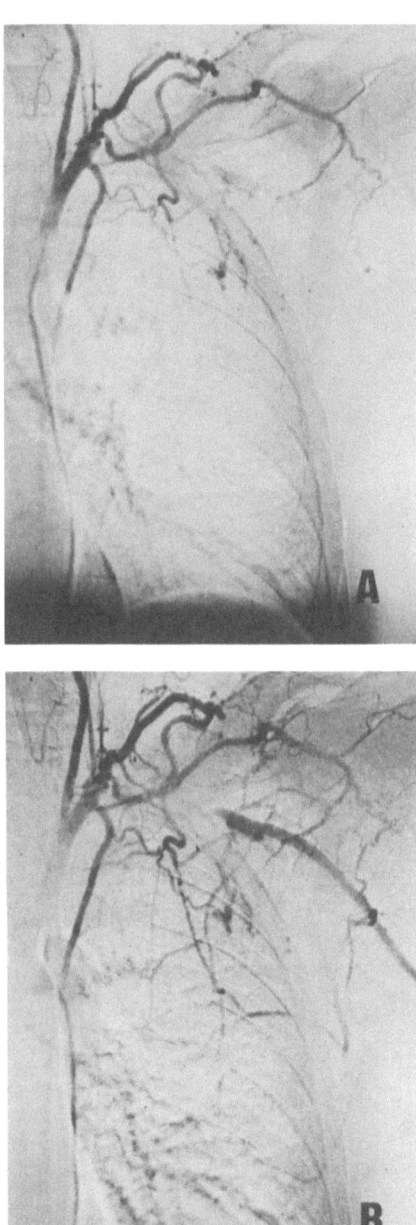

Figure 10*A* Early arterial phase of the left subclavian arteriogram shows a total occlusion of the subclavian artery, as a complication of thoracic outlet compression syndrome.
B Late arterial phase shows filling of the axillary artery through collaterals.

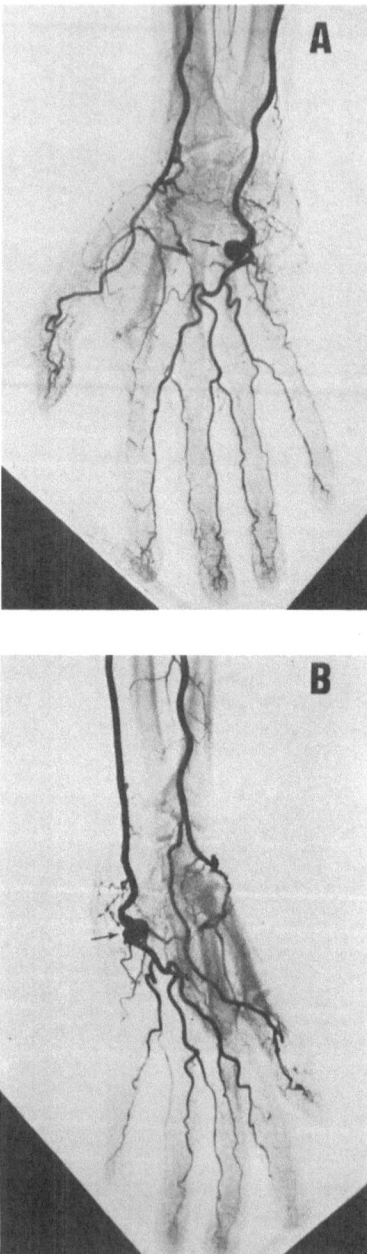

Figure 11. Arterial aneurysm (arrow) at the typical site in patient with history of repetitive blunt trauma to the palm.

The hook of the hamate serves as an anvil against which the ulnar artery is hammered. In the majority of cases the superficial palmar branch of the ulnar artery is the main source of blood to the fingers. An incomplete palmar arch or poor anastomosis between the superficial and the deep palmar arches apparently predisposes to digital ischemia, when trauma to the hand occurs. Thus the presence of ischemic symptoms following occlusion of the ulnar artery, or its superficial palmar branch depends upon the completeness of the arch as well as upon the size and number of collaterals from the terminal branches of the radial artery. An incomplete arch with few collaterals is obviously more vulnerable (34).

The clinical symptoms of ulnar artery occlusion include varying degrees of digital ischemia, numbness, paresthesia, stiffness, coldness, blanching, pain on effort and very rarely atrophic ulcerations of the fingers. The middle and the ring fingers are most frequently involved.

The possibility of hypothenar hammer syndrome should be considered in patients with unilateral Raynaud's phenomenon, ischemia of the fingers, or a hypothenar mass which may or may not be pulsatile. Obtaining an occupational history of chronic palmar trauma, coupled with the presence of a radial artery pulse and evidence of ulnar artery occlusion (positive Allen test) make the diagnosis likely.

The main reason for ulnar artery injury, as I mentioned before is repetitive blunt trauma to the palm, resulting in spasm, thrombosis, or aneurysm formation. Minor repetitive trauma may only produce distal ulnar arterial spasm. Thrombosis of the ulnar artery will occur if the intima is damaged, but if the major site of damage of the arterial wall is the media, then a true palmar aneurysm can develop. Thus, spasm, arterial occlusion, and aneurysm of the distal part of the ulnar artery are the most characteristic angiographic findings in this syndrome (Figures 11 and 12).

Thromboangiitis obliterans (Buerger's disease)

Thromboangiitis obliterans was originally described by Leo Buerger in 1908. The essential observation in this clinical syndrome consists of peripheral limb ischemia very often occurring in male cigarette smokers, with onset in the third or fourth decades of life. Women and nonsmoking men rarely manifest the syndrome. The etiology is unknown.

The pathologic process of Buerger's disease originates in small arteries of the extremities. It is a nonspecific inflammation associated with thrombosis in the vessels. In 42% of the cases the arteries of the upper limbs are involved.

Angiography in patients with Buerger's disease has a certain value, although diagnostically the angiographic pattern of diseased vessels is not entirely specific. The most important arteriographic findings are distal

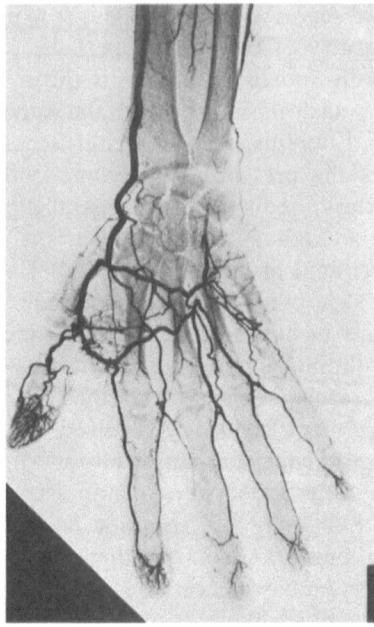

Figure 12. Occlusion of the ulnar artery in the wrist. Only slight digital ischemia (fourth and little) fingers, because of the completeness of the superficial and deep palmar arches.

arterial occlusions associated with small tortuous collaterals. The proximal parts of the occluded vessels and the apparently uninvolved vessels are smooth with regular lumen (Figure 13A).

These angiographic features may also be found in arteriosclerosis. The only difference between thromboangiitis obliterans and arteriosclerosis obliterans rests upon the fact, that arteriosclerosis is a diffuse process with involvement of almost all vessels of the upper extremity. Arteriosclerotic vessels are generally narrowed with irregular lumen and have a tortuous course (Figure 13B). The tortuousity and irregularity of the arterial walls, are the main angiographic differences between these two entities. Nevertheless, arteriosclerosis obliterans remains radiologically the chief problem in the differental diagnosis.

Arterio-venous shunt in hemodialysis (Cimino-Brescia fistula)

Angiography is a readily available examination for evaluation of operatively constructed arterio-venous fistulas in hemodyalisis patients. Brachial angiography is indicated when arterial supply of the hand has to be

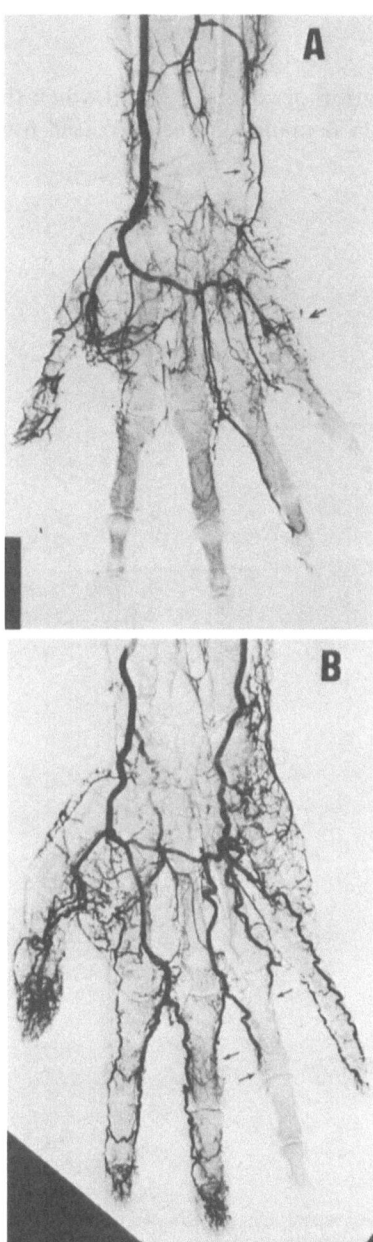

Figure 13.A Right hand arteriogram. Abrupt occlusion of the ulnar artery and almost all proper digital arteries. The proximal portions of the vessels have smooth walls, and regular lumen. Typical small tortuous (corkcrew) collaterals (arrows). They are diagnostically non-specific, we see them often in patients with arteriosclerosis.

B Right hand arteriogram with arteriosclerosis obliterans, occlusion of the proper digital arteries of the third and fourth fingers (arrows). Markedly tortuousity and irregularity of almost all other common and proper digital arteries.

estimated; when cannulation of veins is difficult, when thrombosis is suspected or when a new fistula is planned after decreased function of an old one
(Figure 14).

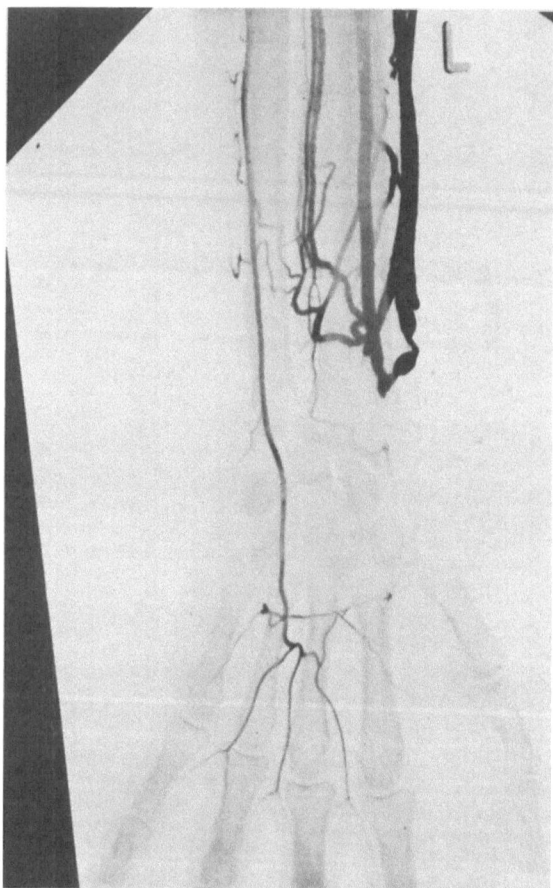

Figure 14. Left brachial angiography. Cimino-Brescia fistula between the radial artery and
cephalic vein. The shunt is functionally good. Note; slight hypertrophy of the radial artery and
a minimal narrowing of the artery proximal to the fistula, may be due to perivascular scarring,
or to angulation of the artery due to elongation. Such artery stenosis does not impair blood
flow significantly.
    The artery distal to the fistula is not filled. Non-filling of this part of the artery might
indicate obstruction of the artery, but is most probably a sign of retrograde flow toward the
fistula by collaterals from the ulnar and interosseous artery.
    There is also a stenosis of the vein a few mm. proximal to the fistula. It is probably caused
by venous spasm or angulation of the vein due to elongation.

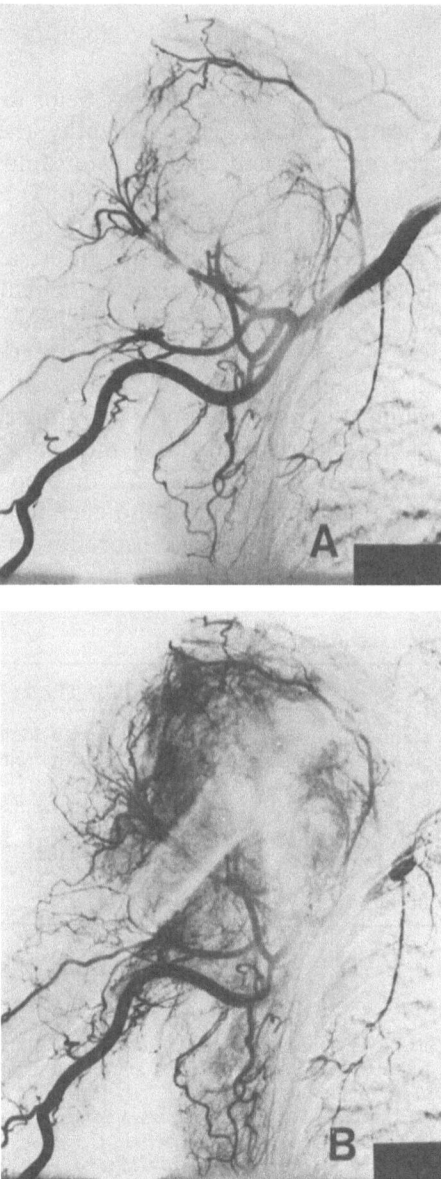

Large hypervascular soft-tissue tumor of the right shoulder.

Figure 15*A* Arterial phase, demonstrates hypertrophic feeding arteries.
   B Capillary phase shows typical capillary stain in the tumor. No arteriovenous shunts within the tumor and no early opacification of the draining veins, these signs suggest benignancy of the tumor. Pathohistologically: Inflammatory tumor, no evidence of malignancy.

Soft-tissue tumors

Angiography in hypervascular soft-tissue tumors, helps to detect the tumor, to define its exact location and extent, to identify the feeding arteries, localize the area to be biopsied and demonstrate tumor recurrence after previous excision.

The hypervascular tumors of the upper extremity can be malignant and benignant. The literature which exists on this subject suggests that angiography although with some limitations, might be helpful in differentiating benign from malignant lesions. The angiographic features of malignancy include demonstration of neovascularity, namely irregular tumor vessels, arterio-venous shunting within the tumor and diffuse vascular staining and rapid filling of the draining veins. The tumor stain in the capillary phase can demonstrate areas of avascularity, due to hemorrhage or necrosis, and provide a guide for selection of an optimal site for biopsy.

Most of these angiographic features have also been found in some benign hypervascular soft-tissue tumors, such as neurofibromas, hemangiomas, absceses, acute and chronic cellulitis and myositis (Figure 15).

Table 1. Hypervascular tumors.

Malignant	Benign
Malignant giant cell tumor	Hemangioma
Fibrosarcoma	Neurofibroma
Liposarcoma	Abscess
Rhabdomyosarcoma	Acute cellulitis
Synoviasarcoma	Chronic cellulitis
Spindle-cell sarcoma	Myositis.
Extraosseous osteogenic sarcoma	
Malignant fibrous histiocytoma	

REFERENCES

1. L. Donald, Arey Jr. Subclavian steal syndrome. J. Florida M.A. 1005–1009.
2. A.P. Vincent Jr., H. LeVeen. The Subclavian Steal Syndrome. Collective Review 9, nr. 1: 51–75, january, 1970
3. G. Knox, R. Howard, E. Robert. The Subclavian Steal Syndrome. Postgraduate Medicine 38: 608–613, 1965
4. C.D. Hafner. Subclavian Steal Syndrome. Arch Surg. 111: 1073–1030.
5. A.E. Van Voorthuisen, T. De Roo, A.G.M. Beelen. Omkering van de bloedstroom in de arteria vertebralis en the "Subclavian Steal Syndrome" Ned. T. Geneesk. 109, II: 1705–1715, 1965
6. O.J. Molloy, E. Wyn Jones. Management of the Subclavian Steal Syndrome Thorax 21: 347–354, 1966
7. Marvin B. Weber; Pitfalls in the Diagnosis of Subclavian Steal IMJ 13, number 3: Sept. 1969

8. J. Allen, J. McCracken. Subclavian Steal Syndrome. The jounral of the Arkansas Medical Society 64: 422–423, 1968
9. N. Finkelstein, A. Byer, B. Rush Jr. Subclavian-Subclavian Bypass for the Subclavian Steal Syndrome Surgery 71: 142–145, 1972
10. S. Marumoto, T. Sawayama. Subclavian Steal Syndrome. Japanene Circulation Journal 30: 379–383, 1966
11. I. Mandelbaum, D. Nahrwold. Spontaneous Resolution of Traumatic Subclavian Steal Syndrome. Annals of Surgery; 314–317, 1967
12. S. Silverblatt. Proximal Subclavian Artery Stenosis. Florida M.A., October 1975; 62: 28–33, 1975
13. K. Clark, O. Perry. Carotid Vertebral Anastomosis: An Alternate Technic for Repair of the Subclavian Steal Syndrome. Annals of Surgery 163: 414–416, 1966
14. M.J. Jennings. A Case of The Subclavian Steal Syndrome. The Medical Journal of Australia; 1149–1151, Dec. 10, 1966
15. P. Nemor Jr., S. Bahabozorgui, D. Wagner. Brachial-basilar Insufficiency and The Subclavian Steal Syndrome. Journal of Thoracic and Cardiovascular Surgery 50 Nr. 4. 534 544, 1965.
16. F. Arevalo, B. Katzen. Bilateral Subclavian Steal Syndrome. Am. J. Roentgenology 127: 668–669, 1976
17. J. Hardy, J.H. Conn, W. Fain. Nonatherosclerotic Occlusive Lesions of Small Arteries. Surgery 57: 1–13, 1965
18. M. Conrad, J. Toole, R. Javeway. Hemodynamics of the Upper Extremities in Subclavian Steal Syndrome. Circulation. 32: 346–351, 1965
19. R.J. Trevino; Thyrocervical Steal Syndrome. Arch Otolaryngology; 92; 177–180, 1970
20. R. Mueller, V. Hinck. Thyrocervical Steal; Radiology. 101 nr. 1, 1967.
21. M. Selman, W. McAlpine, The Thoracic outlet Syndrome, The Ohio State Medical Journal 908–911, Sept. 1969
22. E. Lang. Arteriography and Venography in the Assessment of Thoracic Outlet Syndromes. Southern Medical Journal 65: 129–136, 1972
23. E. Lang. Scalenus Anticus and Pectoralis Minor Syndrome. Journal of The Indiana State Medical Association, pp. 440
24. S. Mathes, A. Salam. Subclavian Artery Aneurysm, sequela of thoractic outlet syndrome. Surgery 3: 506–510, 1974
25. D.S. Mulder, F.A.H. Greenwood. Posttraumatic Thoracic Outlet Syndrome. The Journal of Trauma, 13, nr. 8; pp. 706–715
26. T. Sadler Jr., G. Rauner, G. Twombley. Thoracic Outlet Compression; The American Journal of Surgery 130: 704–706, 1975
27. W. Cox, R. Buker. first rib resection for thoracic outlet compression syndrome; American Family Physician 9: 140–146, 1974
28. T. Tomsick, R. Ahistrand, T. Kiesel. Thoracic Outlet Syndrome associated with rib fusion and cervicothoracic scoliosis. Journal of Canadian Association of Radiologists 25: 211–213, 1974
29. J. Conn. Thoracic Outlet Syndromes. Surgical Clinics of North America 54, No. 1: 155–164, 1974
30. M. Agran, A. Kratzman, M. Lazarek. Thoracic Outlet Syndrome. The Journal of Medical Society of New Jersey; 70, No. 10: 734–735 1973
31. E.D. Telford, S. Mottershead, M. England. Pressure at the Cervico-Brachial Junction. The Journal of Bone and Joint Surgery 30, No. 2, May 1948, 249.
32. E. Lang. Arteriographic Diagnosis of Neurovascular Compresson Syndromes. Journal of Louisiana State Medical Society 121, No. 6: 196–197, 1969
33. R. Kaminski, R. Barnes. Critique of the Allen Test for Continuity of the palmar arch assessed by doppler ultrasound. Surgery, Gynecology & Obstetrics 142: 861–864 1976
34. T. Yao, C. Gourmos. A Method for Assessing Ischemia of the Hand and Fingers. Surgery, Gynecology & Obstetrics, 135: 373–378 1972
35. J. Bergan, J. Conn. Severe Ischemia of the Hand. Annals of Surgery 173 No. 2: 301–307

36. W. Dale, M. Lewis. Management of Ischemia of the Hand and Fingers. Surgery, 67, No. 1: 62–79, 1970
37. S. Shionoya, I. Ban. Diagnosis, Pathology, and Treatment of Buerger's Disease. Surgery 75, No. 5: 685–700 1974
38. S. Wessler. Buerger's Disease Revisited. Surgical Clinics of North America 49, No. 3: 703–713, 1969
39. L. Ekelund, S. Laurin. Comparison of a Vasoconstrictor and a Vasidilator in Pharmaco-angiography of Bone and Soft-Tissue Tumors. Radiology 122: 95–99, 1977
40. D. Levin, D. Gordon. Arteriography of Peripheral Hemangiomas. Radiology 121: 625–630, 1976
41. I. Yaghmai. Malignant Giant Tumor of the Soft Tissue: Angiographic Manifestations. Radiology 120: 329–331, 1976.
42. L. Flores. Dacron arterio-venous shunts for Vascular Access In Hemodialysis Trans. Amer. Soc. Artif. Int. Organs 19: 33, 1973
43. J. Royle, K. Dawborn. The Use of Radiology in The Management of Patients with Arterio-Venous Shunts; The Medical J. of Australia 1: 529-531, 1972
44. G. Abouna. Brachial Arterio-Venous Shunts for Hemodialysis and Extracorporal Procedures, Europ. Surg. Res. 5: 390–400, 1973
45. J. Gothlin, E. Lindstedt. Swelling of The Arm in Patients With Arteriovenous Fistular. British Medical Journal 629–630: Sept. 1974
46. J.A. Bussell, J.A. Abbott. A Radial Steal Syndrome with Arteriovenous Fistula for Hemodialysis. Annals of Internal Medicine 75: 387–394, 1971.
47. K. Benedict, Jr., W. Chang. The Hypothenar Hammer Syndrome; Radiology 111; 57–60, April 1974
48. J. Conn, J. Bergan. Hypothenar Hammer Syndrome: Posttraumatic Digital Ischemia; Surgery 68: 1122–1128, 1970

4. Neurophysiological investigation of the arm

F. SPAANS M.D.*

ABSTRACT

Electromyography and electroneurography (together usually referred to as "EMG") provide us with objective data on muscle and nerve function. The utility of these techniques in patients with complaints of arm and shoulder is explained. The author stresses the need for EMG in patients with long lasting brachialgia, especially when surgical treatment at any level is being considered. Frequently compression of the median nerve in the carpal tunnel causes aspecific complaints which falsely may suggest a lesion at a more proximal level.

INSTRUMENTATION

In electromyography and electroneurography recordings are made of the electrical activity of muscles and nerves. Figure 1 shows the basic components of a typical electromyograph. The muscle or nerve potentials are picked up either by a needle electrode or surface electrodes. The output of the amplifier is connected to different monitoring devices: In the first place an oscilloscope. From the oscilloscope screen recordings can be made with a camera. Registration with penwriters as used in EEG investigations are inefficient, because the frequency response of a pensystem is insufficient for an undisturbed recording of action potentials. Only in kinesiologic investigations can such registrations be used.

In routine EMG the potentials are interpreted from the screen without making a permanent record. Acoustic monitoring of the potentials is an important aid for the investigator.

A special tape recorder may be used to retain the registrations for further analysis or demonstration. The most common electrode used for intramuscular recording is the concentric needle electrode (Figure 2). It consists of an inner platinum wire which is insulated from a hypodermic or intramuscular steel needle surrounding it. The tip of the wire serves as the different electrode and the steel canula as the indifferent electrode. The potential differences between them are registrated.

*Department of Neurophysiology, De Wever Hospital, Heerlen, the Netherlands.

J.M. Greep, H.A.J. Lemmens, D.B. Roos and H.C. Urschel (eds.).
Pain in shoulder and arm: an integrated view, 49–62. All rights reserved.
Copyright © 1979 by Martinus Nijhoff Publishers, The Hague/Boston/London.

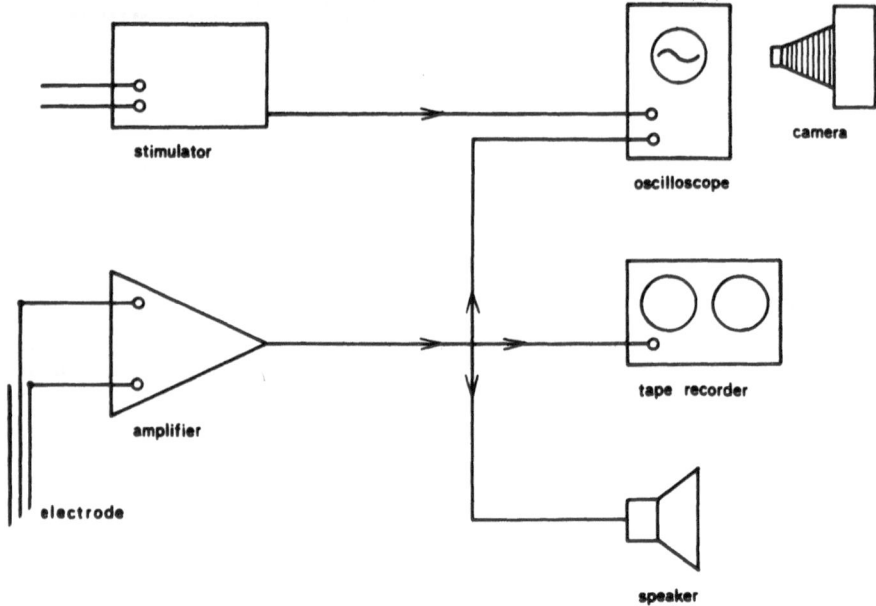

Figure 1. Block diagram of a typical EMG configuration.

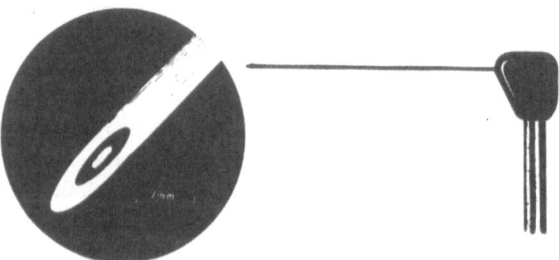

Figure 2. Concentric needle electrode. (DISA 9013–K.0032)

THE ELECTROMYOGRAM

It is obvious that with the needle electrode described above we cannot penetrate a single muscle fibre. The diameter of muscle fibres normally ranges from 25 to 100 micron. The electrode is placed between muscle fibres belonging to a number of anterior horn cells. An anterior horn cell with its axon and the connected muscle fibres is called a "motor unit." When the anterior horn cell fires, all the muscle fibres that belong to the unit will contract almost simultaneously. With the needle electrode we then register a motor unit potential (Figure 3).

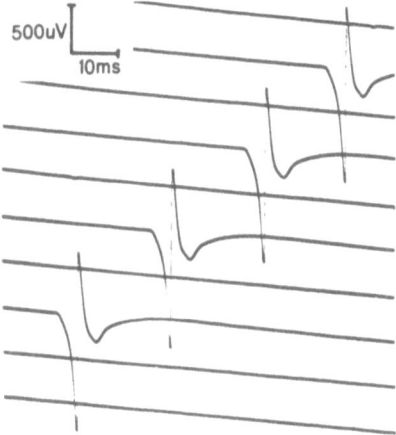

Figure 3. Motor unit potential. The shapes of the consequetive potentials are identical. This proves that the activity of one and the same unit is registered, and that the potential is not the result of the activities of more than one motor unit.

Duration, amplitude and shape of the action potentials can be determined, which is important in several EMG studies, but can be left out of consideration, here.

Normal muscle at rest is electrically silent. On light contraction individual action potentials can be distinguished. During maximal effort no single unit potentials can be identified.

Figure 4 shows the EMG with a slower sweep speed during various rates of muscle contraction. The first trace is called a single pattern, the third trace is an interference pattern and the activity pattern between those two traces is called a mixed pattern. In every normal muscle an interference pattern can be obtained. However this also depends on the cooperation of the patient. Lack of cooperation is not necessarily a matter of malingering. Pain sensations may withhold a patient from optimal contraction.

A very important pathological sign that cannot be influenced by the cooperation of the patient are potentials that may appear in the resting muscle. They have a characteristic shape (Figure 5) and produce characteristic sounds. The small spontaneous potentials are called fibrillation potentials. They are diphasic or triphasic, the third phase being of very small amplitude. Their duration ranges from 1 to 5 m sec and the accompanying sound from the loudspeaker is sharp and crisp.

They are usually combined with positive sharp waves that are often followed by a low negative phase of longer duration. (Positivity is always directed downward in neurophysiology.) The first phase of the fibrillation potential is also positive. The total duration of the positive potentials is longer than that of the fibrillations, usually exceeding 10 msec.

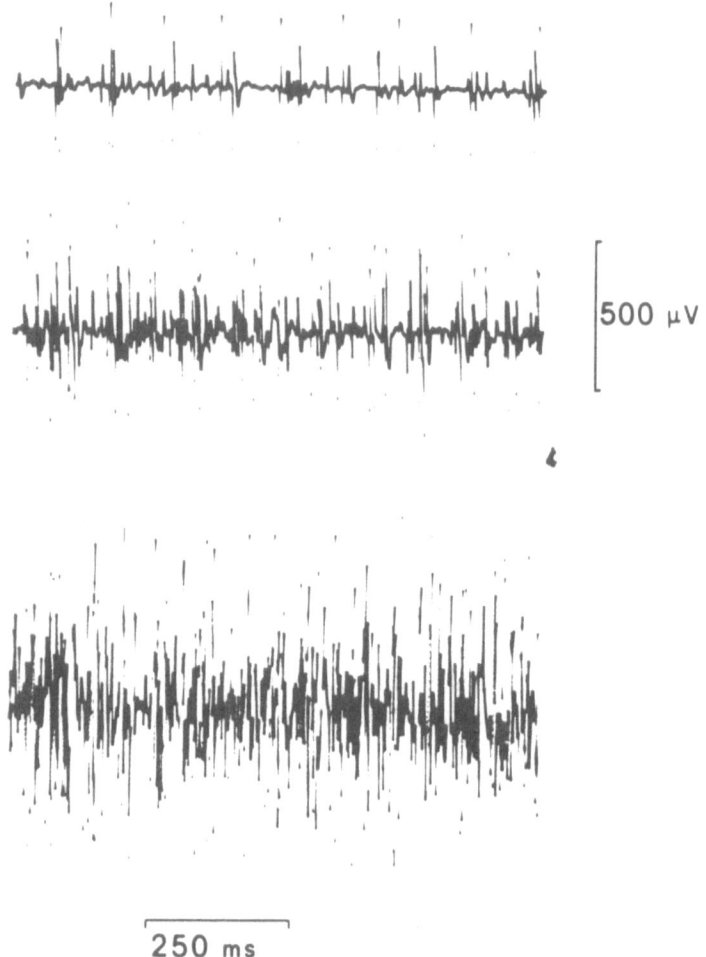

Figure 4. Activity patterns of a normal muscle during slight, moderate and maximal volitional contraction.

Fibrillation potentials and positive sharp waves are usually the results of a degeneration of motor axons. Together they are often called denervation potentials. They are associated with fine twitchings of the muscle fibres which however are not visible through the skin. They may be seen in the tongue in cases where the hypoglossal nerve is damaged, because the mucous membrane covering the tongue muscle is thinner. So the interruption of an axon is not synonymous with complete cessation of the "electrical life" of its muscle fibres. Denervation potentials do not appear at

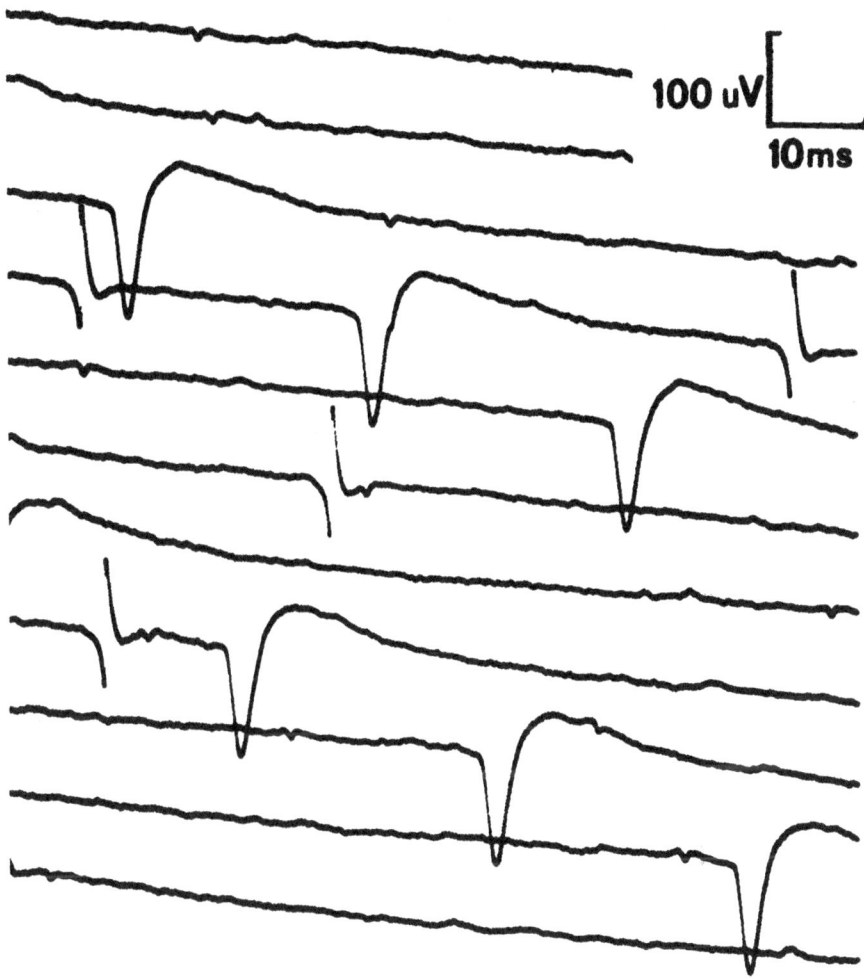

Figure 5. Positive sharp waves and fibrillation potentials.

once, but only 15 to 20 days after the interruption of the axon. They may persist for many years if no reinnervation takes place. Denervation potentials may occur in a number of rare primary muscular diseases, but when we find them in a case of brachialgia we know that there must be axonal damage. From the combination of muscles that show denervation potentials we can often estimate the lowest possible level of the lesion. The lesion must be proximal to the nerve branch of the most proximal affected muscle.

NERVE CONDUCTION MEASUREMENTS

A very important aid in determining the site of the nerve lesion is the testing of nerve conduction in various sections of the nerve. In most nerves motor and sensory fibres are combined. We usually cannot therefore measure motor conduction velocities directly from the nerve. For the estimation of motor conduction velocities we chose an intrinsic hand muscle innervated by that nerve to record the muscle potential evoked by electrical stimulation of the nerve at two sites (Figure 6). The nerve can be stimulated with needle electrodes or with surface electrodes.

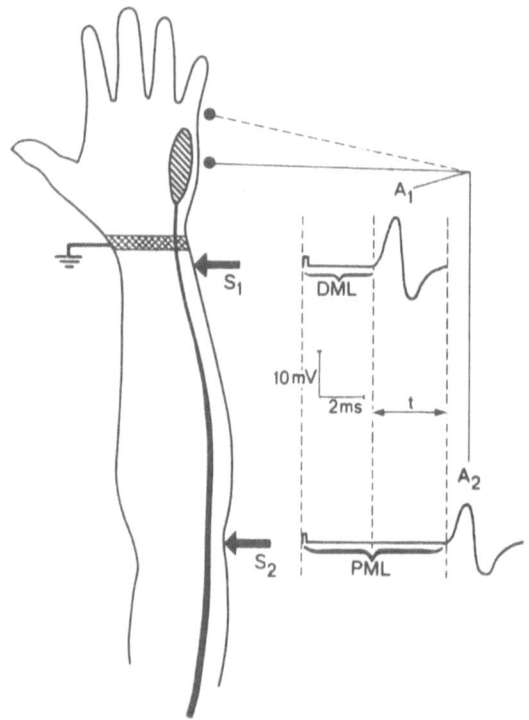

Figure 6. Motor nerve conduction measurement.
A_1 = evoked muscle potential after supramaximal stimulation of a distal point of the nerve (S1)
A_2 = evoked muscle potential after supramaximal stimulation of a proximal point of the nerve (S2).
DML = distal motor latency
PML = proximal motor latency
t = PML − DML = conduction time
$$\frac{\text{distance } S_1 - S_2}{t} = \text{motor conduction velocity in that part of the nerve}$$

Conduction times are measured from the beginning of the electrical stimulus to the beginning of the evoked potential. The interval between stimulation of the nerve at the wrist and the evoked muscle potential is called distal motor latency. This also contains the time needed for the neuromuscular transmission at the motor end-plates which we cannot measure in routine EMG. Therefore we cannot express the motor conduction velocity in this part of the nerve in metres per second.

In order to estimate motor conduction velocity in the forearm we also stimulate the nerve at the elbow and again measure the latency, which may be called proximal motor latency. Proximal latency minus distal latency in milliseconds divided by the distance between the sites of stimulation gives the conduction velocity of the fastest conducting motor fibres in the forearm in metres per second.

The advantage of this method is that we can use the large muscle potential as point of reference. The muscle potential is 300 to 1000 times as high as the nerve action potential. To determine sensory conduction velocities we have to pick up potentials from the nerve itself. The digital nerves are purely sensory and may be used for stimulation as well as for recording. Because nerve potentials are much lower, averaging techniques may be necessary to obtain a response in pathological cases.

In normal cases sensory potentials of the nerve in the forearm can easily be recorded with surface electrodes and without averaging techniques.

Instead of stimulating at the finger and recording from the nerve stem, sensory potentials can also be obtained from the digital nerves when the main stem is stimulated. Because the nerve is conducting the impulse in an opposite direction compaired to the physiological situation this method is called the antidromic method.

The potential obtained from the index finger by stimulation of the median nerve at the elbow is always lower and broader than that obtained by stimulation at the wrist (Figure 7). This is caused by the difference in conduction velocities of the sensory fibres that contribute to this compound potential.

Conduction velocities can be determined in the same way as for the motor fibres. Moreover the conduction velocity in the distal part can be estimated because the distal sensory latency contains no synapse time.

APPLICATION IN BRACHIALGIA

The importance of conduction measurements in the investigation of brachialgia is the fact that local pressure on a nerve causes local decrease in conduction velocity. The pressure may come from the outside or may be caused by structures of the body as in the so-called entrapment neuro-

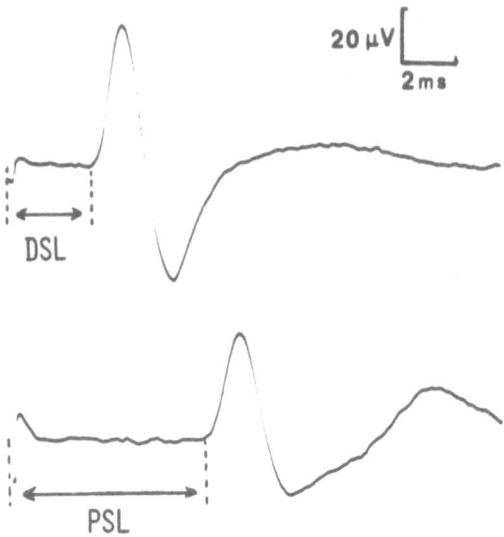

Figure 7. Sensory potentials obtained by stimulation of the median nerve at the wrist and at the elbow and recording from the index finger with ring electrodes.
DSL = distal sensory latency
PSL = proximal sensory latency

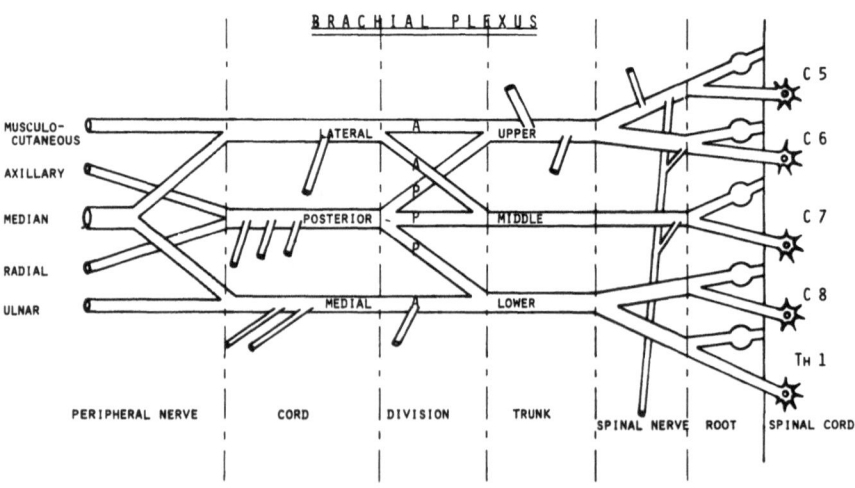

Figure 8. Schematic representation of the brachial plexus. Starting from 5 spinal cord segments, after several rearrangements, the plexus ends in 5 main nerves. A = anterior; P = posterior

pathies. Conduction studies are especially useful to investigate nerve lesions in the peripheral nerves. At the level of the brachial plexus the situation is much more complicated. Figure 8 is a very schematic representation of the brachial plexus. The plexus is formed from the roots C5, 6, 7, 8 and Th1. Non-traumatic root lesion may be caused by a protruding cervical disc or by an osteophyte. If fibres of the motor root are damaged denervation potential may be found in muscles of the corresponding myotome. Because the fibres to the paravertebral muscles are also damaged at this level denervation potentials may also be found in these muscles, which is not the case in plexus lesions.

Whereas degeneration of motor nerve fibres causes denervation potentials in the muscle fibres there is no equivalent that is characteristic for degeneration of sensory fibres. When sensory fibres are interupted distal to the spinal ganglion this will only cause a decrease of the amplitude of the sensory potential. If the interruption takes place proximal to the spinal ganglion the distal sensory fibre remains undisturbed, and the sensory potential stays normal whereas there is a definite sensory disturbance clinically. This is an important differential diagnostic feature, because in plexus lesions loss of sensory nerve potentials may be an early finding.

Compression of the roots and of the brachial plexus may be caused by several kinds of tumors. Malignant tumors especially may cause severe pains in shoulder and arm.

Among the disturbances at the thoracic outlet are included the costoclavicular syndrome, the anterior scalene syndrome, cervical rib and bands. In all such lesions the lower part of the brachial plexus especially may be compressed, that is the lower trunk and the medial cord, with their major outflow through the ulnar nerve.

In cases of cervical ribs and bands Gilliatt et al (1970) found a lowering of sensory nerve potentials of the ulnar nerve and a reduced motor unit pattern on contraction of the thenar muscles.

Urschel and coworkers (1971) state that thoracic outlet syndromes can be diagnosed by conduction studies on the ulnar nerves. This is not the experience of other investigators. Recently the use of the so called F-wave has been recommended for the investigation of these syndromes.

The F-wave is a kind of reflex response conducted exclusively by motor fibres (antidromically and orthodromically respectively). Inouye and Buchthal (1977) registered potentials from cervical spinal nerves after stimulation of the nerves in the arm and in the fingers. These techniques are not generally used at the moment.

The upper part of the brachial plexus is involved in acute cryptogenetic brachial plexus neuropathy, also called Parsonage-Turner syndrome, and in serum- and vaccin-induced brachial plexus neuropathy. There is a rapid onset of severe pain in shoulder and arm, followed in most cases, within the first 2 weeks by muscle weakness and paresis. The axillary and supra-scapular nerves are most commonly affected. Although most patients have unilateral plexus involvement clinically, denervation potentials may also be found on the unaffected side.

In traumatic lesions of the brachial plexus EMG offers a possibility to achieve a rather accurate localisation of the lesion which is of great importance for neurosurgical intervention.

As the brachial plexus starts from 5 roots it ends in 5 major nerves: musculocutaneous, axillary, median, radial and ulnar.

The diagram of the ulnar nerve (Figure 9) shows the preferential sites of compression. The cubital tunnel is the most important site for a lesion of this nerve. There may be a slowed conduction in the nerve segment at the elbow. However it is important to realise that conduction velocity at the elbow may be 10 m/sec lower than in the forearm in subjects without complaints.

A further limitation is that when the distance between the sites of stimulation is short the percentual error in measuring the distance increases, and this influences the accuracy of the conduction velocity. Over larger distances the error is usually less than 10%.

Besides local slowing of nerve conduction there may also be a partial conduction block at the site of the nerve lesion. This results from local demyelination of nerve fibres, whereas the axon remains intact. Stimulation proximal to the lesion will evoke smaller antidromic sensory and ortho-dromic motor potentials than stimulation distal to the lesion. The radial nerve has 3 important sites for compression (Figure 10), the sulcus in the upperarm being the most common. This however is usually not combined with pain. The median nerve has many places where it may be compressed (Figure 11). In the upper arm it may be damaged together with the ulnar and radial nerves for example by pressure of a cuff during operations in the forearm and hand. The pronator syndrome and the anterior interosseous nerve syndrome are rather infrequent, but these possibilities must be remembered, for example in cases of writers cramp. Compression of the median nerve at the wrist, the so called carpal tunnel syndrome is very frequent.

The typical history of this disorder is well known. It is however important to realize that the symptoms may also be aspecific and that the patient may complain of pain in the whole arm and even in the shoulder. It is my experience that too many clinicians search for a cause at a more proximal site without excluding the carpal tunnel syndrome by EMG. We know the EMG criteria for diagnosing the carpal tunnel syndrome better than in any other entrapment of the arm. In the mildest cases only a slight prolongation of the distal sensory latency may be found, or the amplitude of the sensory

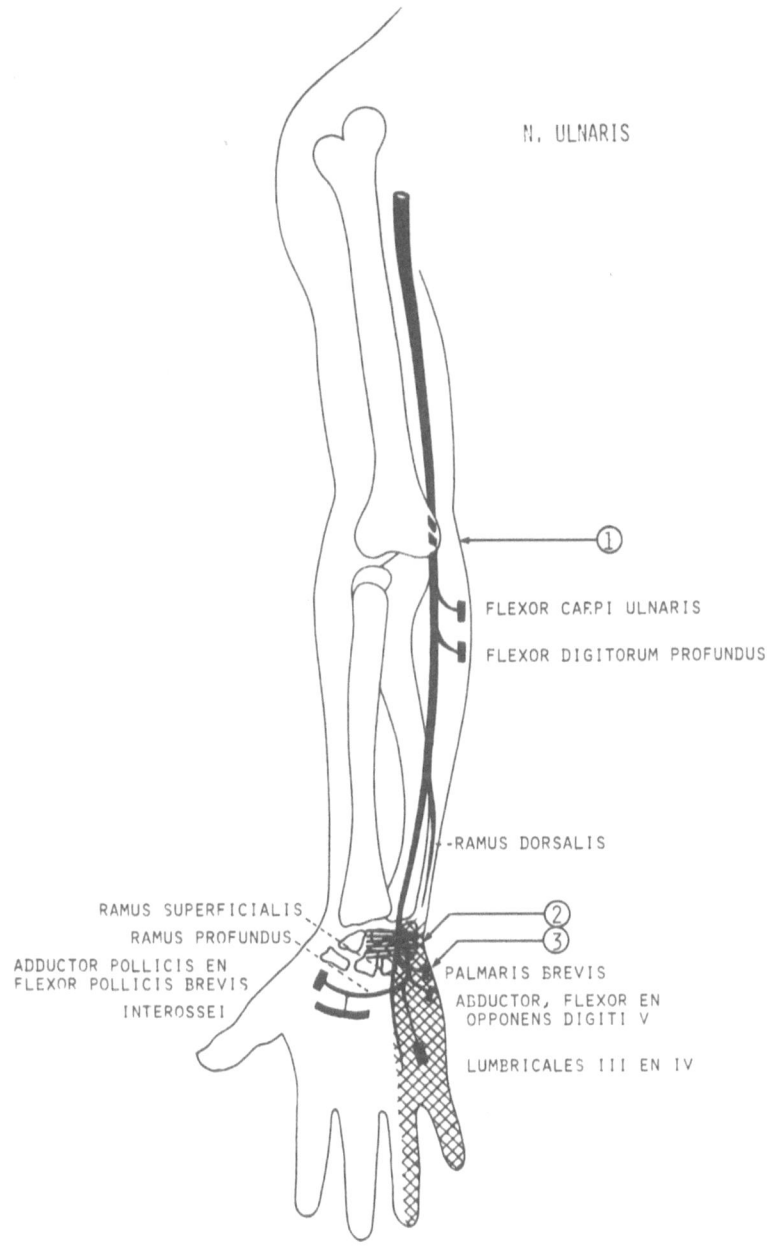

N. ULNARIS

①

FLEXOR CARPI ULNARIS

FLEXOR DIGITORUM PROFUNDUS

-RAMUS DORSALIS

RAMUS SUPERFICIALIS

RAMUS PROFUNDUS

ADDUCTOR POLLICIS EN
FLEXOR POLLICIS BREVIS

INTEROSSEI

②
③

PALMARIS BREVIS

ABDUCTOR, FLEXOR EN
OPPONENS DIGITI V

LUMBRICALES III EN IV

Figure 9. Ulnar nerve (schematic). Arrows indicate the preferential sites where local lesions of the nerve by compression from the outside or from body structures may occur.
////// = volar sensory distribution
\\\\\\ = dorsal sensory distribution

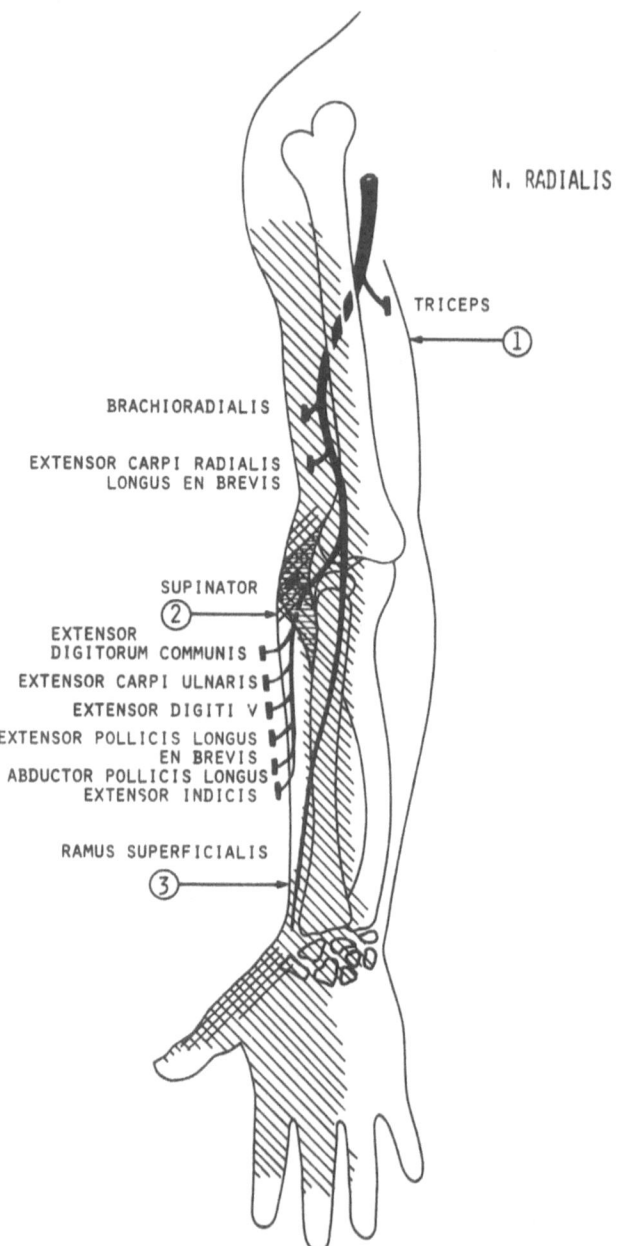

Figure 10. Radial nerve (schematic). Arrows indicate the preferential sites of nerve compression.
////// = volar sensory distribution
\\\\\\ = dorsal sensory distribution

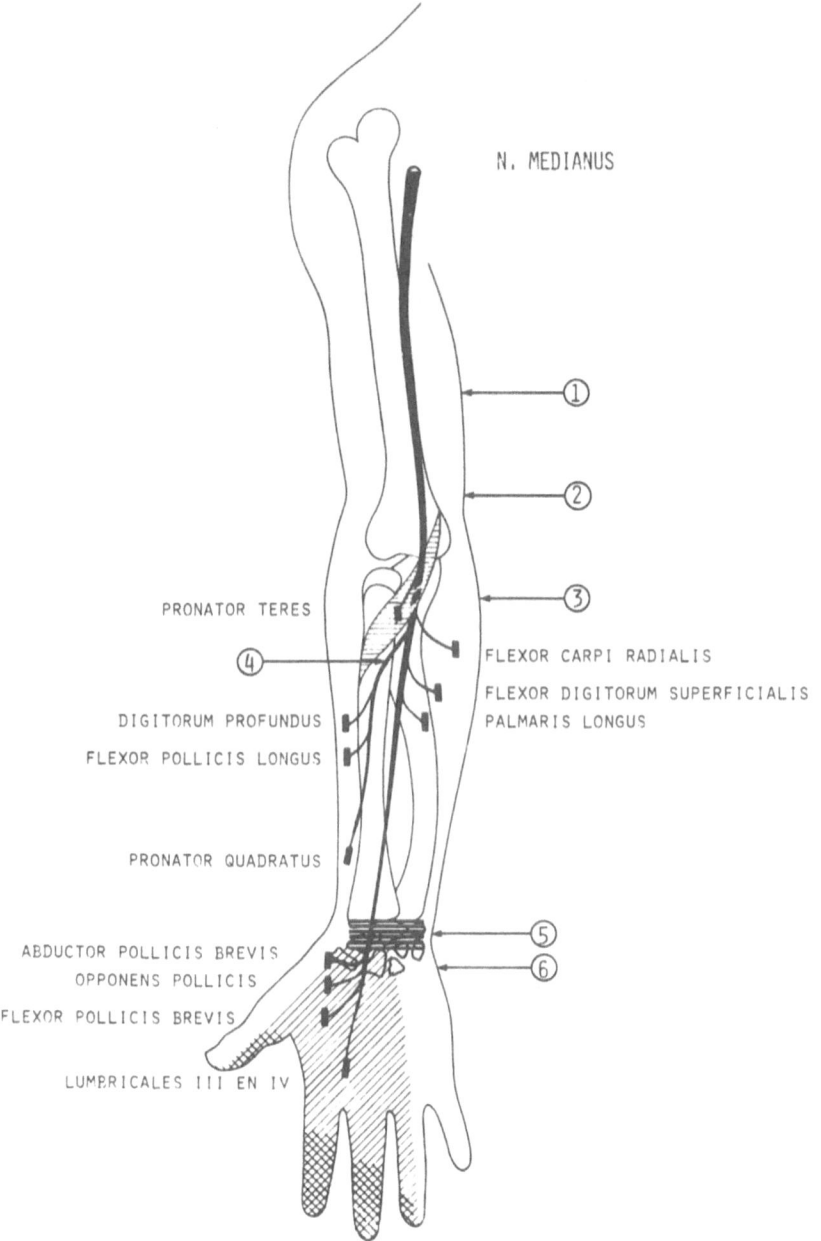

N. MEDIANUS

PRONATOR TERES

FLEXOR CARPI RADIALIS

FLEXOR DIGITORUM SUPERFICIALIS
PALMARIS LONGUS

DIGITORUM PROFUNDUS

FLEXOR POLLICIS LONGUS

PRONATOR QUADRATUS

ABDUCTOR POLLICIS BREVIS
OPPONENS POLLICIS

FLEXOR POLLICIS BREVIS

LUMBRICALES III EN IV

Figure 11. Median nerve (schematic). Arrows indicate the preferential sites of nerve compression.
1. halfway along the upper arm (compression from the outside)
2. ligament of Struthers
3. pronator teres muscle
4. anterior interosseous nerve
5. carpal tunnel
6. palm of the hand
////// = volar sensory distribution
\\\\\\ = dorsal sensory distribution

potential may be found, or the amplitude of the sensory potential may be diminished compared with that of the ulnar nerve or the median nerve of the opposite side.

The upper level for the distal motor latency is 5 msec. In moderate cases distal motor latencies of 7 to 9 msec may be found. In severe cases the sensory potential cannot be obtained without computer averaging and the distal motor latency may become more than 15 msec in some cases. Finally all conductions may be blocked. Denervation potentials may be found in the thenar muscles. Usually they appear only in more severe cases of carpal tunnel syndrome. Clinically at that time there usually also exists a partial thenar atrophy. Decompression of the nerve at that stage will relieve pain and paresthesia, but the muscle atrophy usually remains unchanged. Therefore it is important to decompress the nerve before this atrophy appears.

It is also useful to control patients by EMG after their decompression. Conduction along the nerve at the wrist must show a definite improvement within 3 months after the operation.

Patients that complain after any surgical treatment of the upper limb are not necessarily malingering. The possibility of a neurogenic lesion must always be borne in mind. Brachialgia may have so many causes that needle EMG and nerve conduction studies should not be omitted in patients with incompletely understood long lasting pain in arm and shoulder, especially when surgical treatment at any level is being considered.

REFERENCES

R.W. Gilliatt, P.M. Le Quesne, V. Logue, A.J. Sumner. Wasting of the hand associated with a cervical rib or band. J. Neurol. Neurosurg. Psychiat. 33: 615, 1970
Y. Inouye, F. Buchthal. Segmental sensory innervation studied by the recording of potentials from cervical spinal nerves. Electroenceph. clin. Neurophysiol. 43: 590, 1977
H.G. Urschel, M.A. Razzuk, R.E. Wood, M. Parekh, D.L. Paulson. Objective diagnosis (ulnar) nerve conduction velocity, and current therapy of the thoracic outlet syndrome. Ann. Thorac. Surg. 12: 608, 1971

5. Brachialgia – a differential diagnosis

G. PADBERG, M.D.*

Philologically, it would seem justifiable to translate the word brachialgia, of which the words brakion and algos appear to be the component parts, as pain in the arm.

Many authors use the designation brachialgia to refer to an affection of the brachial plexus. Although brachialgia often proves to result from an affection of the nervous system, it should be borne in mind that, apart from pathological neurogenic dynamic mechanisms, disturbances in the vascular, myogenic, osteogenic, ligamentous and articular functions can be the origin of pain in the arm. From perusal of the extensive literature on the subject, one discovers that there is no uniformity in the use of the terminology. If the term brachialgia is to be reserved for a neural affection, then it is no more than consistent in pertinent cases also to use terms such as vasalgia, myalgia, ostealgia, tenalgia and arthralgia. As a rule, however, factors of diverse origin play a role in the pathogenesis of brachialgia. In our opinion, therefore, it is simpler, clearer and also more meaningful to define brachialgia as any sensory disturbance characterized by pain in and about the shoulders, radiating to the arms, regardless of its cause.

ETIOLOGICAL FACTORS

The problems of brachialgia are closely related, not only with the function and structure of the spine and its encompassed parts of the nervous system with its surrounding membranes, but also with the function and structure of certain muscles and vessels, the peripheral somatic and autonomic nervous system, and the static and locomotor apparatus.

We believe ourselves justified in omitting a discussion of the structural and physiological relations of the above mentioned body parts, which can be regarded as generally known. But we do wish to stress the fact that a number of anatomical factors, in combination with certain postures and movements, can be of influence in the occurence of pain in the arm.

*Department of neurology, St. Annadal Ziekenhuis, Maastricht, The Netherlands.

J.M. Greep, H.A.J. Lemmens, D.B. Roos and H.C. Urschel (eds.).
Pain in shoulder and arm; an integrated view, 63–72.

Besides the brachial plexus, vascular structures can also be subject to
pressure. It is a fact established by experience that the symptoms produced
by pressure as a rule do not become manifest until the subject is over
20 years of age. This means that possible congenital anomalies have produced no symptoms until that age. Consequently, there must be some other
factor which later begins to play a role in the pathogenesis of pressure symptoms.

Todd investigated the gradual descent of the humeroscapular joint region
after birth, and his findings are of importance in this context. The following
factors, separately or in combination, can be decisive.

1. Compression of the nerve fibres as they pass between the anterior and
   the middle scalenus muscle; variations in insertion are of influence in
   this respect.
2. The nerve fibres and the subclavian artery can be compressed as they
   cross the normal first rib or a cervical rib; or they may be compressed
   between either of these and the clavicle.
3. The first ribs can be unusually high, or very large, or of irregular
   curvature.
4. The tubercle of the scalenus muscle on the first rib can be greatly
   enlarged.
5. The anterior scalenus muscle, merely by an abnormal structure and
   insertions or by these anomalies in combination with a cervical rib, can
   irritate the sympathetic and the vasomotor nerves of the subclavian
   artery, giving rise to vascular lesions.
6. Developmental defects may have altered the course of the nerve fibres
   relative to the scalenus muscles and the normal ribs or cervical ribs.
   Not only can the brachial plexus derive one segment higher or lower,
   but it may also show variations in the combination of its branches.
7. The course of vessels may be anomalous. The right subclavian artery
   can originate directly from the aorta; the subclavian artery or vein can
   pass in front of, behind or through, the anterior scalenus muscle. The
   transverse artery of the neck may take its course over, through or
   beneath the brachial plexus.
8. Thoracic skeletal deformities can alter the lateral diameter of the upper
   thoracic aperture.
9. A direct or indirect injury can affect the anterior scalenus muscle, with
   consequent haemorrhage and swelling, and later fibrosis, resulting in
   compression of the nerve fibres and the subclavian artery.
10. Acute infections can give rise to myositis in the scalenus muscle.
11. Curvatures of the spine can give rise to anomalous traction on the first
    rib or a cervical rib.
12. The physiological shoulder descent.
13. Postural influences (Jackson; Nelson; Todd).

INFLUENCE OF AUTONOMIC NERVOUS SYSTEM

No aspect of the pain problem, including that focussed on brachialgia, can be considered in its entirety unless it is clearly borne in mind that the autonomic nervous system, too, is involved in pain perception. This view is supported by numerous physiological and clinical experiments (Pick). A discussion of all these experiments would exceed the scope of this paper. Considering, from an anatomical point of view, the central organization of the autonomic nervous system within the spinal cord, we find that both a viscero-receptive and a viscero-motor part can be distinguished in the intermedio-lateral nucleus.

The viscero-receptive part receives the afferent impulses from the autonomically innervated body-parts, and practical experience teaches us that these impulses can appear in the human consciousness, among other things, as sensations of unpleasure and pain. It has been established neuronographically that pain stimuli produced in the autonomic viscera under experimental conditions, can effect cerebral activities in some cortical areas of the ventral telencephalon, i.e., in the phylogenetically older parts of the telencephalic organizations, more specifically in the visceral-emotional brain (Gastaut and Lammers; McLean; Pick; Pribram and McLean; Wall and Davis).

The last mentioned part of the brain is known to function as the biological condition par excellence of pleasure-unpleasure moods and pleasure-unpleasure feelings. All this indicates that pain stimuli from the external environment or from the human organism itself can travel to the cortex of the visceral-emotional brain via viscero-receptive and other afferent autonomic systems, there to give rise to pleasure-unpleasure experiences and sensations (e.g. pain).

PATHOGENESIS

Primary physical causes of pain in the arms and shoulders may be found in the nervous system, the skeletal system with its capsules and ligaments; the tendinous system and the vascular system. Intrathoracic processes may also exert an influence, as can intra-abdominal processes in as much as they cause irritation of the diaphragm. Table I presents a survey of the various possibilities. In computing this table we have been aware of imperfections inherent to this type of classification.

It is not our intention to present detailed discussion of all these circumstances mentioned in the table. Many of these are relatively rare causes of brachialgia. It must be sufficient to refer to the pertinent literature. Now

Table 1. Causes of brachialgia.

A. Visceral causes	B. Vascular causes

I. Lesions of the superior pulmonary sulcus
  1. malignant tumours
  2. neurofibromata
  3. inflammations
	I. Acute arterial occlusion
	II. Chronic occlusive arterial affection
	III. Raynaud's disease and related
	  affections
	IV. Erythromelalgia and related

II. Oesophagus spasm	affections V. Aneurysms VI. Arteriovenous fistula

III. Heart
  1. coronary sclerosis
  2. acute coronary occlusion
  3. syphilitic aortitis
  4. dissecting aortic aneurysm
  5. pericarditis
  6. paroxysmal tachycardia
	VII. Acute thrombophlebitis
	VIII. Chronic venous failure
	IX. Acute diffuse lymphangitis
	X. Chronic lymphoedema

IV. Mediastinum
  1. tumour
  2. inflammation	

V. Diaphragm
  1. hiatal hernia
  2. diaphragmatic pleurisy
  3. pulmonary embolism
  4. subphrenic processes	

a. radiating to the *left* shoulder
      splenic lesion
      pancreatitis
	C. Myogenic causes

pancreatic carcinoma
      ruptured peptic ulcer
    b. radiating to the *right* shoulder
      cholecystopathy
      hepatopathy
      subdiaphragmatic abscess
      ruptured peptic ulcer
	I. Inflammations
	II. Metabolic disorders
	III. Traumatic myopathies
	IV. Circulatory disorders
	V. Tumours
	VI. Myospasms
	VII. The "stiff man" syndrome

follows a brief discussion of 4 conditions and circumstances which are decisive in a large number of cases of brachial pain.

1. Cardiac conditions

Pain radiating from the heart more frequently extends to the arms than to any other part of the body. The pain impulses have their beginning in the nerve ends, ascend via the cardiac plexus and, via the superior and the inferior cardiac nerve, reach the various ganglia i.e., the superior cervical ganglion and the stellate ganglion. From these ganglia, the impulses descend in the sympathetic trunk and, via the rami communicantes albi C8–

Table 1 continued.

D. *Neurogenic causes*	

I. Lesions of the central nervous system
1. tumours, cysts, vasopathies
2. degenerative affections
   a. syringomyelia
   b. amyotrophic lateral sclerosis
   c. paralysis agitans
   d. multiple sclerosis
3. inflammations
4. circulatory disorders
5. mechanical-traumatic lesions
6. cervical myelopathy

II. Lesions of nerve radices
1. tumors
   a. extramedullary tumors
   b. tumours of the roots
2. perineural radicular cyst
3. cervical discopathy
4. mechanical-static factors
5. inflammations
6. circulatory disorders

III. Lesions of the brachial plexus
1. tumours
2. inflammations and toxic factors
3. circulatory disorders
4. mechanical-traumatic lesions
   a. exogenous violence
   b. compression-traction
      cervical rib
      scalenus syndrome
      aneurysm
      costoclavicular syndrome
      first thoracic rib syndrome
      subcoracoid-pectoralis-minor
         or hyperabduction syndrome
   c. various static influences
5. idiopathic nocturnal dysaesthesia

IV. Peripheral nerve lesions
1. trauma associated with:
   a. luxation
   b. fracture
   c. rupture
   d. penetrating wounds
2. pressure
   a. cubital tunnel (ulnar nerve)
   b. carpal tunnel syndrome (median
      nerve)

D. *Neurogenic causes* (continued)
3. neuroma formation
4. tumour
5. inflammation
6. Sluder's Vidianus' neuralgia
7. neurogenic muscular atrophy
8. reflexogenic sympathetic dystrophy
   and causalgia
9. glomus tumour (glomangioma)

E. *Orthopedic causes*

I. Lesions of the cervical vertebrae
A. *Traumatic*
   1. fractures
   2. dislocation
   3. distortion
   4. arthritis

B. *Non-traumatic*
   1. arthritis
   2. disc infection
   3. osteomyelitis
   4. tuberculosis
   5. syphilis
   6. tumours

II. Lesions of the shoulder and -region
A. *Traumatic*
   1. fractures
   2. dislocation
   3. distortion
   4. tendon ruptures
   5. bursitis
   6. haemarthrosis

B. *Non-traumatic*
   1. acute lymphadenitis
   2. arthritis
   3. osteomyelitis
   4. tuberculosis
   5. neurogenic arthropathy
   6. tenosynovitis
   7. periarthritis
   8. fibrositis
   9. tumours

Th4 (sometimes Th1–Th5) and the corresponding posterior roots, reach the spinal cord. Here, the impulses cross the contralateral side, to reach the cerebral cortex via the spinothalamic tract. A number of pain impulses pass directly from the cardiac plexus to the first 5–7 thoracic nerves and, via the uncrossed anterolateral fasciculus, to the cerebral cortex.

The problem is why the pain, which arises in the heart, should give the impression of being localized in the arm. An explanation might be that the pain impulses which arise in the heart, on their way to higher brain centres, pass through the same cord segments as pain impulses originating from the arms.

The pain can be felt in both arms simultaneously, sometimes only in the right, but as a rule in the left arm. The pain is of a tenebrant, sometimes paroxysmal character.

When the ascending part of the aortic arch is affected, the pain can be perceived in the right cervical region and shoulder. Pain originating in the transverse or the descending part of the aortic arch is localized more often in the left cervical region and shoulder. As regards the localization in the arm, it can be stated that the pain is felt on the inside of the upper arm as far as the elbow. The pain often stops at the elbow while, nervertheless, simultaneously felt in the wrist. As a rule there is no continuous pain throughout the arm. The pain sometimes extends into the fingertips but, if this is the case, its character usually changes.

The pain in the fingers is described by many patients as burning and tingling. The pain can affect all the fingers, but is usually confined to the fourth and fifth. The most characteristic feature of this pain is that it is provoked by effort. It occurs while the effort is being made, not afterwards.

It has been established that interruption of the pain conduction can be effected by extirpation or destruction of the left stellate ganglion, and by anaesthesia or severance of the rami communicantes or the dorsal roots of the proximal five thoracic nerves.

The stellate ganglion is the main junction not only for impulses travelling towards but also for those travelling from the heart. Stimulation of this ganglion produces pain very similar to that which occurs in attacks of angina pectoris. This pain can be arrested, however, by blocking the stellate ganglion, e.g. with the aid of procaine.

2. *Various static influences*

For some time it has been clear to us from personal clinical observations that brachialgia, regardless of whether this is peracute or more gradual onset, can become manifest in persons who spend many hours a day carrying out certain activities in a tense, more or less immobile attitude. A number of such activities come under domestic headings such as peeling potatoes, knitting, sewing and making beds. But also activities as writing, typing, reading, watching TV and, last but not least, driving a motor vehicle, can be associated with protracted flexion or hyperextension of the cervical column; this, in association with abnormal muscle contractions and a degenerative affection of the cervical column, can give rise to pain in the neck, shoulder and arm. (Jackson; Nelson; Padberg).

3. *Humeroscapular periarthritis*

This term was coined by Duplay, who used it in reference to posttraumatic painful stiffness of the shoulder. He thought that dessication and calcification of the subdeltoid bursa were the primary causes of this condition. There is a tedious pain in the anterior aspect of the shoulder at the approximate site of insertion of the tendon of the supraspinatus muscle on the greater tuberosity, or slightly lower near the insertion of the deltoid muscle. The pain is most intense during the night.

Examination discloses limitation of movement in the humeroscapular joint, with marked impairment especially of abduction and rotation. Later, various factors were accepted as possible causes of the syndrome which, it was found, is not always preceded by a simple macroscopic injury.

It was established that, apart from acute inflammation, specific processes and tumours, there are several other conditions which show the same syndrome; those syndromes, too, were verified by pathological-anatomical examinations. In the course of time, reports were published on degeneration and rupture of the tendon of the supraspinatus, muscle, coracoiditis, arthritis deformans of the acromio-clavicular joint and of the intertubercular sulcus, changes of the synovial bursa, degeneration of the long biceps tendon, inflammations of the greater and lesser tuberosity, detachment of the limbus from the shoulder socket, and stiffness of the shoulders as a result of protracted rest.

Some authors believe that affections of the supraspinatus muscle constitute by far the most important cause, followed by affections of the long biceps tendon, which are much less frequent (Armstrong; Exner).

A trend developed in favour of replacing the indifferent collective concept "humeroscapular periarthritis," for clinical usage, by more specific diagnoses on an anatomical basis. This produced designations such as supraspinatus and biceps syndrome, and supraspinatus tendinitis (Brown; Jones; Withers).

In fact there are investigators who regard humeroscapular periarthritis as part of the cervical vertebral syndrome (Gutzeit; Reischauer). A slipped cervical disc can be associated with acute stiffness of the shoulder in which even calcium deposits may occur. The syndrome could be controlled by blocking the stellate ganglion; even the calcium deposits then disappeared.

These observations indicate the existence of a form of shoulder stiffness to be interpreted as a sequelae of changes in the neurovegetative state, resulting from irritation of the sympathetic in the cervical column region. In our opinion sharp distinction must be made between painful stiffness of the shoulder based on a variety of pathogenic factors still to be discussed, and the stiff painful shoulder as a neural symptom. Numerous affections of the bones, joints and soft parts of the shoulder and the axilla, ruptures, haemorrhages and injuries resulting from overstraining the tendon insertions, contractures of the shoulder muscles from any cause, lesions due to metastatic, focal-toxic and allergic processes, and degenerate conditions of the humeroscapular joints and its adjacent parts – all these can be conditional factors for painful shoulder stiffness.

The stiff, painful shoulder as a neural symptom, however, produces special, characteristic clinical features characterized by intermittence, certain age limits, the nature of the stiffness and particularly the nature of the pain experience, which unmistakably reveals the intensive emotional involvement of the entire person in the disease picture.

Many authors consider such an attack of shoulder pain the consequence of a vegetative-neural irritation, taking its course in crises, in the region governed by the stellate ganglion (Gutzeit; Morgenstern; Reischauer; Zülch). The question whether the stiff, painful shoulder as a neural symptom can be provoked exclusively from the cervical vertebral region, is still open to discussion. Several authors have presented a number of strong clinical arguments in the affirmative (Gutzeit; Morgenstern; Reischauer; Schaer). They maintain that the intermittent occurrence of the pain and the fact that most patients of this description are between 40 and 60 years of age, are not explained by a calcium opacity in the shoulder angle, if any. These authors also found that 15% of their patients had a past history which included a typical cervical syndrome with acute painful stiffness of the shoulder. Nearly all these patients also complained of paresthesia, and many showed a Sudeck syndrome throughout the arm, which could not be explained on the basis of other diseases. In all these cases, a stellate ganglion block proved to have a supreme therapeutic effect. Our findings point in the same direction (Padberg). In many patients with a cervical discopathy we observed painful shoulder stiffness which showed a strikingly favourable response to stellate ganglion block. It can be maintained that many cases of painful shoulder stiffness have an unmistakable neural signature, and are provoked from the cervical vertebral column.

4. Compression syndromes

There are several places in the body where nerves and vessels are vulnerable to compression or entrapment. These are narrow and rigid compartments the boundaries of which are formed by tendons, bones and musculofibrous tissue. As regards the upper extremities these points are the cervical root canals, the thoracic outlet, the costoclavicular space, the point of insertion of the pectoralis minor tendon, the cubital tunnel and the carpal tunnel.

There may be three types of syndromes: cases with mainly neurological symptoms, cases with mainly vascular symptoms and cases with a combination of both. All these syndromes will be dealt with in other parts of this book.

CONCLUSIONS

Summarizing these considerations, we would maintain that pain in the arm can be produced by a wide variety of causes and circumstances. In some cases pain in the arm can be an initial symptom of a severe affection, but in the majority of cases it is based on a benign process. Where the various causes can produce the same symptoms and because of the fact that pain and paresthesias of the hands and arms often prove to be psychogenic in origin (Mayfield) it is obvious that the differential diagnosis may be difficult.

On the basis of my own experience however, I feel that the cervical column and the carpal tunnel are by far the most common sources of pain and dysesthesias in the hands and arms, and that the autonomic nervous system plays an important role.

REFERENCES

1. J.R. Armstrong. Report British Orthopaedic Association. Annual Meeting 1948. The Painful Shoulder. J. Bone J. Bone Jt. Surg. 31 B: 133, 1949
2. J.R. Armstrong. Excision of the acromion in treatment of the supraspinatus syndrome. J. Bone Jt. Surg. 31 B: 436, 1949
3. J.T. Brown. Report British Orthopaedic Association. Annual Meeting 1948. The painful shoulder. J. Bone Jt. Surg. 31 B: 133, 1949
4. J.T. Brown. Early assessment of supraspinatus Tears. J. Bone Jt. Surg. 423, 1949
5. S. Duplay. De la péri-arthrite scapulo-humeral et des raideurs de l'épaule qui en sont la conséquence. Arch. gén. Méd. 2: 513, 1872
6. G. Exner. Die Halswirbelsäule. Stuttgart, G. Thieme, 1954
7. H. Gastaut, H.J. Lammers. Anatomie du rhinencéphale. In: Les grandes activités du rhinencéphale. Vol. 1. Ed. T. Alajouanine. Paris, Masson, 1961
8. K. Gutzeit. Wirbelsäule als Krankeitsfaktor. Dtsch. med. Wschr. 76: 44, 1951
9. R. Jackson. The cervical Syndrome. 2nd edn. Springfield, Ill., Charles C. Thomas 1958
10. G.B. Jones. Report British Orthopaedic Association. Annual Meeting 1948
   . The Painful Shoulder. J. Bone Jt. Surg. 31 B: 133, 1949
11. G.B. Jones. Painful Shoulder. Calcification of the Supraspinatus Tendon. J. Bone Jt. Surg. 31 B: 433, 1949
12. F.H. Mayfield. Neural and vascular compression syndromes of the shoulder girdles and arms. In: Handbook of clinical Neurology. Vol. 7. Diseases of Nerves. Part I. Ed. by P.J. Vinken and G.W. Bruyn. Amsterdam, North-Holland Publ. Cie., 430.

13. P.D. McLean. The limbic system and its hippocampal formation. Studies in animals and their possible application to man. J. Neurosurg. 11: 29, 1954
14. V. Morgenstern. Periarthritis humero-scapularis als neurales Symptom. In: F. Reischauer, Ed. Die cervicalen Vertebralsyndrome. Stuttgart, G. Thieme, 1955
15. P.A. Nelson. Treatment of Patients with cervicodorsal outlet syndrome. J.A.M.A. 163: 1570, 1957
16. G. Padberg. Brachialgia. Psychiat. Neurol. Neurochir. (Amst.) 67: 406, 1964
17. J. Pick. The Autonomic Nervous System. J.B. Lippincott Company, Philadelphia-Toronto, 1970
18. K.H. Pribram, P.D. McLean. Neuronographic Analysis of Medial and Basal Cerebral Cortex. I. Cat. J. Neurophysiol. 16: 312, 1953
19. F. Reischauer. Konservative Behandlung des Cervical-Syndroms. In: F. Reischauer, Ed. Die cervicalen Vertebralsyndrome. Stuttgart, G. Thieme, 1955
20. H. Schaer. Die Periarthritis humero-scapularis. Ergeb. Chi. u. Orth. 29: 211, 1936
21. T.W. Todd. The Descent of the Shoulder after Birth. Its significance in the production of pressure symptoms on the lowest brachial trunk. Anat. Anzeiger, 41: 385, 1912
22. T.W. Todd. Posture and the Cervical Rib Syndrome. Ann Surg. 75: 105, 1922
23. P.D. Wall, G.C. Davis. Three cerebral cortical systems affecting autonomic function. J. Neurophysiol. 14. 507, 1951
24. R.J.W. Withers. Report British Orthopaedic Association. Annual Meeting 1948. The Painful Shoulder. J. Bone Jt. Surg. 31 B: 133, 1949
25. R.J.W. Withers. The Painful Shoulder. Review of one hundred personal cases with remarks on the pathology. J. Bone Jt. Surg. 31 B: 414, 1949
26. K.J. Zülch. Zur Genese der neurologischen Symptome bei cervicular Osteochondrose. In: F. Reischauer, Ed. Die cervicalen Vertebralsyndrome. Stuttgart, G. Thieme, 1955

Part II

Causes of pain in the shoulder and arm

6. Shoulder pain as a rheumatologic problem

J.K. VAN DER KORST M.D.*

ABSTRACT

The rheumatologist is often confronted with a painful limitation of both shoulder joints in elderly people. This might be due to rheumatoid arthritis, polymyalgia rheumatica, bilateral shoulder-hand syndrome or adhesive capsulitis. Based on a follow-up study of 75 cases of shoulder-hand syndrome the course of this clinical entity is described.

Some drugs, especially phenobarbital and isoniazide, can probably induce sympathic dystrophy, although decisive evidence is still lacking.

Shoulder problems in rheumatological practice are numerous and manifold. On the whole, the shoulder problems the rheumatologist is confronted with, are not so different from those the orthopaedic surgeon and the neurologist see. The acute and the chronic painful shoulder, the frozen shoulder and cervicobrachialgia belong to the daily routine of the consulting rheumatologist and occasionally a thoracic outlet syndrome, thrombosis of the subclavian or axillar vein or an arterial lesion of the shoulder region might find its errant way into the consulting room of the rheumatologist.

If there is some sort of selection of shoulder problems which can be designated as more or less specific rheumatological shoulder disease, then that might be chronic pain of both shoulders. Perhaps rheumatologists see more bilateral shoulder complaints than the other specialists already mentioned. The chance that a patient with a painful condition of both shoulders will end up in the rheumatological clinic will increase as his sedimentation rate increases and if he has complaints or abnormalities of other joints, and especially of the hands. Based on these considerations one could name as typical rheumatological shoulder conditions: Rheumatoid arthritis (with involvement of both shoulder joints), polymyalgia rheumatica and the shoulder-hand syndrome (especially so if bilateral).

*Amsterdam Center for Rheumatic Diseases

J.M. Greep, H.A.J. Lemmens, D.B. Roos and H.C. Urschel (eds.).
Pain in shoulder and arm: an integrated view, 75 – 81. All rights reserved.
Copyright © 1979 by Martinus Nijhoff Publishers, The Hague/Boston/London.

RHEUMATOID ARTHRITIS

Shoulder complaints due to rheumatoid arthritis are often easy to recognize. Most often there are already more or less typical changes of the more peripheral joints when the shoulders are involved. Rheumatoid arthritis is – schematically speaking – a disease with a symmetrical and centripetal distribution of peripheral joint involvement. One would therefore expect that the shoulder joint would become affected late in the course of the disease. That is often true. The shoulder, however, is involved more frequently and mostly earlier than the hip joint. The reason for this is not clear. Anyhow, in most cases of rheumatoid arthritis of some years' duration there is a painful limitation of shoulder movements. This might increase the – already existing – burden of functional incapacity of the upper extremity, due to deformation of the hands and painful limitation of the wrists and elbows.

How great is the risk that an isolated painful limitation of one shoulder is the precursor or an initial symptom of rheumatoid arthritis? To my knowledge this risk is very small. Having so far seen hundreds and hundreds of cases of rheumatoid arthritis I can recall only one patient originally presenting with what was supposed to be an acute periarthritis of one shoulder, evolving to a fullblown rheumatoid arthritis. This experience is in agreement with the literature. Probably, no more than five percent of the cases of rheumatoid arthritis have a monarticular onset. Among these involvement of one knee joint or a finger joint is much more frequent than involvement of one shoulder joint. There is one more reason not to worry so much about rheumatoid arthritis in regard to the differential diagnosis of unilateral shoulder pain. In general, rheumatoid arthritis with monarticular onset – including that of the shoulder – has a relatively good prognosis from the statistical point of view. Therefore we should not be too reproachful if unexpectedly a humeroscapular periarthritis evolves to rheumatoid arthritis.

POLYMYALGIA RHEUMATICA

One of the problems in the diagnostic examination of the shoulder region is that the humeroscapular joint is surrounded by massive muscles. Therefore – in contrast with e.g. the knee joint – physical diagnosis of humeroscapular arthritis is almost always impossible. This can sometimes make the differential diagnosis between rheumatoid arthritis and polymyalgia rheumatica very difficult. Both syndromes can cause painful limitation of both shoulder joints as the dominant complaint. In both conditions the sedimentation rate will be markedly increased and whether the patient suffers from either rheumatoid arthritis or polymyalgia rheumatica, he will suffer from general malaise. As polymyalgia rheumatica is a pathological condition, which is almost always confined to senescence, the risk of false-positive rheumatoid factor test is in the order of about four percent, being the percentage in which rheumatoid factor has been demonstrated in elderly healthy people. The problem with polymyalgia rheumatica is that it is most often a diagnosis by exclusion. A temporal artery biopsy, showing definite signs of giant cell arteritis can be obtained in no more than one third of the cases. Some years ago there was a suggestion that arteriography of the temporal artery eventually followed by selective arterial biopsy might enhance the chance of a positive diagnosis. I have been discouraged by the radiologists of my acquaintance from using this technique, as being too risky in elderly patients. So, for the moment, distinguishing between polymyalgia rheumatica and rheumatoid arthritis in elderly patients seems to depend entirely on the weighing of all the data gathered from complete physical examination, laboratory findings and X-rays.

To my knowledge there is a certain tendency to overdiagnose polymyalgia rheumatica. We are in need of well-defined diagnostic criteria. For the time being the diagnosis of polymyalgia rheumatica should be reserved for those patients over 60, who have a very painful restriction of at least the shoulder girdle, bilaterally, and with no sign of polyarthritis, but with at least a sedimentation rate of over 50 mm in the first hour and/or histologically proven giant cell arteritis.

SHOULDER-HAND SYNDROME

Another condition which might be confused with rheumatoid arthritis is shoulder-hand syndrome, whether unilateral or bilateral, because it not only causes painful limitation of the shoulder, but also deformity and functional incapacity of the hand. Often there is severe and rapidly progressive flexion contracture of the fingers. Confusion with rheumatoid arthritis is increased by the fact that there might be a severely irregular decalcification, which might simulate rheumatoid erosions and cysts. Remarkably, the radiographic changes, which can be designated as Sudeck's dystrophy, are mostly confined to the hand and wrist. There is a great variation in the extent of the radiographic changes, which do not seem to be related to the severity of the clinical signs. I have very little experience in posttraumatic Sudeck's dystrophy. But I have the idea that in spontaneous sympathic dystrophy of the upper extremity – which is just another name for the shoulder-hand syndrome – the radiographic signs are in general less pronounced than in posttraumatic sympathic dystrophy.

Cases in which there is a severe Sudeck dystrophy not only of the hand but also of the elbow and shoulder joint, mimicking destructive or erosive arthropathy are very rare. Several years ago we made a retrospective study of the course of the shoulder-hand syndrome in 75 patients. In 59 cases x-ray pictures of the hands were available; 37 showed typical abnormalities in contrast with 22 without such changes. (See Table 1). There was no definite relationship between the presence of such changes and the duration of the clinical symptoms although radiological signs were most frequently found five to six months after onset of the disease. Relatively few radiographic changes were found if the hand x-rays were taken within one month from the onset of the disease. X-rays of the shoulder were even less helpful in diagnosis of the shoulder-hand syndrome. Only 12 out of 43 showed spotty decalcification. The small number of shoulder radiographs taken, suggests that the clinicians were aware of the low significance of shoulder x-rays in diagnosing spontaneous reflex dystrophy of the upper extremity.

Table 1. Radiological signs of Sudeck's dystrophy in patients with should-hand syndrome.

Months after onset of symptoms	Hand		Shoulder	
	Radiologic dystrophy	Normal	Radiologic dystrophy	Normal
1	3	8	2	9
2	2	1	1	1
3	3	3	0	6
4	4	0	1	1
5	8	0	1	6
6	4	2	3	2
7	2	1	–	–
8	2	1	2	2
9	2	4	1	2
10	2	0	1	–
11	0	1	–	–
12	1	0	–	–
> 12	4	1	0	2
Total	37	22	12	31

From this study of 75 consecutive cases of shoulder-hand syndrome we learned several other things of which I will mention only some salient points. Somewhat to our amazement spontaneous reflex dystrophy was found to be predominantly a disease of elderly people. Although the average age was found to be 58.5 years, the peak incidence was found in the age group 60–70 years, the There was no significant difference between bilateral and unilateral cases. The number of bilateral cases was somewhat more than 30 percent, namely 29 against 46 unilateral cases.

The relatively greater age of patients with the shoulder-hand syndrome becomes even more remarkable when it is compared to the age distribution of a series of patients with cervicobrachialgia or humeroscapular periarthritis. Like the patients with shoulder-hand syndrome the two other series were consecutive series of patients diagnosed in a rheumatological out-patients clinic. In both the other conditions the peak incidence is below the age of 60, whereas that of shoulder-hand syndrome is above the age of 60.

We also tried to establish the course of shoulder-hand syndrome. Out of the 75 cases diagnosed 37 patients were seen at regular intervals so that we were able to establish the development of the syndrome. After one year 32 out of the original 37 were still complaining about pain and/or stiffness. However, in the second year about half of the patients became symptom free. There was no obvious difference in the course of the condition between the bilateral and the unilateral cases. Pain both of the shoulder and the hand disappeared first, in most cases between 6 and 12 month after onset (See Table 2). At the same time the diffuse swelling – accompanied by hyperemia and hyperhydrosis – of the hands, disappeared. However the limitation of movement of shoulder and hand persisted. After two years 15 out of the original 37 patients still had marked limitation of finger movements. After the diffuse swelling of the hands had disappeared the hand often became white and cold with a marked atrophy of the skin and subcutis, which might even mimick scleroderma. We postulated two stages in the course of the shoulder-hand syndrome based on these findings.

First there is the *hypertrophic stage*, lasting a half to a full year and being characterized by diffuse warm swelling of the hand and pain both of the hand and the shoulder. After the hypertrophic stage subsides, there is a more or less marked *atrophic stage*, mainly characterized by a white, tight and cold skin mainly of the fingers. The atrophic stage is far less painful than the hypertrophic stage, although the limitation of the shoulder and the fingers, which occur early in the hypertrophic stage, do often persist. The atrophic stage was observed in only one third of our patients.

Although the exact cause of shoulder-hand syndrome is unknown, in many cases a concomitant disease can be found, as we already know since Steinbrocker conceived the shoulder-hand syndrome in 1948 (Table 3). In

Table 2. Course of shoulder-hand syndrome in 37 patients.

Months after onset	0	3	6	12	18	24
Shoulder pain	37	29	24	6	5	4
Hand pain	37	22	15	6	3	3
Limited movements shoulder	37	26	21	17	7	7
Limited movements hand	37	29	29	21	17	15
Swelling hands	37	24	17	3	2	1
Atrophy hands	–	3	9	11	12	10

some cases it is very tempting to assume a causal relationship as e.g. when the shoulder-hand syndrome occurs after thoracotomy for bronchial carcinoma on the same side, or cervical herpes zoster, or cervical lymphoma, or myocardial infarction, but these connections are very rarely observed in the series of patients so far published. I feel that one should not think too much of a relationship, as has been postulated, with cervical spondylosis. As the shoulder-hand syndrome is mainly a condition found in elderly people one could expect at least a coincidental occurrence with degenerative changes of the cervical spine.

Table 3. Concomitant diseases in patients with shoulder-hand syndrome.

	Steinbrocker 1948 (n = 43)	Thompson 1961 (n = 17)	Graham and Ross 1962 (n = 73)	Own series (n = 75)
Epilepsy	–	6	–	9
Psychosis/neurosis	–	–	–	6
Hemiplegia/Paraplegia	5	1	4	–
Cerebrovascular accident	–	–	7	2
Cerebral tumor	–	–	1	1
Meningo-encephalitis	–	1	–	–
Pulmonary tuberculosis	–	–	1	3
Generalized arteritis	2	–	–	–
Cervical lymphoma	2	1	1	1
Herpes zoster (cervical)	2	2	–	1
Infectious arthritis (shoulder)	1	–	–	–
Weber-Christian disease	1	–	–	–
Myodegeneratio cordis	9[1]	2[1]	29	10
Cervical discopathy	2	1	10	(28/43)
Trauma	5	1	6	1
None	15	2	14	(27)

1) Myocardial infarction only.

A remarkably high incidence of epilepsy as well as psychotic and neurotic conditions was found in our patients. In the three earlier series published, only Thompson has observed a high incidence of epilepsy. With only one exception in the patients with epilepsy or psychosis and neurosis was the shoulder-hand syndrome bilateral. For reasons, which are too extensive to give here and which have already been published, we think that not these conditions, but their treatment, might induce the shoulder-hand syndrome. In fact we think that phenobarbital might – especially in older people – induce a reflex dystrophy, most often bilateral, of the upper extremity. In fact 19 out of 29 patients with bilateral shoulder-hand syndrome were found to be taking phenobarbital at the onset of the syndrome. Other drugs, especially isoniazide, have been thought, by other authors, to induce the shoulder-hand syndrome. I readily admit that there is no conclusive evidence with regard to the causative role of drugs in shoulder-hand syndrome, but we should keep in mind that some drugs – especially phenobarbital and isoniazide – might possibly be a cause of bilateral reflex dystrophy in elderly people.

SUMMARY

I have been trying to show you a number of conditions which might induce painful limitation of both shoulders especially in elderly people, namely rheumatoid arthritis, polymyalgia rheumatica and presumably drug-induced shoulder-hand syndrome. I did not of course cover all aspects of shoulder problems from the rheumatological point of view. So something is left for the next postgraduate to do.

REFERENCES

A.E. Good, R.A. Green, J.C. Zanafonetis. Rheumatic symptoms during tuberculosis therapy. Ann. intern. Med. 63: 800, 1965

W. Graham, P. Rosen. The shoulder-hand syndrome. Bull. rheum. Dis. 12: 277, 1962

J.K. van der Korst, A. Cats. Het schouder-hand syndroom. Een retrospectief onderzoek van 75 gevallen. Ned. T. Geneesk. 111: 723, 1967

J.K. van der Korst, H. Colenbrander, A. Cats. Phenobarbital and shoulder-hand syndrome. Ann. rheum. Dis. 25: 1553, 1966

O. Steinbrocker, N. Spitzer, H.H. Friedman. The shoulder-hand syndrome in reflex dystrophy of the upper extremity. Ann. inter. med. 29: 22, 1948

M. Thompson. Shoulder-hand syndrome. Proc. roy. Soc. Med. 54: 679, 1961

7. Radiological changes of the shoulder joint in rheumatoid arthritis and humero-scapular periarthritis

KATHARINA A.E. MEIJERS M.D.*

ABSTRACT

In a study of 250 pairs of shoulder radiographs taken from 55 patients suffering from rheumatoid arthritis three types of abnormalities were consistently detected, and affected:
1. cranio-lateral part of humerus,
2. gleno-humeral joint space and surroundings,
3. acromio-clavicular joint.
Comparison with a group of 54 patients suffering from humero-scapular periarthritis revealed that both groups show irregularities of the cranio-lateral part of the humerus; these occur more frequently in rheumatoid arthritis. Calcification was found only in the HSP group. The gleno-humeral joint space may be narrowed in the rheumatoid arthritis group, but this was not seen in the humero-scapular periarthritis group. The acromio-clavicular joint space can show a marked widening in RA but this was not encountered in the HSP group.

INTRODUCTION

Shoulder complaints are frequently encountered. Beside the physical examination, radiographs are regularly taken. The question arises whether a radiograph of the shoulder can contribute to the diagnosis; in particular in differentiating between rheumatoid and non rheumatoid lesions. For this purpose standard X-rays of patients with rheumatoid arthritis (RA) were compared with a group of patients with painful shoulders. A radiograph of the shoulder will show the humerus, the scapula and the clavicle together with the humero-scapular and acromio-clavicular joint spaces.

METHOD

In this study a standard method was used for the radiological examination of the shoulder joint. In this procedure the patient lies supine, the arms along the body in maximal exortation. The beam of X-rays is directed cranio-caudally at an angle of 15°–30° from the perpendicular. Unfortunately RA patients with shoulder involvement tend to have a

*University Medical Centre, Leiden, The Netherlands.

J.M. Greep, H.A.J. Lemmens, D.B. Roos and H.C. Urschel (eds.).
Pain in shoulder and arm: an integrated view, 83–95. All rights reserved.
Copyright © 1979 by Martinus Nijhoff Publishers, The Hague/Boston/London.

limitation of movement of the humerus. The projection of this bone may therefore vary. Knowledge of different projections of the humerus will be essential for a good interpretation of a radiograph. To elucidate this point radiographs of a loose humerus were taken in the following four positions (Figure 1), extreme exorotation, moderate exorotation, mid-position (in this position the upper- and lower arm are both lying in a saggital plane and this is the position most RA patients can achieve), and endorotation.

In exorotation – extreme or moderate – the greater tubercle is projecting on the cranio-lateral side; in mid-position it is somewhat flattened, while in endorotation it is projected upon the humeral head (and its dorsal part will form the lateral side of the humerus).

The projection of the lesser tubercle also varies. In extreme exorotation it will be visible as a triangle on the lateral side; in a less pronounced exorotation as a straight dense line, in mid-position it is a scarcely visible line on the medial aspect of the humerus, and in internal rotation it again appears as a triangle but this time on the medial aspect of the humerus. Between the greater and the lesser tubercle lies the intertubercular groove. A wire in this groove demonstrates the changes in position of the long tendon of the m. biceps in the above mentioned positions (Figure 2). The other wire occupies the frontal part of the anatomical neck in extreme external rotation. It visualizes the changes of this part in the various positions. The humeral head is situated on the medio-cranial part of the humerus and its full circumference is seen in extreme external rotation; on internal rotation the caudal border of the head will be turned dorsally. One should be cautious in interpreting this phenomenon as an elevation of the humerus. This can easily be demonstrated on a radiograph (Figure 3) taken of the same person in moderate exorotation (on the left), and in endorotation (on the right), while the scapula is not altered in the two positions. Although in endorotation the caudal border seems to be elevated in relation to the glenoid cavity, the space between the cranial part of the humerus and the acromion remains the same. This will result in an apparent elevation towards the glenoid cavity. In a standing subject the scapula makes an angle of about 30° with the frontal plane, and is tilted forward about 10–15°. The supine position does not much alter this position [1].

When radiographs are taken with the beam perpendicular to the body the lower part of the acromion is merged with the cranial part of the humerus (Figure 4). When the beam is at an angle of 15–30° with the perpendicular the view of the inferior part of the acromion is diminished. The acromion and the superior part of the humerus are no longer seen together; on the contrary, space is now visible between the two bones allowing a better view of the cranio-lateral part of the humerus. In this

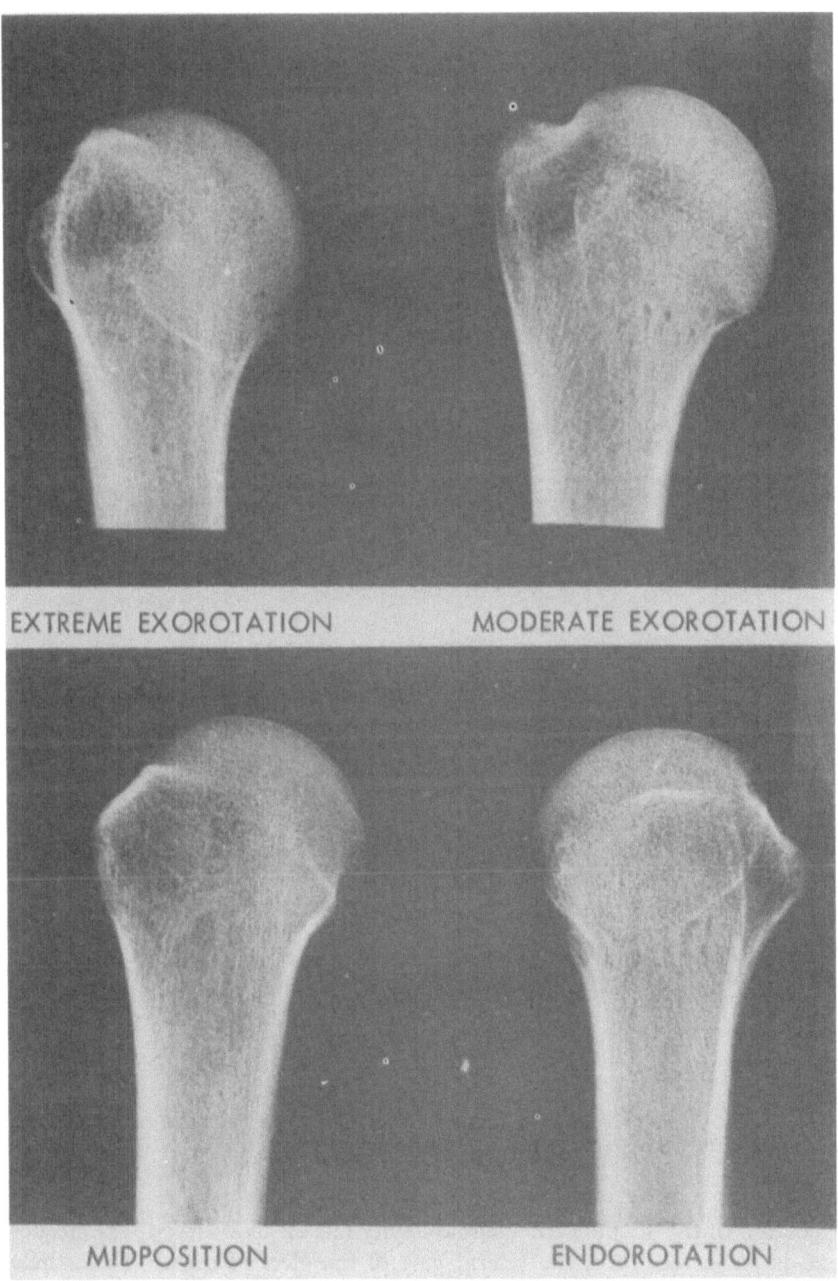

Figure 1. The four positions of the humerus.

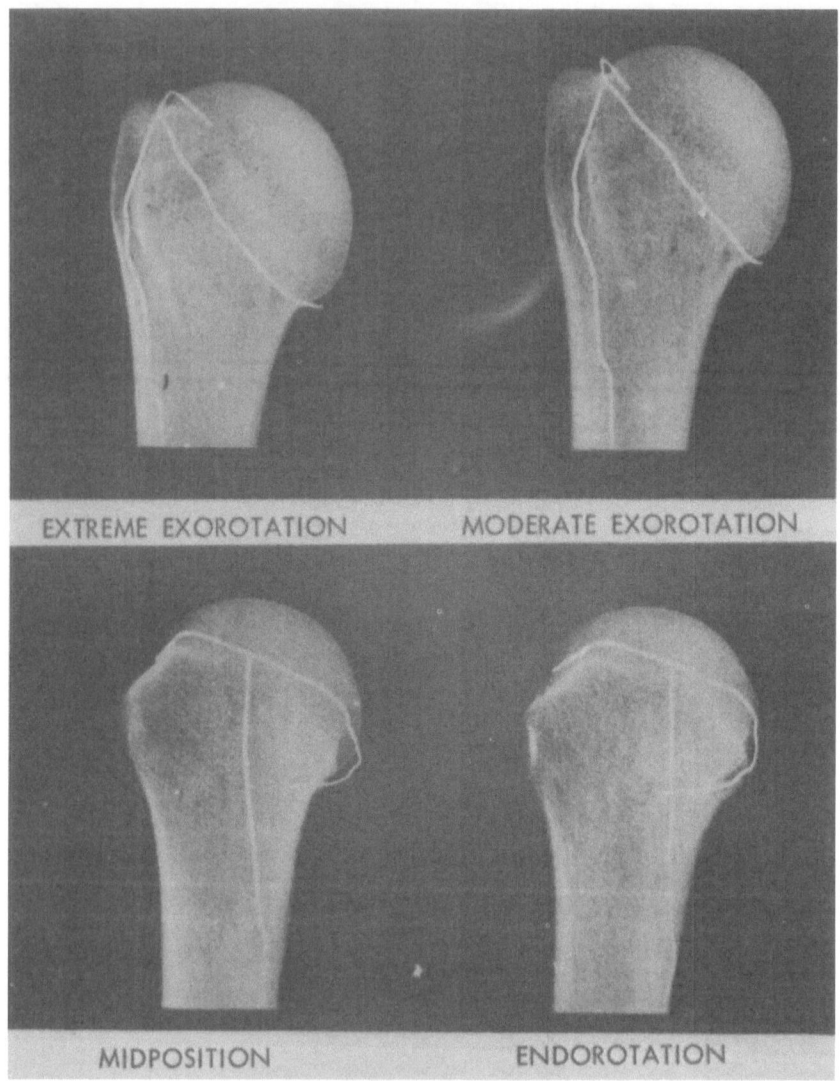

Figure 2. Humerus in four positions with a wire occupying the frontal part of the anatomical neck and a vertical wire lying in the intertubercular groove.

projection of the scapula the glenoid cavity has an oval shape. The humeral head is projected upon the lateral part of the glenoid cavity. Nevertheless the anterior and posterior rims of the glenoid cavity, the humeral head and the joint space are easily discernable.

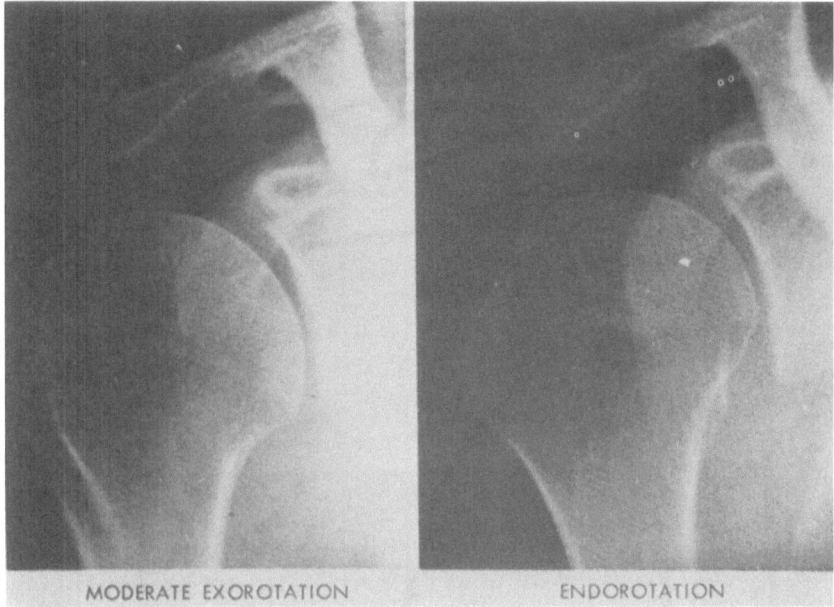

MODERATE EXOROTATION   ENDOROTATION

Figure 3. On the left side the humeral head is in moderate exorotation, on the right side in endorotation with apparent elevation towards the glenoid cavity. On both films the distance between the cranial part of the humerus and the acromion is the same.

MATERIAL

Films from patients suffering from RA and those with humero-scapular periarthritis (HSP) were studied for abnormalities and the differences between the 2 groups were recorded later.

Of 55 patients suffering from definite RA according to the ARA criteria [2] 250 pairs of radiographs were available. The duration of the disease before the first radiograph of the shoulder was taken ranged from one to 31 years, with an average of 10 years. Usually it was not possible to determine for how long the patient had been suffering from shoulder complaints as only a few were seen in the outpatient department at the onset of the disease, and this study was made in retrospect.

The average follow-up period of these shoulder films was three and a half years. In 2/3 of the group the follow-up was possible up to 5 years and in 1/4 of the group longer follow-up, with an average duration of 8 years was possible.

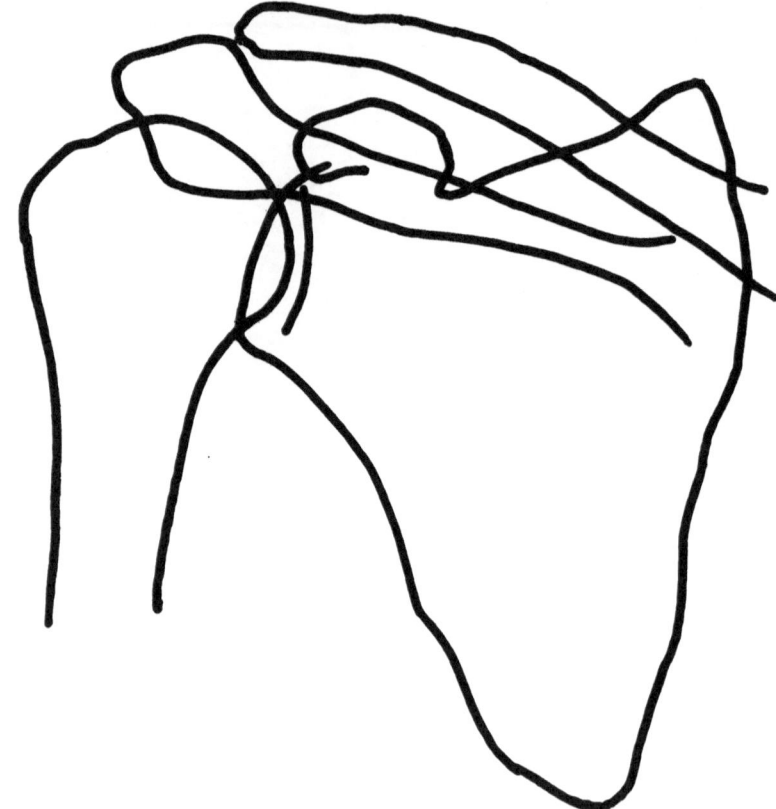

Figure 4. Drawing showing the overlap of the lower part of the acromion and the head of the humerus, when the X-ray beam is perpendicular to the body.

RESULTS

Abnormalities found in these rheumatoid patients can be localized in 3 regions:
1. on the cranio-lateral part of the humerus
2. at the gleno-humeral joint
3. at the acromio-clavicular joint.
    1. Several types of lesions of the cranio-lateral part of the humerus can be distinguished:
a. definite erosions at the anatomical neck, an extension of these erosions towards the humeral head is seen as the disease progresses (Figure 5),
b. superficial lesions of the anatomical neck with an extension towards the superior part of the humeral head (Figure 6),

c. severe destructive lesions of the anatomical neck, greater tuberosity and superior part of the humeral head; these lesions may sometimes be accompanied by new bone formation (Figure 7).

2. Abnormalities of the gleno-humeral joint are characterised by narrowing of the joint space (Figure 8). This finding is usually accompanied by erosions and sclerosis of the humeral head, and to a lesser degree of the glenoid cavity. Sometimes marked osteophytosis of both glenoid cavity and humeral head is visible, with a remodelling of the head (Figure 9). In this series, narrowing of the joint space is usually accompanied by abnormalities of the cranio-lateral part of the humerus. Figure 10 illustrates progressive change in a patient aged 54 years, who had had rheumatoid arthritis for 15 years.

3. Acromio-clavicular joint. Erosions and marked widening of the joint space are found in this joint. They occur less frequently than the lesions referred to at the gleno-humeral joint. Figures 11 and 12 illustrate normal and abnormal acromio-clavicular joints.

DISCUSSION

At this point the question arises: are these lesions specific for rheumatoid arthritis? To answer this, radiographs were taken of 54 consecutive out patients who were not suffering from rheumatoid arthritis, tuberculous arthritis or suppurative arthritis. They belong to the group of painful shoulders, or humero-scapular periarthritis (HSP). They are all characterised by one or more abnormalities around the shoulder joint, localized in the supraspinatous tendon, subacromial bursa or in the whole musculotendinous cuff. The films were read for the same changes as mentioned above for the RA group. In comparing the 2 groups (Table 1) there are more females in the RA than in the HSP group. The age was equally divided in the 2 groups (Table 2). The disease duration was in both groups difficult to estimate.

In both groups (RA and HSP) the cranio-lateral part of the humerus was normal in some and showed irregularities in others. The radiographs from both groups were read several times, and although irregularities occur more frequently in the RA group, statistical analysis did not reveal any significant difference. Besides the irregularities, calcification was seen in this area, but this is confined to the HSP group.

When we compared the two groups for localization of the abnormalities it was found that the distribution of the lesions varied. In the rheumatoid group the anatomical neck and the superior part of the humeral head were more frequently affected, whereas in the HSP group the greater tuberosity was more frequently affected, and to a much lesser degree the anatomical

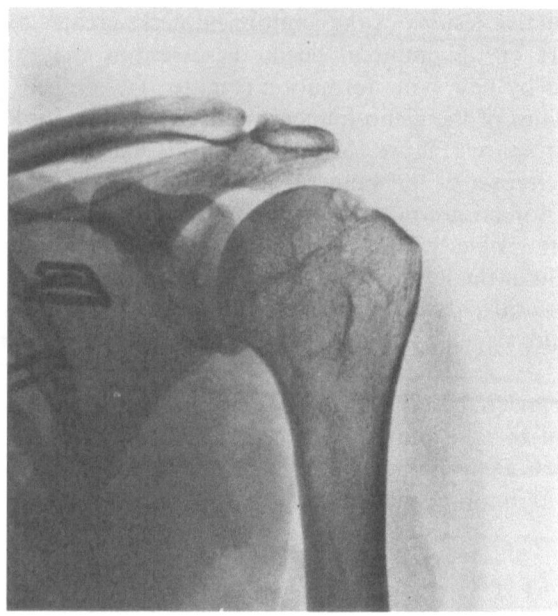

Figure 5. Radiograph of shoulder showing definite erosions at the anatomical neck.

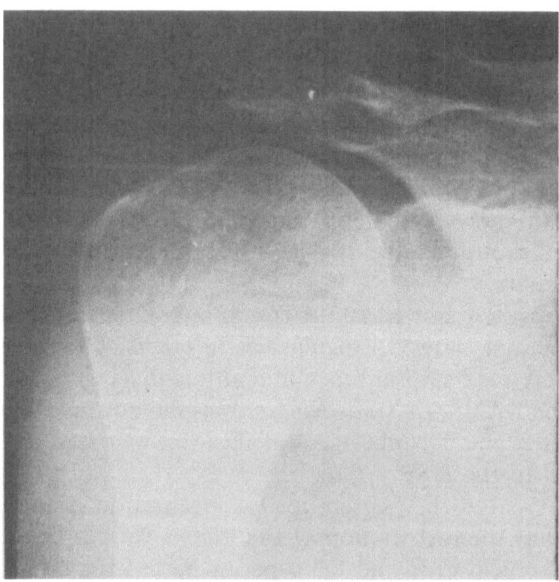

Figure 6. Radiograph of shoulder showing superficial lesions of the anatomical neck with an extension towards the cranial part of the humeral head.

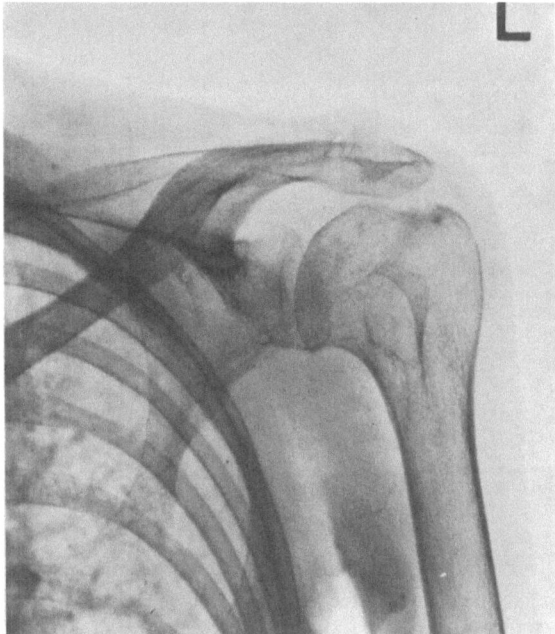

Figure 7. Severe destructive lesions of the anatomical neck, the greater tuberosity and the humeral head.

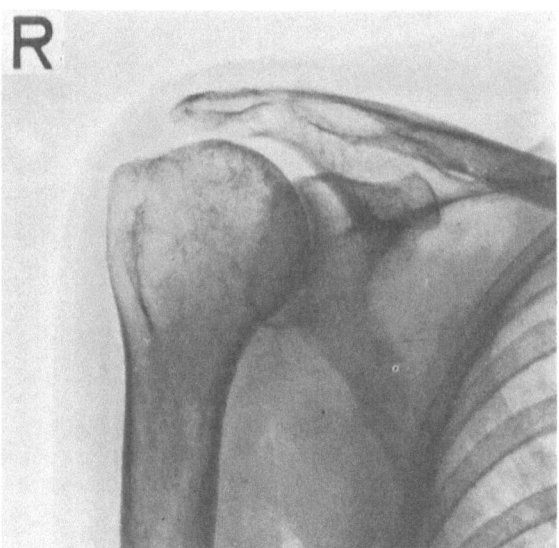

Figure 8. Narrowing of the humero-scapular joint space.

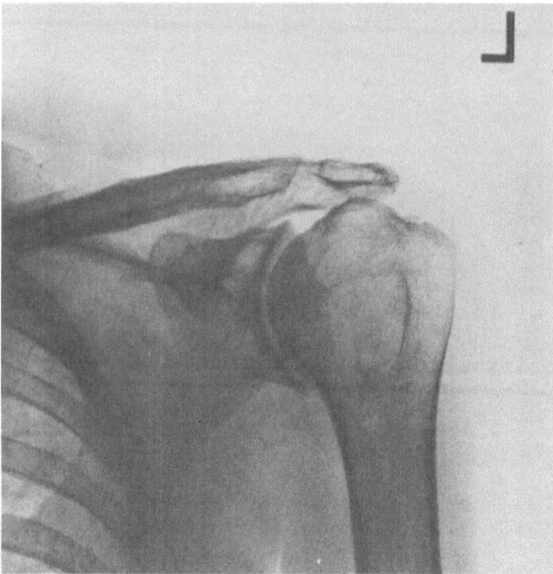

Figure 9. Radiograph of shoulder, showing remodelling of the humeral head and narrowing of joint space with osteophytosis.

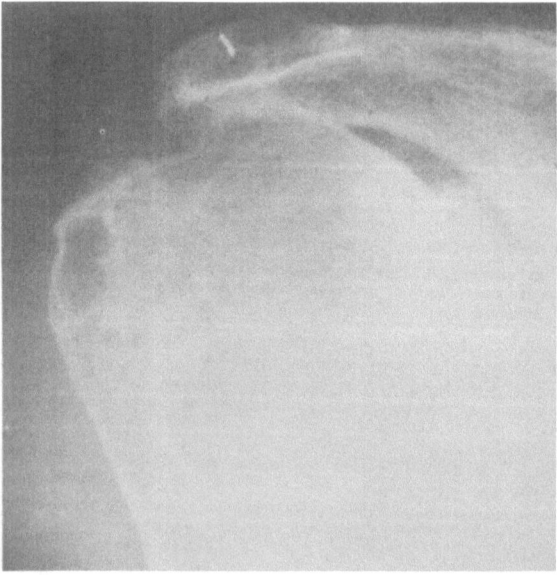

Figure 10. Radiograph of shoulder illustrating severe change in a patient aged 54 years, who had had rheumatoid arthritis for 15 years.

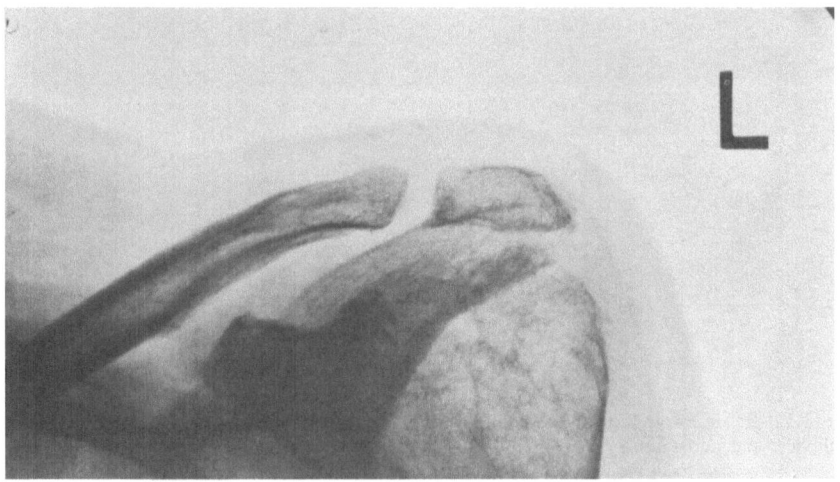

Figure 11. Radiograph of normal acromio-clavicular joint.

neck and the head of the humerus. The gleno-humeral joint. Radiographs were read for width of the joint space and allocated to three categories:
a. normal
b. narrowed space
c. doubtful narrowing.
With radiographs taken under previously described conditions, narrowing of joint space was found in some instances in the rheumatoid group, but not in the HSP group.

Narrowing of joint space was first estimated with the naked eye. Later it was measured by placing a ruler horizontally at the mid-point of the dome of the glenoid cavity, thus measuring the distance between the humeral head and the anterior rim of the glenoid cavity. The joint space in the HSP group ranged between 3.5 and 6 mm., the most common measurements falling between 4 and 5 mm. Narrowing of the space was thereafter defined as measuring 3 mm. or less. Repeated readings and measurements were made and confirmed narrowing of joint space in rheumatoid arthritis, but none was seen in the HSP group.

It is of importance to mention that all films studied were taken as described above. Films taken with the scapula more or less parallel to the plane of projection – also available in the HSP group – showed an empty or nearly empty joint space. Measurements of the joint space showed a much greater variability, probably due to the difficulty of accurate positioning of

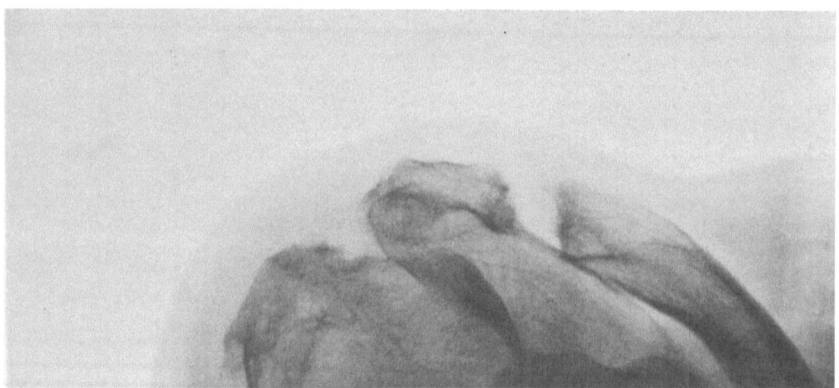

Figure 12. Radiograph showing widening of the acromio-clavicular joint space with erosions of clavicle and acromion.

Table 1. Sex incidence in two groups of patients suffering from rheumatoid arthritis or humero-scapular periarthritis.

Sex	Rheumatoid Arthritis (RA)	Humero-scapular periarthritis (HSP)
Male	17	28
Female	38	26
Total	55	54

Table 2. Age distribution in two groups of patients suffering from rheumatoid arthritis or humero-scapular periarthritis.

Age (Yrs)	RA	HSP
< 30	1	–
30–39	5	5
40–49	13	10
50–59	18	18
60–69	13	15
70–79	5	4
80+	–	2
	55	54

Table 3. Number of patients with or without involvement at cranio-lateral part of humerus; comparison of two groups (RA and HSP).

State of cranio-lateral part of humerus	RA	HSP
Normal	17	28
Irregularities	37	26
Doubtful	1	–
Total	55	54
Calcification	–	10

Table 4. Localization of irregularities at cranio-lateral part of the humerus in two groups of patients with rheumatoid arthritis or with humero-scapular periarthritis.

Cranio-lateral part of humerus	RA	HSP
Greater tuberosity	23	25
Anatomical neck	33	14
Head of humerus	30	6
Total	37	26

the scapula. We therefore are in favour of using the single film taken as described above in RA patients, which makes a good follow-up possible.

In the HSP group detection of calcium deposits can sometimes be promoted by taking films in various positions of humerus and scapula. Changes in the acromio-clavicular joint such as marked widening of joint space and erosions were found only in the RA group and not in the HSP group.

REFERENCES

1. K.A.E. Meijers. Een studie over de articulatie van de schouder. Proefschrift, Leiden, 1961
2. M.W. Ropes, G.A. Bennett, S. Cobb, R. Jacox, R.A. Jesser. Revision of diagnostic criteria for rheumatoid arthritis. Bull on the Rheum. Dis. IX, 4: 175–176, 1958

8. Orthopedic diagnosis in shoulder and arm pain

H. CLAESSENS, D. UYTTENDAELE and N. DE STOOP*

ABSTRACT

The authors stress the importance of a careful case history and clinical examination in the orthopedic diagnosis of shoulder and arm pain.

The possible technical investigations are mentioned and their indication and value in establishing a proper diagnosis are examined.

It must be taken into consideration that pain syndromes of shoulder girdle and arm can be equally vascular, nervous, orthopedic or traumatic in origin and that all these aspects call for simultaneous investigation. Clinical and technical investigations should not be limited to the shoulder girdle exclusively, since pain may also originate in abnormalities of the trunk and cervical spine in particular, and in more distal disturbances of the upper limb.

As in all other fields, correct diagnosis in orthopedics depends largely on careful history taking and thorough clinical examination, combined with the necessary technical investigations.

ANAMNESIS

The time of onset, the type and localization of the pain, together with the kind of dysfunction, are interesting data, enabling us to seek the correct diagnosis in a certain direction.

Congenital anomalies are mostly responsible for decreased mobility, abnormal anatomical configurations, muscular atrophy and weakness, but they are only rarely accompanied by pain syndromes.

A sudden onset of severe pain and dysfunction is to be attributed either to trauma or acute nerve root compression, or also to an acute inflammatory process, including either a bacterial or an aseptic arthritis, as in the case of chondrocalcinosis and bursitis subsequent to calcified tendinitis.

*From the Department of Physical Medicine and Orthopedic Surgery, University Hospital, De Pintelaan 135, B-9000 Gent (Belgium).

J.M. Greep, H.A.J. Lemmens, D.B. Roos and H.C. Urschel (eds.).
Pain in shoulder and arm: an integrated view, 97–101. All rights reserved.
Copyright © 1979 by Martinus Nijhoff Publishers, The Hague/Boston/London.

Chronic or aching pain with minimal or no dysfunction, localized in the shoulder-neck or in the scapular or interscapular region, is in the first place suggestive of cervical spine lesions and cervical arthrosis in particular, secondly of disturbances in the scapulothoracic mechanism or may in the third place be due to postural defects with fibrositis or secondary muscle spasm.

Pain radiating from the neck into the arm or hand often accompanies a cervical root syndrome, whilst pain with bipolar localization in shoulder and hand suggests a shoulder-hand syndrome.

When the patient localizes the pain by means of a 'shoulder grasp,' the discomfort mainly arises from articular lesions, either of the glenohumeral or acromioclavicular joint, or from affections of the bone, such as tumours. It may also be due to periarthritis. Such periarthritic lesions are very common and account for 50% of all causes of shoulder pain.

CLINICAL EXAMINATION

Inspection and palpation reveal possible abnormalities in the anatomical configurations, muscular atrophy, postural disturbances and palpation-induced pain.

Examination of the mobility about the shoulder girdle is of extreme importance in establishing a correct diagnosis. The initial restriction of mobility is nearly always encountered in external rotation with adducted arm, in internal rotation with abducted arm or in the hand-back movement. In case of intact rotation movements, the existence of limited passive elevation of the arm can hardly be accepted. Reduction of mobility, both actively and passively, is indicative of joint lesions with incongruence of articular surfaces, or capsular retraction, as can be found in osteoarthritis, chronic infections, post-traumatic sequelae or frozen shoulder.

Normal passive mobility associated with lack of active movement, leads to a diagnosis of muscular weakness or inhibition due to painful movements. Muscular weakness is encountered in nerve and muscle diseases or in musculotendinous avulsion.

The exact moment at which movement induces a sensation of pain is of utmost importance in diagnosing the lesion. Abduction normally amounts to 180 degrees, two thirds of which are accounted for by the glenohumeral joint and one third by the scapulothoracic system. Throughout the entire motion, the displacements of arm and scapula progress very smoothly as there exists a constant relation between them during the complete abduction movement, i.e. 3 degrees of abduction comprise 2 degrees of motion in the glenohumeral joint and 1 degree in the scapulothoracic system. Gliding of the scapula around the thoracic wall is possible thanks to a 20 degree motion range in the acromioclavicular joint and one of 40 degrees in the sternoclavicular joint. Motion in the latter only occurs after 90 degrees of abduction. Pathological changes in this smooth movement give rise to the following conclusions with regard to diagnosis:

1. In case of mere scapular displacement without motion in the glenohumeral joint, frozen shoulder is the most proper diagnosis. Abduction is then limited to some 60 or 70 degrees.

2. Scapular displacement with the arm remaining in adduction, indicates weakness in the scapulohumeral junction, as encountered in paralysis of deltoid muscle or complete avulsion of the rotator cuff.

3. When abduction becomes painful above 90 degrees and when from this point on, further movement is mainly restricted to the scapulothoracic system, an affection of the acromioclavicular joint is often the cause.

4. An alteration of the smooth scapulohumeral displacement is very frequently observed during elevation between 75 and 120 degrees and is encountered in cases of periarthritis due to lesions of the rotator cuff or the long head of the biceps. This alteration results from the fact that, at about 75 degrees of abduction, the greater tuberosity with the insertions of the rotator cuff muscles and underlying biceps tendon is compressed under the thoracoacromial osteoligamentous roof, causing pain. In an attempt to avoid this painful condition, further movement will be limited to the scapulothoracic system, which is apparent by excessive motion of the scapula during this period. Once no further scapular bascule is possible, the greater tuberosity will still be forced to tilt underneath the thoracoacromial arch, which occurs at about 120 to 130 degrees. Further elevation movement will then be painless in the glenohumeral joint. Such alterations in the humeroscapular rhythm, called a positive abduction arch, indicate the existence of a painful lesion at the insertion of the rotator cuff muscles or underlying biceps tendon.

TECHNICAL INVESTIGATIONS

1. *Laboratory investigations* are imperative when shoulder pain is part of a polyarticular affection, in acute inflammatory conditions or in cases of possible tumor.

2. *Puncture of the joint* and *examination of the synovial fluid* are necessary in cases with articular swelling or inflammatory signs. This will permit the differentiation between mechanical and inflammatory fluid on the basis of the number of cells present and the ratio between lymphocytes and granulocytes. The presence of crystals may confirm a suspicion of chondrocalcinosis. Bacteriological investigation of the fluid permits an early diagnosis of septic arthritis.

3. *Scintigraphy* is useful in the objective evaluation of the organic nature of pain complaints or in the early detection of progressive bone tumors.

4. *X-rays* are indicated whenever pain results from traumatic events. In conjunction with standard anteroposterior roentgenograms, transthoracic and axial views are often necessary to reveal e.g. a posterior dislocation. In case of periarthritic affections X-rays do not furnish direct information, unless a calcium deposit is present in one of the rotator cuff tendons. There are some abnormalities indirectly suggesting a lesion of the rotator cuff, particularly narrowing of the subacromial space with cranial displacement of the humeral head and, to a lesser extent, also geode formation, eburnation or osteophytic reaction about the greater tuberosity. To visualize these, radiographs with the arm in internal and external rotation must be taken, making sure that the incident X-ray beams run parallel with the lower face of the acromion.

5. *Arthrographic examination* of the shoulder joint can give us interesting information in various pathological conditions. It permits assessment of the relation of the humeral head to the glenoid cavity and enables us to determine the smoothness of the articular capsule (helpful in villinodular pigmented synovitis) and to visualize possible ruptures of capsule and rotator cuff. A rupture at the inferior recess provides evidence of a sustained dislocation.

A pathologically broad junction with the subcoracoid recess is observed in cases of recurrent dislocation of the shoulder, subsequent to rupture of the medial glenohumeral ligament or laxity of the glenoid lip.

Too large an inferior recess is encountered in habitual dislocation. Lack of filling of the various recesses and of the normally shaped synovial folds points to sclerosis of the capsule and reveals the anatomical basis of a frozen shoulder syndrome. The fact that the surface of the articular cartilage is sharply delineated, permits visualization of abnormalities or erosions.

Lesions of the long head of the M. Bicipitis and its sheath can be demonstrated directly and indirectly, which is extremely important when this tendon is to be used in stabilizing the shoulder (Nicola procedure).

The examination allows evaluation of the soundness and thickness of the insertion tendons of the short rotators and detection of a possible defect. In addition, it yields accurate data on the extent of the tendon rupture.

In epiphyseal growth disturbances and congenital shoulder lesions, arthrography reveals the shape and congruence of the cartilaginous humeral head.

CONCLUSION

Although periarthritic lesions are by far the most common cause of shoulder pain in the orthopedic field, it should however be noted that there exists in addition a variety of musculoskeletal and nervous disorders, which may provoke a pain syndrome in arm and shoulder. Careful history taking, meticulous clinical examination and properly chosen technical investigations are necessary to establish the correct diagnosis.

REFERENCES

J.C. Adams. An Outline of Orthopaedics. First edition, p. 217. London and Edinburgh: E & S Livingstone 1955
H. Claessens. De pijnlijke schouder. Leiden; Stafleu, 1969
Watson, M. Lipmann Kessel, The Painful Arc Syndrome. Clinical Classification as a Guide to Management J. Bone Jt. Surg. 59B: 166–172, 1977
I. Macnab. Rotator Cuff Tendinitis. Ann. R. Coll. Surg. Engl. 53: 271–287, 1973
H.F. Moseley. Shoulder Lesions. Paul B. Hoeber Inc., Medical Book Department of Harper & Brothers, 1953

9. Traumatology of the shoulder region

ANDREW A. McBEATH. M.D.*

ABSTRACT

Acute injuries to the shoulder region have been described for nearly 5000 years. This paper deals primarily with pathophysiology, diagnosis and treatment of glenohumeral and acromio-clavicular dislocations.

Ninety-eight percent of glenohumeral dislocations are anterior. Physical examination or the anterior-posterior radiograph are usually diagnostic. Following reduction of the initial dislocation the patient's shoulder is immobilized for three to six weeks to minimize a chance of recurrent dislocation. Generally, the greater the initial trauma the less the chance of recurrence. Patients under twenty years of age with an anterior dislocation have an 80–90% chance of recurrent dislocation while the risk for those over forty drops to 10–15%. Posterior glenohumeral dislocations are rare and frequently not diagnosed. Diagnostic error is due to the near normal appearance of the anterior-posterior radiograph, therefore a second view is essential. Several views are available but the axillary view is the most easily interpreted. Treatment of the initial dislocation is again immobilization. External rotation of the humerus may be necessary to maintain reduction. Surgical procedures exist to treat the recurrent form of both types of glenohumeral dislocation. The actual repair performed is tailored to fit the existing pathology.

In acromioclavicular dislocations the treatment for first and second degree lesions is clearly nonoperative. Third degree lesions are treated both operatively and nonoperatively, but the author favors closed treatment for most cases as no study has shown surgical treatment to give superior functional end results. The most common late complication of acromioclavicular separation is arthritis of the acromioclavicular joint, and the most interesting complication is osteolysis of the distal clavicle. Both these sequella may, if troublesome, be treated by resection of the distal clavicle.

Although diagnostic and therapeutic progress has been made, challenges still exist to find more effective therapy for shoulder injuries.

Acute injuries of the shoulder region were described as long ago as 3000 B.C., in the Edwin Smith Papyrus. The following discussion deals with such injuries. Emphasis is placed on glenohumeral and acromioclavicular dislocations.

*Professor and Chairman, Division of Orthopedic Surgery, University of Wisconsin Medical School, Madison, Wisconsin, USA.

J.M. Greep, H.A.J. Lemmens, D.B. Roos and H.C. Urschel (eds.).
Pain in shoulder and arm: an integrated view, 103–109. All rights reserved.
Copyright © 1979 by Martinus Nijhoff Publishers, The Hague/Boston/London.

ANTERIOR GLENOHUMERAL DISLOCATION

A drawing from 1200 B.C. found in the tomb of Upay depicted the reduction of an anterior dislocation by the method of Kocher. In 460 B.C. Hippocrates described the lesion well and indicated the severity of the recurrent form when he mentioned that it caused some individuals to give up gymnastics and others to perish in war because of ineptness.

The subcoracoid type is the most common anterior glenohumeral dislocation. It can be caused by a posterior blow but is more frequently caused by forced abduction and external rotation.

The patient presents with shoulder pain and holds the humerus slightly abducted and externally rotated. The contour of the shoulder is pathopneumonic. There is a sharp drop off at the tip of the acromion. The lateral deltoid muscle as viewed from the front or back shows a straight or concave contour instead of the normally convex contour. The head of the humerus is generally palpable in the subcoracoid region. The examination before and after reduction must include the neurovascular status of the extremity. The axillary and musculocutaneous nerves are the ones most commonly damaged. Circulatory damage is more common in elderly patients. Physical findings of vessel damage would be hematoma formation in the axilla and ischemia in the limb. The anterior-posterior radiograph is usually diagnostic.

If the patient is seen within 20–30 minutes of the injury the dislocation can often be reduced without medication but after this time period the administration of an analgesic and a muscle relaxant is necessary. Infrequently, general anesthesia is needed. Through the ages many methods, often brutal, have been utilized to reduce the dislocation. Reduction involves traction. A physician with an assistant can apply traction to the arm while the assistant applies counter traction by means of a sheet wrapped around the patient's thorax. If no assistant is available, the Hippocratic method is useful. The unshod foot that provides the counter traction can also be used to push the humeral head laterally. The Stimson manoeuver is often effective and is ideal for physicians who do not treat the problem often as it requires minimal manipulative intervention. If weights are used they must be attached to the patient's arm rather than having him grip them, as gripping inhibits muscle relaxation and thereby impedes reduction. The Kocher maneuver carries some risk of fracturing to the humerus but it may be the only effective maneuver. After reduction the arm is immobilized with a sling and swath for three to six weeks after the first dislocation. This is followed by a rehabilitation program. Subsequent dislocations are immobilized only as long as discomfort persists.

RECURRENT FORM OF GLENOHUMERAL DISLOCATION

The most important factor in determining whether or not an individual will suffer from recurrent anterior glenohumeral dislocation is the age of the patient at the time of the initial dislocation. If the original injury occurs before the age of 20 years the patient has an 80–90% chance of subsequent dislocations. If the patient is over 40 years old at the time of the initial injury, the chance of recurrence drops to 10–15%. The greater the initial trauma, the less the chance of recurrence. The length of immobilization after the initial dislocation is a debated factor.

The two most consistently found pathological alterations seen in the recurrent form were well noted before 1900. The defect in the posterior lateral aspect of the humeral head is a crush fracture from impingement on the anterior glenoid. The capsule avulsed from the anterior scapula offers little restraint to anterior displacement of the humeral head. Other defects less commonly seen include attenuation of the subscapularis muscle, excessive anteversion of the glenoid, a small glenoid or an anterior erosion of the glenoid.

The recurrent form can be controlled with a restraint strap between the thorax and the humerus, but corrective treatment is surgical. Since Hippocrates delineated the fine points of applying a hot iron, more than 100 surgical procedures have been advocated to treat this problem. Such drastic procedures as humeral head resection and shoulder arthrodesis have been done.

Current operative procedures can be grouped according to the structure being attacked. Often elements of two or more methods are combined to adequately treat existing pathology in a given shoulder. Reapproximation of the avulsed anterior capsule to the scapula is most often done by the method of Bankart. Drilling the proper holes can be difficult. Reapproximation with the staple has also been advocated. In the pure form this type of repair does not limit external rotation. Modification of the subscapularis muscle is either an imbrication as in the Putti-Platt procedure or a lateral transfer of the insertion as in the Magneson Stack procedure. Either modification will decrease external rotation which is felt to be important when a Hill-Sachs defect exists. Glenoid alterations include anterior augmentation with a bone graft as advocated by Eden and Hybbinette, and scapular neck osteotomy to decrease excessive glenoid anteversion.

A currently popular procedure in the United States is the modified Bristow operation. This procedure is felt to provide a dynamic anterior inferior muscle sling, a bone block, and subscapularis retention to prevent dislocation.

Originally this was favored for throwing athletes as it was thought not to limit external rotation, but a follow-up study has shown limitation of external rotation [1].

Osteotomy in the proximal humerus to increase humeral retroversion has been advocated. This procedure places the head defect away from the glenoid.

The terres minor muscle can be placed into the humeral head defect. Transfer of the latissimus dorsi to the region of the infraspinatus has also been advocated.

Follow-up studies of the major procedures indicate success rates of 90+% or better [2].

The author most often uses a combination of Bankart and Putti-Platt methods with an axillary skin incision. Men appreciate an inconspicuous scar as much as women. After the indicated period of immobilization a vigorous program of motion and strengthening exercises is necessary.

POSTERIOR GLENOHUMERAL DISLOCATION

Posterior glenohumeral dislocations constitute only 2% of all glenohumeral dislocations. The subacromial type is the most common. This rare dislocation is important because it is difficult to diagnose and therefore the diagnosis is often missed. It is missed because the dislocation is rare, the physical examination is not striking and the anterior-posterior radiograph appears quite normal.

Posterior glenohumeral dislocation may be produced by an anterior blow, it may follow a grand mal seizure or an electric shock. It may occur as a result of a forced internal rotation adduction and flexion as would be sustained in a fall on the outstretched hand.

The patient presents himself with pain. The humerus is held in adduction and internal rotation. A thin patient and an astute examiner are necessary to appreciate the minimal posterior displacement of the humerus and the increased prominence of the coracoid.

The anterior-posterior radiograph is not helpful to most viewers. Careful interpretation by a skilled observer will reveal absence of the eliptical overlap, a vacant glenoid or a globular shaped humeral head due to the internal rotation of the humerus. Because these findings are only suggestive, a second projection is imperative for precise diagnosis. A transthoracic lateral view is nearly worthless. A tangential view of the scapula is helpful in skilled hands. An axillary view is the best view and it is easiest to interpret. If the patient cannot abduct the humerus effectively for a conventional axillary view to be taken, the valpaux modification can be obtained. This is accomplished by having the patient lean back over the X-ray table with the cassette beneath the elbow while the camera is placed above the shoulder. Only slight humeral abduction is necessary to delineate the meaningful glenohumeral relationship.

For reduction of posterior dislocation more relaxation is usually necessary than for reduction of an anterior glenohumeral dislocation. Traction is used while pressure is applied over the posterior aspect of the shoulder. Slight internal rotation may be necessary to dislodge the impacted humeral head. If the reduction is stable with the arm across the chest sling and swath immobilization is sufficient. If the reduction is not stable in this position the humerus must be immobilized in external rotation. This requires plaster on the arm fixed to plaster around the trunk.

A posterior glenohumeral dislocation may also go on to a recurrent form. If so, procedures analogous to those for anterior dislocation are available.

ACROMIOCLAVICULAR DISLOCATION OR SHOULDER SEPARATION

Hippocrates also spoke of this problem. He noted that physicians confused it with anterior glenohumeral dislocation. He stated that little impediment but tumification will result from this injury. Both of these latter points are well illustrated in a recent Time magazine photograph of Joe Namath, an American professional football quarterback, with a tumification located on his throwing arm.

Classification of acromioclavicular dislocation is based on an understanding of the functions of the acromioclavicular and coricoclavicular ligaments. The acromioclavicular ligaments are felt to be mainly responsible for ventraldorsal stability of the acromioclavicular joint while the coricoclavicular ligaments prevent cephaloid displacement of the clavicle. In the first degree injury only the acromioclavicular ligaments are stretched. In a second degree injury the acromioclavicular ligaments may have a second or third degree sprain, but the coricoclavicular ligaments are intact. There is little or no cephaloid displacement of the clavicle. In a third degree injury both the coricoclavicular and acromioclavicular ligaments are completely torn.

The injury is most frequently incurred as a result of falling and landing on the point of the shoulder. In a third degree separation the diagnostic step off deformity is seen, tenderness exists both superior to the acromion and over the acromioclavicular joint. The distal clavicle is ballotable without crepitation. In first and second degree separations tenderness exists only over the acromioclavicular joint

When taking radiographs of the acromioclavicular joint, the exposure must be decreased so that the distal clavicle is not overexposed. Weighted films can be helpful to definitely diagnose third degree separations.

The treatment for first and second degree lesions is clearly nonoperative. Debate exists whether or not third degree lesions should be treated operatively or nonoperatively. The literature fails to document superiority of either form of treatment. The manufactured devices for the closed treatment of this lesion have made closed treatment more effective and convenient. Elderly individuals should be treated for comfort only.

Because the most effective operation involves resection of the distal clavicle, the author favors closed treatment for most cases. If this fails the distal clavicle is excised. If the clavicle is high riding, it is stabilized by inserting the detached acromial end of the corico-acromial ligament into the distal clavicle [3].

If primary open repair is undertaken a multitude of procedures are available. When selecting a procedure the surgeon should ideally select one that accomplishes the following: (1) adequate debridement of the acromio-clavicular joint including removal of the meniscus if it is torn, (2) adequate reduction – the anterior posterior reduction is usually the more difficult, (3) good fixation; this should not damage the articular surface and should not permanently rigidly fix the clavicle to the scapula, (4) repair of the corico-clavicular ligaments and the acromioclavicular ligaments, (5) repair of the avulsed trapezius and deltoid muscles.

The most common late complication is arthritis of the acromioclavicular joint. The most interesting complication is post-traumatic osteolysis of the distal clavicle. It is most commonly seen after first and second degree lesions. This lysis can cause confusion on subsequent radiographs as both tumor and infection may be suspected. If either of these sequelae become symptomatic they are effectively treated by resection of the distal clavicle.

FRACTURE OF THE CLAVICLE

Most of these fractures are best treated closed. The commercially available dressings are convenient and generally eliminate the need for a plaster reinforced dressing. When treating adults a sling applied on the involved side is a very advantageous addition to the "figure 8" dressing, even though it is not often used. The sling transfers much of the arm weight directly to the neck and diminishes the tendency of the figure 8 to bind the axilla.

FRACTURE DISLOCATION OF THE GLENOHUMERAL JOINT

These will be mentioned only to refer the reader to the classic work of Neer that details a classification and a rational plan of treatment [4].

Even though we have made progress on the diagnosis and treatment of these shoulder injuries since Hippocrates was confronted with them, challenges still exist to find more effective therapy.

REFERENCES

1. S.J. Lombardo, R.K. Kerlan, F.M. Jobe, V.S. Carter, M.E. Blazina, C.L. Shields Jr. The modified bristow procedure for recurrent dislocation of the shoulder. J. Bone and Joint Surg. 58-A: 256, 1976
2. C.A. Rockwood Jr. Rockwood and Green-fractures. Philadelphia, J.B. Lippincott, 672–673, 1975
3. J.K. Weaver, H.K. Dunn. Treatment of acromioclavicular injuries, especially complete acromioclavicular separation. J. Bone and Joint Surg. 54-A: 1187, 1972
4. C.S. Neer II. Displaced proximal humeral fractures-parts I and II. J. Bone and Joint Surg, 52-A: 1077, 1970

10. Thrombosis of the axillary-subclavian vein

J. DREWES M.D.*

ABSTRACT

One must differentiate between the *primary* or spontaneous thrombosis of the subclavian/axillary vein, the so-called Paget-v.-Schroetter syndrome and the *secondary* or symptomatic thrombosis.

We had a total of 109 patients. The Paget-v.-Schroetter syndrome was observed in 85 cases, while symptomatic thrombosis occurred in only 24 patients.

Since the clinical symptoms and the phlebographic findings are similar in both conditions, the differentiation between the two forms of thrombosis requires an exact case – history taking and a thorough general examination.

The *phlebogram* most frequently shows a complete, less frequently a partial closure and seldom a stenosis. The position of the occlusion is very variable. With the help of the phlebography – especially later control phlebography – it may also be demonstrated, that the occlusion of the vessel is really caused by a thrombosis.

As regards *aetiology*, in symptomatic thrombosis, it is the primary desease which plays the most important role, while in Paget-v.-Schroetter syndrome several causative factors have been discussed.

The *prognosis* of Paget-v.-Schroetter syndrome is very good, quoad vitam. Fatal pulmonary embolism occurs very seldom. However functional hindrance of the involved arm is not uncommon, especially in patients who have not undergone early *treatment* with thrombolytic therapy or a thrombectomy. The latter may be combined with a partial resection of the first rib or a scalenotomy. In patients with remaining severe post-thrombotic symptoms a venous by-pass should be considered.

Pain of the shoulder and arm is comparatively seldom caused by venous deseases. Doubtless the thrombosis of the axillary-subclavian vein is the most important among these venous diseases.

The acute phase of the axillary-subclavian thrombosis begins only occasionally with sudden stabbing pain in the shoulder respectively in the axilla. A remarkable pain at rest is not the rule. When, however, the involved arm is used, there occur cramplike pains and early tiredness, combined with a feeling of weakness and heaviness. These symptoms occur regularly in all acute cases, though in the later stages of the disease they are found only in a small percentage. These complaints are named by some authors as "claudicatio intermittens venosa".

The clinical picture of axillary-subclavian thrombosis is characterized by

*Surgical University Clinic, Düsseldorf, West Germany.

J.M. Greep, H.A.J. Lemmens, D.B. Roos and H.C. Urschel (eds.).
Pain in shoulder and arm: an integrated view, 111–128. All rights reserved.
Copyright © 1979 by Martinus Nijhoff Publishers, The Hague/Boston/London.

swelling, bluish discolouration and also venous marbling of the skin. The swelling extends, as Figure 1 shows, along the whole arm and can be of considerable degree. If the disease has been present for some time, the swelling is often moderate or just minimal. The bluish or blue-reddish discolouration of the skin is often only clearly seen at the peripheral parts, especially at the hand and more so, if the arm is hanging down (Figure 2). In Figure 3 it can be seen, that the venous marbling mostly develops at the upper arm, the shoulder and the upper anterior part of the thoracic wall.

If the arms are put up above the head, the veins of the involved arm empty themselves more slowly than those of the opposite arm. Occasionally one could palpate a cord-like painful induration in the axilla.

Among the special investigations venous-pressure determination and especially phlebography are the most important. Most often phlebography shows a complete closure of the main vein-stem, though less frequently we can see a partial closure and even more seldom we see a stenosis. These are always combined with an evident collateral circulation.

The position of the closure is very variable. Figures 4a and b show a high closure of the subclavian vein. In these cases the filling defect of the contrast medium is very short. Such short filling defects have especially been observed in long standing cases.

In the two phlebograms, which are to be seen in Figures 5a and b, the closure of the vessel is more peripheral. Figure 5a shows the stoppage of the

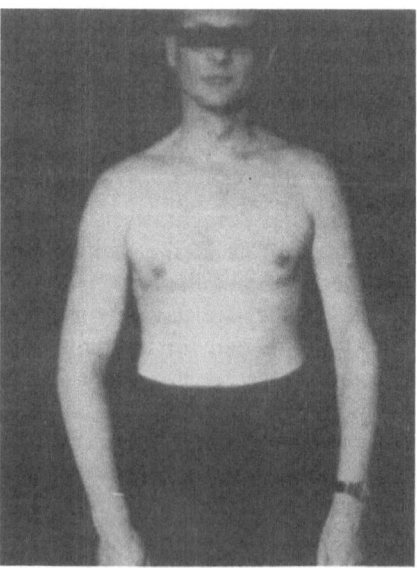

Figure 1. Remarkable swelling of the right arm in a patient with spontaneous thrombosis of the subclavian vein (= Paget-v.-Schrötter syndrome).

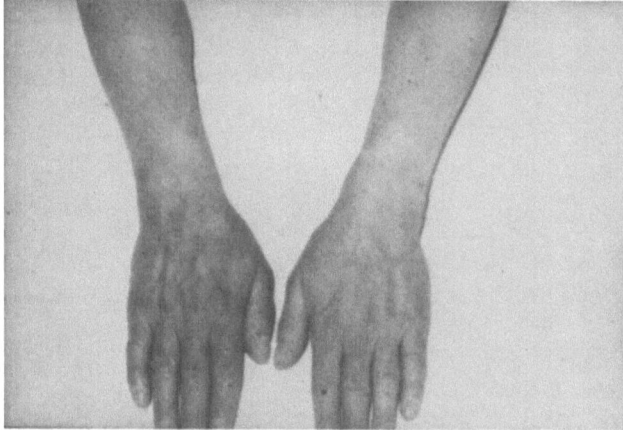

Figure 2. Bluish discolouration of the hand and the forearm on the involved side.

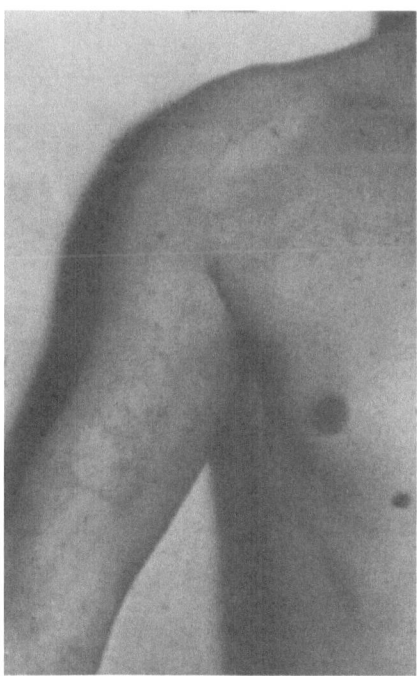

Figure 3. Distended superficial veins (venous marbling) of the upper arm, shoulder and upper part of the thoracic wall.

114

J. Drewes

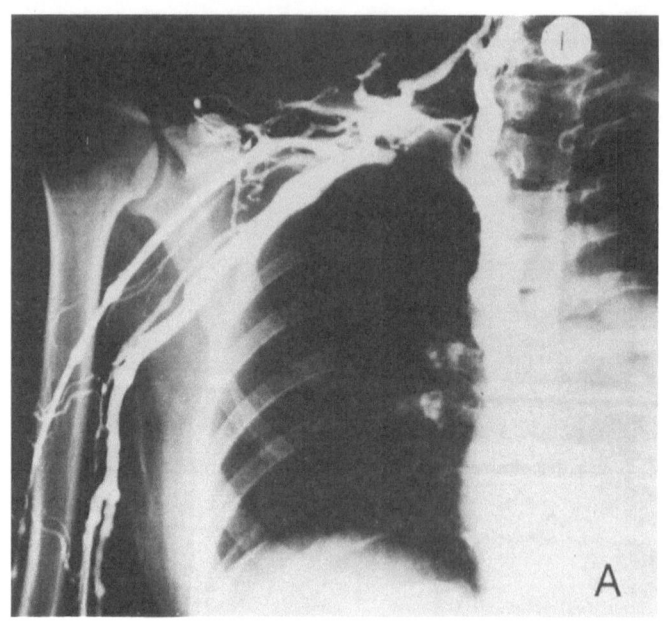

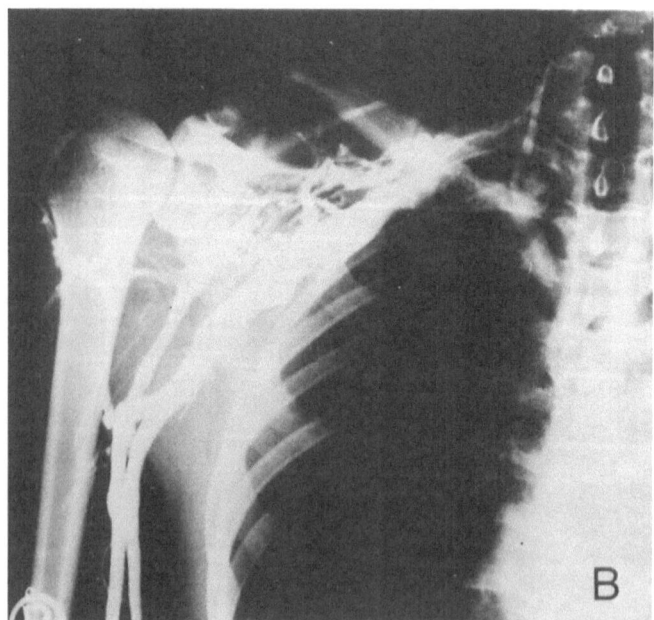

Figures 4A and B. Two examples of a blockage of the subclavian vein.

contrast medium at the middle of the axillary vein. In Figure 5b the closure occurs even more distally, that is in the region of the brachial veins or of the basilic vein. These large filling defects of the contrast medium were observed mostly in early thromboses.

An example of a stenosis of the subclavian vein is seen in Figure 6. In all these phlebograms, an evident collateral circulation can be observed. But there is a remarkable difference with regard to the number, the calibre and the direction of the collateral vessels in the individual cases.

Phlebography not only shows the site of the closure of the vessel, but may also demonstrate, that this closure is really caused by a thrombosis. This can be proved by later control phlebograms. In Figure 7a the initial phlebogram can be seen. One can see a complete stop in the distal part of the axillary vein. The phlebogram in Figure 7b was performed 5 months later. One sees, that the axillary vein is again open. However at the subclavian vein there is still a partial closure or rather a stenosis, whose organic character is mainly demonstrated by the permanence of the collateral circulation.

Because the subclavian vein generally remains partially or totally blocked in the control-phlebograms of patients, who have not undergone a thrombolytic therapy, we have to conclude, that the initial grey thrombus starts in the subclavian vein itself and not in the axillary vein. As is known the grey thrombus is dissolved with more difficulty than the red thrombus.

Because of the characteristic symptoms the diagnosis of the axillary-subclavian vein thrombosis provides no difficulty. One must however differentiate between the spontaneous thrombosis of the axillary-subclavian vein, the so-called Paget-v.-Schrötter syndrome, and the secondary or symptomatic thrombosis. In the latter group we include for instance the post-operative, postpartal and posttraumatic thromboses, as well as those thromboses resulting from a large cervical rib or a deformity of the clavicular bone and those caused by inflammatory or neoplastic lymph-node swellings, by a retrosternal goitre, by an aneurysm and by benign or malignant tumors and finally those resulting from cardiac failure or from progressive peripheral thrombophlebitis.

In my series the Paget-v.-Schrötter syndrome was observed in 85 patients, while symptomatic thromboses occurred in only 24 patients. In these 24 cases I have not included iatrogenically caused thromboses, that is, those occurring after intravenous pace-maker implantation or caval-catheterization, which currently form the largest group of secondary thromboses.

The Paget-v.-Schrötter syndrome, that is the spontaneous thrombosis of the axillary-subclavian vein, is our main interest. It is remarkable, that the Paget-v.-Schrötter syndrome mostly occurs in young and healthy indi-

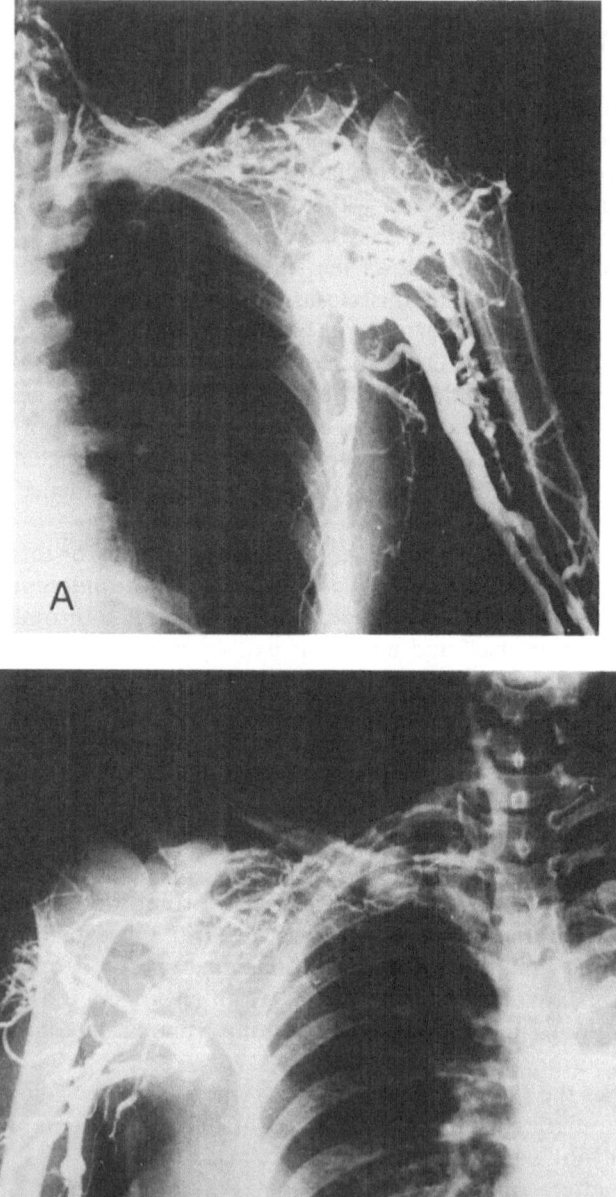

Figures 5*A* and *B*. Two examples of a more peripheral blockage of the vessel, *A*) in the middle of the axillary vein, *B*) in the basilic vein.

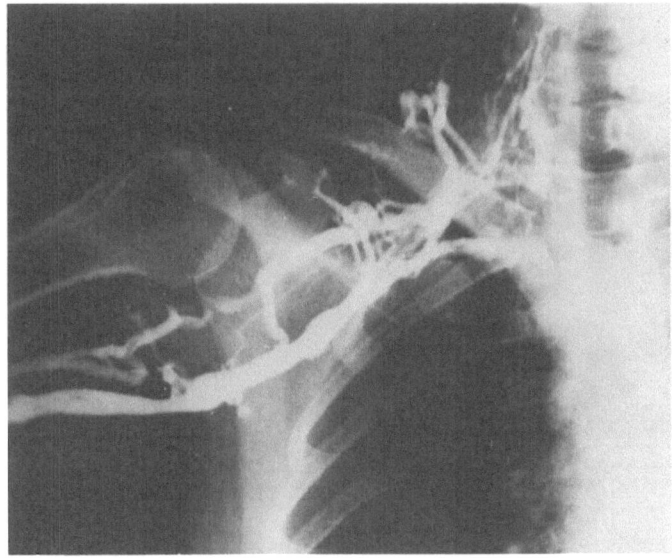

Figure 6. Postthrombotic stenosis of the subclavian vein.

viduals – the majority of the patients are in the twenties and thirties – and that two-thirds of the patients are males and also that the syndrome often occurs in the arm which is mostly used.

Differentiation between the Paget-v.-Schrötter syndrome and symptomatic thrombosis requires an exact case history taking and a thorough general examination, which should be supplemented with radiological examination of the thorax and cervical vertebrae. From the phlebogram one cannot differentiate between the Paget-v.-Schrötter syndrome and symptomatic thrombosis. This, too, I would like to demonstrate with the help of three examples. All the phlebograms, which have already been shown, are from patients with Paget-v.-Schrötter syndrome. In Figure 8 we see a closure of the subclavian vein, produced by lymphnode metastases from a bronchial carcinoma. Figure 9 shows an extensive closure of the main vein stem in a 73 year old man suffering from heart failure. And in Figure 10 there can be seen a thrombosis of the subclavian vein from a patient, who had undergone a pacemaker implantation.

I would like now to go quickly over the aetiology of the axillary-subclavian vein thrombosis. In the symptomatic form, which is practically a secondary disease, the basic disease without questions plays an important role. The question is however, how the Paget-v.-Schrötter syndrome comes about.

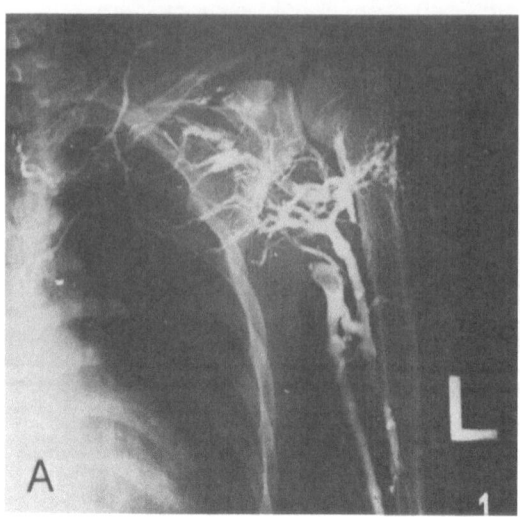

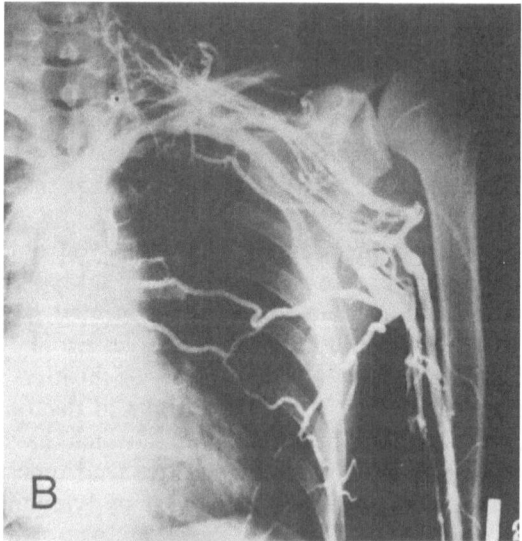

Figure 7A. Complete blockage of the axillary vein.
    B. Controlphlebogram 5 months later. The axillary vein is again open but there still exists
a partial closure of the subclavian vein.

This question has been much discussed. Some hold, that the cause is a
primary, segmentary venous spasm – an opinion which was expressed by
Cottalorda [7]. Most authorities hold, that the thrombosis results from a
mechanical injury to the vein wall arising from certain movements or through

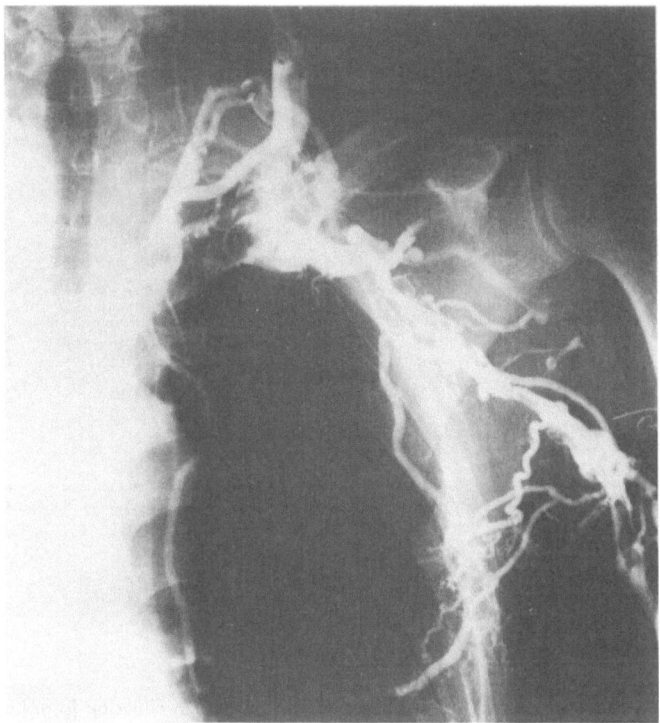

Figure 8. Closure of the subclavian vein produced by a lymphnode metastasis from a bronchial carcinoma.

special anatomical structures. It is quite clear, that during certain movements the subclavian vein can be compressed as it passes through the narrow costoclavicular space or – that because of its tight strut to the periosteum of the first rib and the fascia of the subclavian muscle it can be overextended or stretched.

In my opinion there is yet another causal possibility which can be put forward, that is, damage of the terminal valve of the subclavian vein. In the Valsalva manoeuvre or during forced espiration the terminal valve of the subclavian vein is the first barrier which the return blood flow meets. I hold as possible that the pressure strain can produce small fissures in the delicate valve cusps, and these together with special flow effects – temporary stasis and turbulent flow – may result in the initiation of thromboses.

Before I pass on to the treatment, I would like to say a few words about prognosis. Quoad vitam the prognosis of Paget-v.-Schrötter syndrome is very good. Pulmonary embolism occurs relatively seldom. Only 2 of our 85 patients suffered a pulmonary infarction. Fatal embolism is an extreme rarity. To my knowledge there are only reports from Hermann (1957) [24]

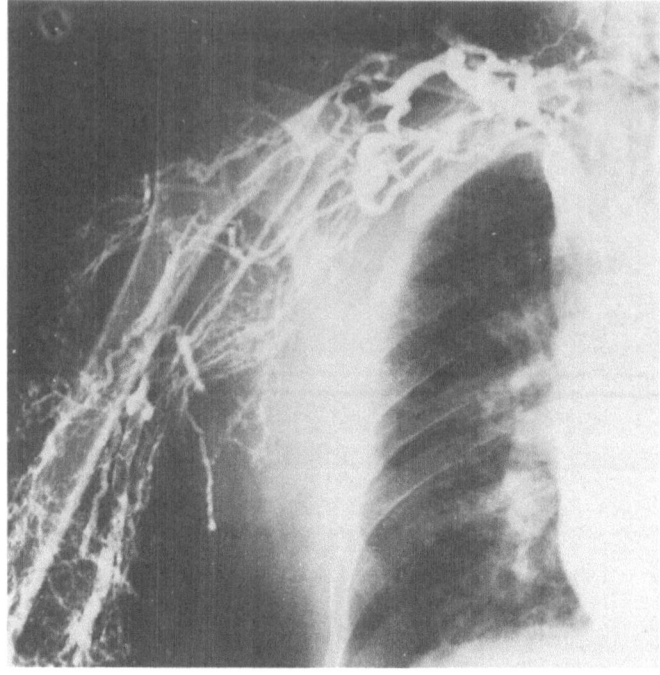

Figure 9. Extensive closure of the main vein stem in a patient suffering from heart failure.

and Uehlinger (1964) [37]. A recurrance is on the other hand not uncommon. According to our experience one could reckon with a recurrence in about 10% of the cases.

Quoad functionem the prognoses could likewise be very good. Unfortunatly till now it hasn't been so, because even today many of the patients come at a late stage of the disease for thrombectomy or thrombolytic treatment and so a total restitution cannot be achieved. In these cases, the severity of the remaining symptoms and the severity of the complaints on using the arm is dependent on the effectiveness of the collateral circulation.

Eventually in the involved patients, the existing inborn vascular channels, through which the main flow blockage could be bypassed, could be of greater importance. This applies especially in certain variations of the cephalic vein. Figure 11 shows a normal finding. The cephalic vein totally empties in the end-part of the axillary vein. In Figure 12 we observe that the cephalic vein divides into two branches, the lower emptying at the normal site, while the upper empties into the angulus venosus. In Figure 13, too, a division of the cephalic vein can be seen. In this case the upper branch joins

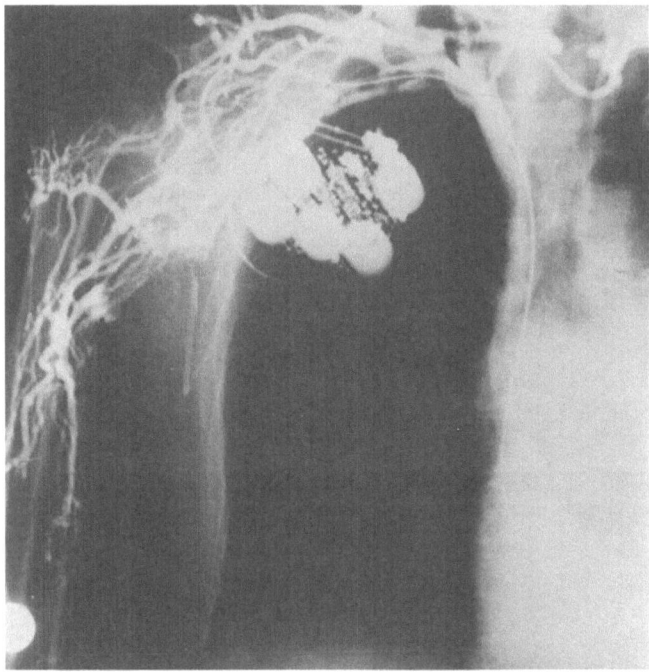

Figure 10. Partial closure of the subclavian vein in a patient who underwent a pace-maker implantation.

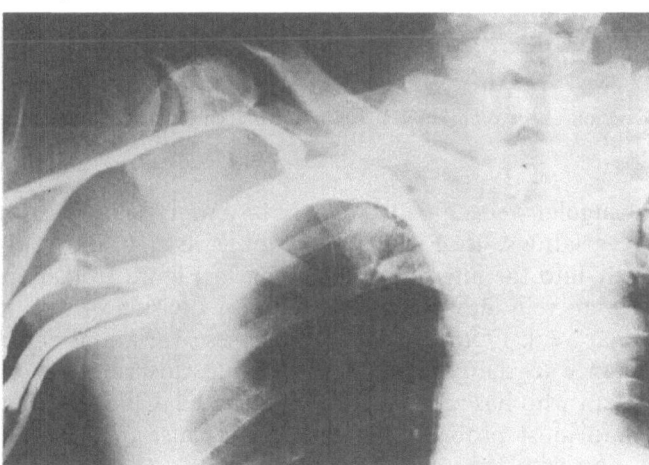

Figure 11. Normal course of the cephalic vein, which totally empties into the end-part of the axillary vein.

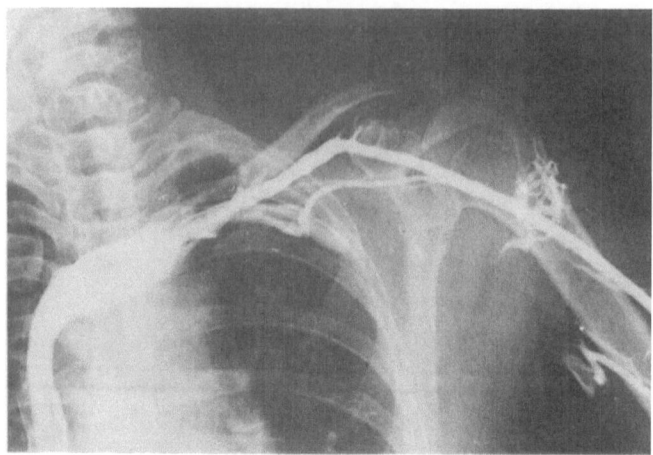

Figure 12. Division of the cephalic vein into two branches, the lower emptying at the normal site, while the upper empties into the angulus venosus.

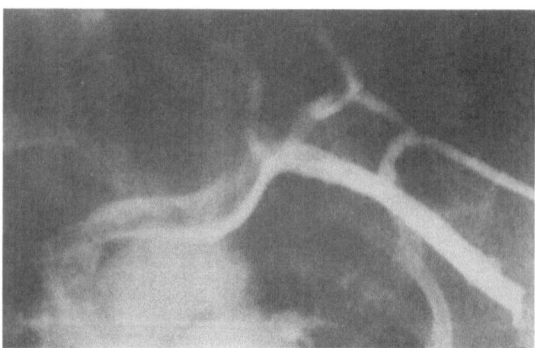

Figure 13. Division of the cephalic vein. The upper branch joins the external jugular vein.

the external jugular vein. Finally Figures 14 and 15 show two other very uncommon variations. In Figure 14 we observe that the cephalic vein empties totally into the internal jugular vein. In Figure 15 there is division of the subclavian vein into two parts, the upper division of which joins the internal jugular vein. Figure 16 shows, that these variations could, indeed, be of importance to the patients. A thrombotic closure of the subclavian vein in a patient who has a pacemaker is illustrated. Clinically the blockage was slilent and most probably remained so because of the presence of a wide connection with the internal jugular vein.

Now we pass on to treatment. In the early stage of the disease, there are two methods of treatment, that is thrombectomy and thrombolytic therapy.

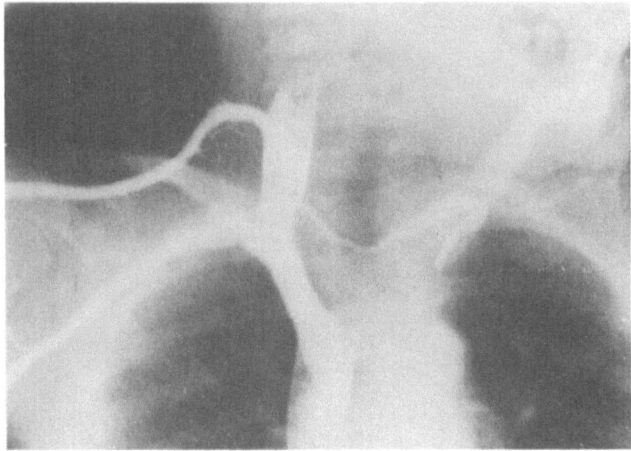

Figure 14. The **cephalic vein flows** totally into the **internal jugular** vein.

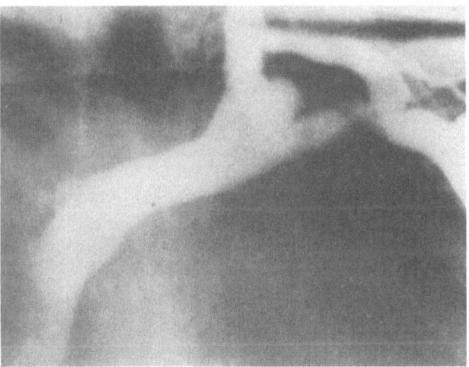

Figure 15. Division of the subclavian vein. The upper branch joins the internal jugular vein.

We follow the latter, with which, I must say, we have obtained very good results. Indeed, a real cure, and so a complete lysis of the thrombus, generally can be obtained only when the treatment is started within the first 48, or at the latest, 72 hours. X-ray evidence of a complete restitution should include not only a completely renewed passage through the channel but also the disappearance of the collateral circulation. Figure 17 shows an example after successful thrombolytic therapy. The initial phlebogram (Figure 17a) was performed two days after the onset of the condition. There is an extensive distal blockage of the main vessel stem with numerous collateral channels. In Figure 17b we have the control phlebogram after therapy with streptokinase. The axillary and the subclavian vein are again totally open and the collateral circulation has disappeared.

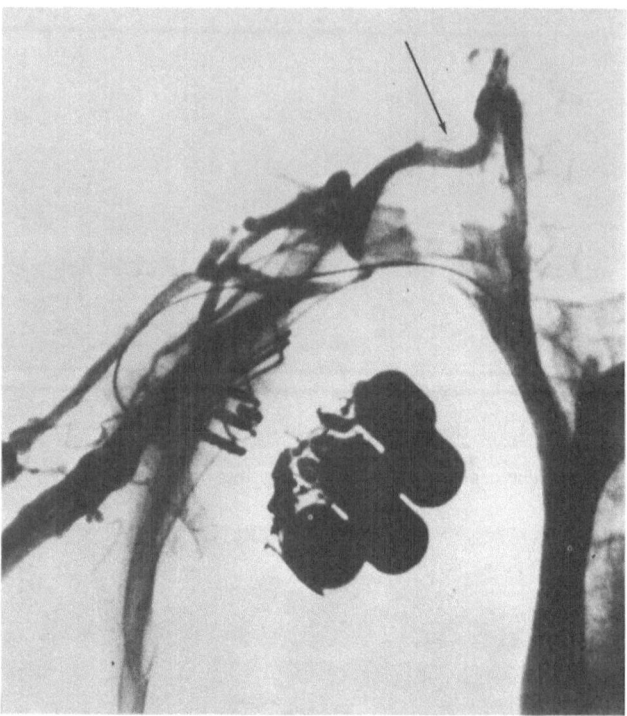

Figure 16. Blockage of the subclavian vein occurring after the transvenous introduction of pace-maker electrodes. The blockage was clinically silent because of the wide connection (→) to the internal jugular vein.

As is the case for thrombolytic therapy, the success of thrombectomy depends on its being performed as early as possible. Because of the danger of rethrombosis, thrombectomy performed later than five days after onset of symptoms, is hardly worthwhile.

When the patients come to us too late for a thrombectomy or a thrombolytic therapy we put them on anticoagulant therapy for about two to three years to prevent an apposition thrombosis. We also elevate the arm for a transient period, apply heparin ointment, and also possibly a compression bandage. This is done with the hope that through the formation of an effective collateral circulation we may achieve a satisfactory improvement, and very often this is luckily the case.

When, however the collateral circulation remains ineffective, with resulting considerable functional hindrance of the arm, which prevents the patient from performing his previous work, then one should consider the question of operative treatment.

The previously performed operations like veinlysis, veinresection, partial

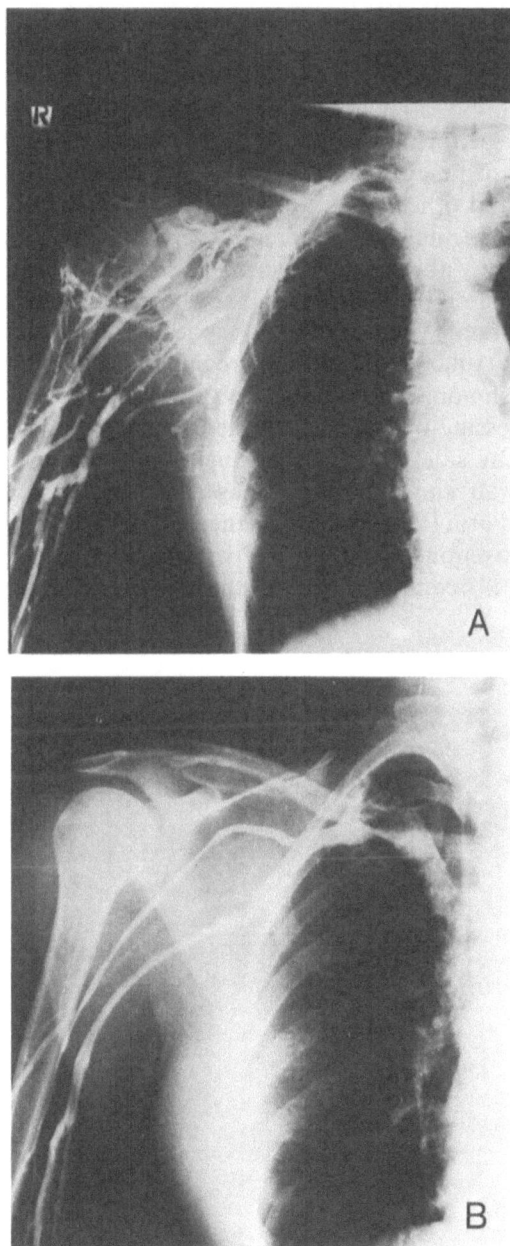

Figure 17*A*, Initial phlebogramm. There is an extensive blockage of the main vessel stem with numerous collateral vessels.

B. Controlphlebogramm after thrombolytic therapy. The axillary and subclavian vein are again totally open. The collateral circulation has disappeared.

resection of the first rib, division of the scalenus anterior or the subclavius muscle or of the tendon of the pectoralis minor have not fulfilled expectations. Nevertheless, if after a succesful thrombolytic therapy or thrombectomy the possibility of a recurrence due to special causal factors exists, one should think of performing some of these operations, for example the partial resection of first rib or a scalenotomy (Dunant [15, 16], Schulze-Bergmann [35] and others).

Nowadays, in patients with remaining severe post-thrombotic symptoms, it is practically only the venous bypass which is involved. This was put forward by Carstensen in 1968 [6]. Rabinowitz and Goldfarb [33] and also Passl and co-workers [32] applied a saphenal vein-bypass between the distal part of the axillary vein and the proximal part of the internal jugular vein. In 1976 Hashmonai and co-workers [22] performed – as in the Palma operation – a crossing-over bypass of the cephalic vein. Here the cephalic vein of the healthy side is directed through a subcutaneous tunnel at the upper thoracic wall and then anastomosed with the cephalic vein of the opposite involved arm (Figure 18). Together with these by-pass operations a temporary arteriovenous fistula is also performed.

Although these operations are in themselves an enrichment in our

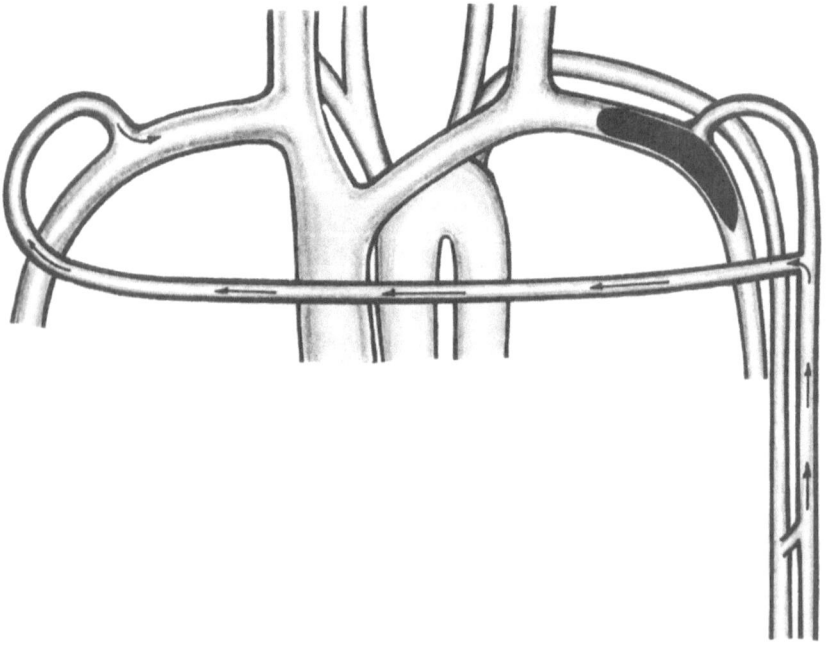

Figure 18. Schematic figure of a crossing-over bypass of the cephalic vein (performed by Hashmonai and co-workers [22]).

therapeutic possibilities, we must ensure that patients are referred, as early as possible, to a hospital where either a thrombectomy or a thrombolytic therapy can be undertaken so that the chances of a complete restitution can be offered.

REFERENCES

1. J.T. Adams, R.M. Mc Evoy, J.A. de Weese. Primary deep venous thrombosis of the upper extremity. Arch. Surg. 91: 29, 1965
2. J.T. Adams, J.A. de Weese, E.B. Mahoney, Ch. G. Rob. Intermittent subclavia vein obstruction without thrombosis. Surgery 63: 147, 1968
3. J. Balau, K.H. Buysch, E. Marx, A. Seling, H.-J. Knieriem. Thrombose der Vena subclavia nach transvenöser Schrittmacherimplantation. Der Radiologe 11: 50, 1971
4. M. Biebl. Thrombektomie bei blander Thrombose der V. axillaris und subclavia. Zbl. Chir. 66: 1560, 1939
5. H. Brandt, Der Achselvenenstau. Bruns Beitr. klin. Chir. 177: 231, 1948
6. G. Carstensen. Jahrestagung der Deutschen Gesellschaft für Angiologie e.V. 1968, Düsseldorf. Ergebnisse der Angiologie, Band 2, herausgegeben von N. Klüfen, Stuttgart-New York 1969. p.49
7. J. Cottalorda. La thrombophlébite par effort. Lyon Chir. 29: 169, 1932
8. J. Drewes. Phlebographische Befunde bei der Venensperre der oberen Extremität (Paget-von-Schroetter-Syndrom). Fortschr. Röntgenstr. 80: 34, 1954
9. J. Drewes. Die Phlebographie der oberen Körperhälfte. Springer, Berlin-Göttingen-Heidelberg 1963
10. J. Drewes. Varietäten der V. cephalica im Phlebogramm. Fortschr. Röntgenstr. 100:490, 1964
11. J. Drewes. Echte und scheinbare Stenosen und Verschlüsse im Kontrastbild der Vena subclavia. Chirurg 37: 105, 1966
12. J. Drewes. Bemerkungen zur Ätiologie des Paget-von-Schroetter-Syndroms. Fortschr. Röntgenstr. 105: 865, 1966
13. J. Drewes. Das Paget-von-Schroetter-Syndrom. – Ergebnisse der Angiologie. Bd. II. Stuttgart-New York: K.F. Schattauer 1969
14. J. Drewes. Besondere Venenerkrankungen. Klinisches Ärzteblatt 71 Jg., 1977, S. 446–455
15. J.H. Dunant. Die primäre akute Thrombose der V. subclavia. Vasa 3: 461, 1974
16. J.H. Dunant. Venendruckmessungen im Arm zur Beurteilung von Kompressionserscheinunge beim Schultergürtel-syndrom. Vasa 3: 418, 1974
17. O. Eylau. Die primär spastische Venensperre der oberen Extremität (Paget-von-Schroetter-Syndrom). Med. Klin. 52: 1291, 1957
18. M.A. Falconer, G. Weddell. Costoclavicular compression of the subclavian artery and vein; relation to scalenus anticus syndrome. Lancet II: 539, 1943
19. R. Fontaine, L. Tuchmann. Die venöse Thrombektomie in der Behandlung der tiefen frischen Fernthrombosen. Langenbecks Arch. klin. Chir. 304: 113, 1963
20. B.A. Glass. The relationship of axillary venous thrombosis to the thoracic outlet compression syndrome. Ann. of thorac. surg. 19: 613, 1975
21. E.P. Gould, D.H. Patey. Primary thrombosis of the axillary vein. Brit. J. Surg. 16: 208, 1928
22. M. Hashmonai, A. Schramek, J. Farbstein. Cephalic vein cross-over bypass for subclavian vein thrombosis: A case report. Surgery 80: 563, 1976
23. O. Henningsen. Venenwandverletzungen als Ursache der akuten Achselvenenstauung. Langenbecks Arch. klin. Chir. 199: 439, 1940
24. S.F. Hermann. Discussion after Loe, R.H. Primary subclavian vein occlusion. Amer.J. Surg. 94: 165, 1957.
25. E.S.R. Hughes. Venous obstruction in the upper extremity (Paget-Schroetter Syndrome). A Review of 320 Cases. Surg. Gynec. Obstet. Suppl. 88: 89, 1949

26. W. Löhr Über die sogenannte "traumatische" Thrombose der V. axillaris und subclavia. Dtsch. Z. Chir. 214: 263, 1929
27. W. Löhr. Die Claudicatio venosa intermittens der oberen Extremität. Ein kritischer Beitrag zur sog. traumatischen Thrombose der Vena axillaris und subclavia (Thrombose par effort). Langenbecks Arch. klin. Chir. 176: 701, 1933
28. K.E. Loose, Beitrag zum Krankheitsbild des Achselvenenstaus. Die Medizinische I: 220, 1952
29. P.S. Lowenstein. Thrombosis of the axillary vein. An anatomic study. J. Amer. med. Ass. 82: 852, 1924
30. R.S. Mc Cleery., J.E. Kesterton, J.A. Kirtley, R.B. Love. Subclavius and anterior scalene muscle compression as a cause of intermittent obstruction of the subclavian vein. Ann. Surg. 133: 588, 1951.
31. P. Ollinger. Die "nichtthrombotische Venensperre der oberen Extremität" und die Bedeutung der Venendruckmessung für die Frage der Diagnose and Ätiologie. Langenbecks Arch. klin. Chir. 260: 277, 1948
32. R. Passl, M. Staudacher, S. Szalay, G. Kobienia, H. Martinek. Zur Problematik und chirurgischen Therapie des veralteten Paget-v.-Schrötter Syndroms. Hefte Unfallheilk. 126: 170, 1976
33. R. Rabinowitz, D. Goldfarb. Surgical treatment of axillosubclavian venous thrombosis: A case report. Surgery 70: 703, 1971
34. J.J. Sampson, J.B. de L.M. Saunders, C.S. Capp. Compression of the subclavian vein by the first rib and clavicle, with special reference to the prominence of chest veins as a sign of collateral circulation. Amer. Heart J. 19: 292, 1940
35. G. Schulze-Bergmann. Das Paget-v.-Schroetter Syndrome. Med. Welt 26: 1952, 1975
36. I.M. Stevenson, E.W. Parry. Radiological study of the aetiological factors in venous obstruction of the upper limb. J. Cardiovas. Surg. 16: 580, 1975
37. E. Uehlinger. Bericht in Selecta 6: 1348, 1964.
38. J.R. Veal, E.M. Mc Fetridge. Primary thrombosis of the axillary vein. An anatomic and roentgenologic study of certain etiologic factors and a consideration of venography as a diagnostic measure. Arch. Surg. 31: 271, 1935
39. I.S. Wright. Neurovascular syndrome produced by hyperabduction of the arm. Amer. Heart J. 29: 1, 1945

11. Primary axillary-subclavian vein thrombosis

E. PARRY*

INCIDENCE

Primary Axillary Subclavian Vein Thrombosis is a rare clinical condition. It arouses little interest because the general impression has been, and probably still is, that they should be left well alone and they "all do well." The rarity is such that few general surgeons will see even one case in a year. If secondary thrombosis following thrombophlebitis of arm veins, malignant axillary glands and mediastinal tumours are included, the condition is still rare.

Tilney, Griffiths & Edwards in 1970 published a series collected from two hospitals in Boston, including the Peter Bent Brigham Hospital. Over a 25 year period they found 48 cases and in only 17 patients was the condition a primary or spontaneous thrombosis. The impression that this is an every-day problem is false and the impression that they "all do well" is equally false.

Seventy per cent of the cases have significant residual symptoms and more than half have disabling symptoms enforcing a change of occupation and sometimes inability to carry out any manual work. These facts are important in that 80–90% of cases are male and the dominant arm is affected in most cases. It is also interesting that the average age of these patients is under 40 years.

In 1974–75 we investigated this problem to see what relationship existed between external compression and intermittent venous obstruction as well a primary of spontaneous thrombosis. The impression that this is an every-

Group I

Patients with clinical evidence of intermittent venous obstruction in one or both upper limbs. The symptoms consisted of swelling, cyanosis, paraes-thesiae and aching of the affected limbs without any evidence of previous venous thrombosis.

* Broadgreen Hospital, Liverpool, England.

J.M. Greep, H.A.J. Lemmens, D.B. Roos and H.C. Urschel (eds.).
Pain in shoulder and arm: an integrated view, 129–132. All rights reserved.
Copyright © 1979 by Martinus Nijhoff Publishers, The Hague/Boston/London.

Group II

Patients with previous clinical and radiological evidence of axillary-subclavian vein thrombosis in one or both upper limbs.

Group III

A casual group of patients exhibiting no previous evidence of venous obstruction of the upper limbs.

Subclavian venography was carried out using Cardio-Conray. The radio-opaque medium was injected into a forearm vein and its progress through the axillary-subclavian venous system followed radiologically via an image intensifier.

Venograms of the arms were taken with the limbs by the patients side — adduction film.

Further venograms with the arm abducted 120° at the shoulder joint were taken – abduction film. Venous compression was regarded as positive when there was –

1. Narrowing of the axillary-subclavian vein in the root of the neck accompanied by
2. Radiological "hold up" in the passage of the radio-opaque medium on screening
3. Dilatation of the vein proximal to the site of venous narrowing

RESULTS

Group I. (Intermittent venous obstruction)
4 patients
3 Experienced unilateral symptoms
1 Experienced bilateral symptom
Results of bilateral subclavian venograms
All showed bilateral venous compression in abduction
2 Showed bilateral venous compression in adduction
1 Showed unilateral venous compression in adduction

Group II. (Previous acute axillary-subclavian vein thrombosis)
8 patients
Side of thrombosis: Right (5 patients), Left (3 patients)
Results of subclavian venogram on affected sides
All showed post-thrombotic axillary-subclavian vein occlusion with collateral formation
Results of subclavian venogram on unaffected sides

All showed venous compression in abduction
4 Showed venous compression in adduction

Group III. (Control Group)
10 patients
Side of subclavian venograms: Left (6 patients), Right (4 patients)
Results of subclavian venograms
All patients showed normal venographic appearances both in abduction and adduction

These results lead one to the conclusion that only patients with demonstrable venous outlet compression are at risk in developing acute venous thrombosis of the axillary-subclavian veins.

There is no long term follow-up of patients with clinical and radiological evidence of intermittent venous obstruction and we have no information as to whether or not they are more prone to develop thrombosis.

It is recorded that the subclavian vein has been explored on a presumed diagnosis of thrombosis and no clot has been found. Numerous anatomical compression sites have been listed:
1. Costo-clavicular
2. Costo-subclavian muscle
3. Anomalous muscle band between pectoralis major and latissimus dorsi
4. Space between the tendon of pectoralis minor and the coracoid process
5. Space between the subscapularis muscle and the head of the heumerus
6. Costo-coracoid ligament
7. Pre-venous phrenic nerve

This long list of possible compression is analogous to the pre-Rob and Standeven era with arterial compression and we must adopt the same general term of thoracic outlet compression because I have no doubt that the major point of compression is between the 1st rib and the clavicle and the subclavius muscle or tendon.

MANAGEMENT

1. *Chronic and intermittent venous obstruction*

These patients have congestion and swelling causing stiffness and clumsiness of movements of the fingers amounting to a real disability. Four women with this problem have been cured by the transaxilliary resection of the 1st rib as described by Roos.

2. *Venous thrombosis*

These cases present with sudden onset of severe pain, dull ache, gross oedema and cyanosis of the arm.

Management

a. Rest and arm elevation will allow gradual resolution over a few weeks with residual permanent disability. Most cases are treated initially at home by this method. When they are admitted to hospital it is often too late to offer more active treatment.

b. *Anticoagulants*   Heparin for 10 days is standard therapy and is followed by Warfarin or Sinthrone for three months. If started early this treatment will limit the thrombosis and possibly accelerate resolution. The incidence of pulmonary embolism, although rare, is reduced.

c. *Fibrinolysis*   This has not been successful in our hands and the mechanical obstruction at the site of origin of the thrombosis may account for this.

d. *Thrombectomy*   Good results are obtained by early thrombectomy but this must be accompanied by 1st rib resection to remove the compression on the subclavian vein.
  One of three surgical approaches can be used.
1. Transaxillary excision of the 1st rib followed by thrombectomy (Roos).
2. Supraclavicular exposure of the subclavian vein. This involves dividing the clavicle in its middle third
3. Infraclavicular incision. This allows excellent exposure of the subclavian vein after dividing the clavicular attachment of the pectoralis major muscle. The anterior two thirds of the 1st rib causing venous compression can be removed at the same time.

3. *Post phlebitic arm*

There is some evidence that excising the 1st rib lessens the disability in the late cases and may reduce the risk of further thrombosis.

REFERENCES

1. N.L. Tilney, H.J.G. Griffiths, E.A. Edwards. Natural history of major venous thrombosis of the upper extremity. Arch. Surg. 101: 792, 1970
2. C.G. Robb, A. Standeven. Arterial occlusion complicating thoracic outlet compression syndrome. Brit. Med. J. 2: 709, 1958
3. D.B. Roos, J.C. Owens. Thoracic outlet syndrome Arch. Surg. 93: 71, 1966
4. I.M. Stevenson, E.W. Parry. Radiological study of the aetiological factors in venous obstruction of the upper limb. Journal of Cardiovas. Surg. 16: 580, 1975

12. Surgical therapy and results in arterial occlusive disease of the upper extremities

H. DENCK M.D., G. KOBINA M.D.
AND P. WEIDINGER M.D.*

Vascular disorders of the upper extremitiy differ from those of the lower extremity in respect to anatomy, sexual distribution and hemodynamic, vasomotoric and pathogenetic factors. In addition except for central subclavian artery lesions a mainly peripheral localization of the occlusions can be found (Table 1). As can be seen in Figure 1 the main sites of the vessel lesions are, as stated, the central part of the subclavian artery, to a certain extent the costoclavicular narrowing and the periphery respectively the digital arteries.

In the years 1862 and 1874 Raynaud described a syndrome of vascular disease of the upper extremities with bilateral, peripheral, attackwise appearance for all cases in which no pathogenetic substance could be found. For many years now next to every vascular disease of the upper extremities was named Morbus Raynaud which was wrong both in the sense of the first description as of the pathogenesis assumed. Lemmens who has dealt with this problem for many years advised a nomenclature in 1976 which according to clinical and angiographic parameters differs between the attackwise appearing Raynaud Phenomenon, the Asphyxia Manus et Digitorum and the Digitus Moriens. We believe that the terminus Morbus Raynaud should be restricted to those cases with unknown pathogenesis whereas the terminus Raynaud Phenomenon is reserved for the cases with

Table 1. Disturbed arterial blood supply disorders of the upper extremities.

Specialities
1. Anatomy (collateral circulation)
2. Haemodynamic (steal mechanism)
3. Vasomotricity (sympathetic nerve!!! peripheral resistance at rest extremely high)
4. Sex distribution
5. Pathogenetic factors (immunopathy – rheology – compression syndrome)
6. Mostly peripheral location of the occlusion

*Surgical Department of the Vienna City Hospital, Lainz, Austria, and the Ludwig Boltzmann Institute for Cerebrovascular Research.

J.M. Greep, H.A.J. Lemmens, D.B. Roos and H.C. Urschel (eds.).
Pain in shoulder and arm: an integrated view, 133–150. *All rights reserved.*
Copyright © 1979 by Martinus Nijhoff Publishers, The Hague/Boston/London.

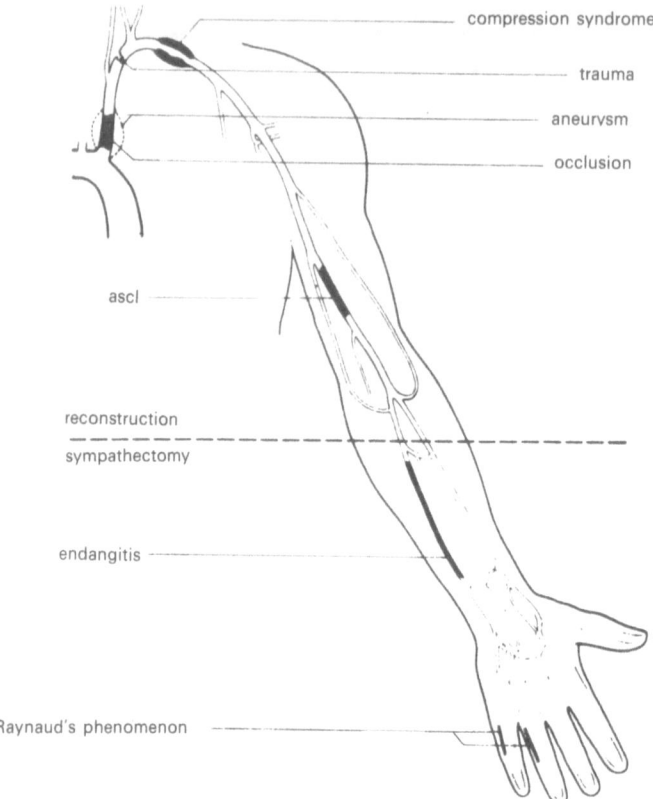

Figure 1. Causes of disturbed arterial blood supply of the upper extremities and a treatment proposal.

attackwise usually bilateral appearance with known pathogenesis (Tables 2 and 3).

In Table 3 an attempt has been made to match the pathogenetic factors with the clinical stages of the arterial lesion and it can be seen that finding

Table 2. Raynaud syndrome (1862–1874).

Paroxysmal
Bilateral
Acral ischemia
Low temperature stimulus-emotion

Nomenclature of Lemmens (1976) in respect to clinical and angiographic pictures
Phenomenon of Raynaud
Asphyxia manus et digitorum
Digitus moriens

M. Raynaud (unknown pathogenesis)
Phenomenon of Raynaud (known pathogenesis)

Table 3. Pathogenetic factors of arterial blood supply disorders of the upper extremity.

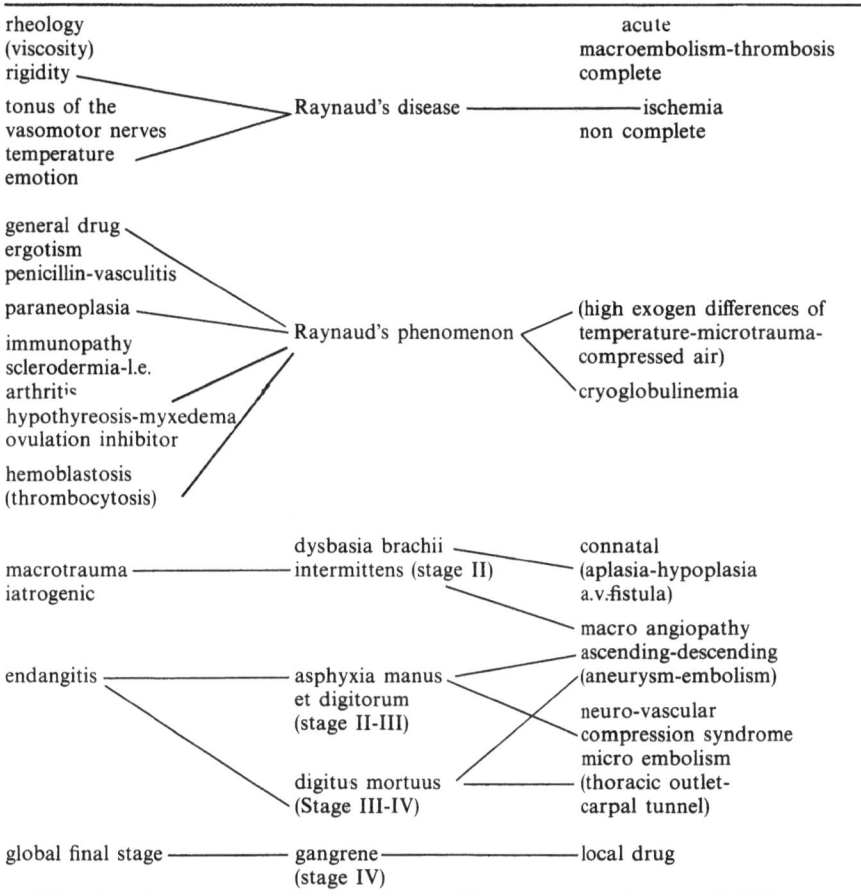

the right diagnosis of an upper extremity vascular disorder quite often resembles a criminalistic puzzle game. If we want to apply Fontaines scheme for the lower extremities also to the upper extremities we have to say that the attacks of Morbus Raynaud and Raynaud Phenomenon according to the stage II Dysbasia Intermittens have to be differentiated from stage II-III, respectively the Asphyxia Manus et Digitorum, from stage III, the Digitus Moriens and from stage IV, the frank necrosis and gangrene (Table 4).

The following discussion of the problems of vascular disease of the upper extremities is based on our own patients material (Table 5). Acute vascular disorders mainly were caused by embolism (Table 6), localized primarily at

Table 4. Experiment of a nomenclature. Disturbed arterial blood supply of the upper extremities.

1. Attack	("Raynaud")
2. Stage II	Dysbasia intermittens
	Asphyxiamanus et digitorum
III	"Digitus moriens"
IV	Necrosis
	Gangrene (mostly acral)

Table 5. Number of cases I. Surgical department of the city hospital of Vienna Lainz (1957–1977).

Disturbed blood supply of the upper extremities	
Acute	260
Chronic	381
	641 = 6% of all disturbed arterial blood supply

the axillary and cubital artery. Acute thrombosis, trauma and iatrogenous lesions as underlying factors were rare.

From Table 6 it also can be seen that due to the routine use of the Fogarty-catheter from the cubital artery with selective catheterization of both the radial and ulnar artery the amputation rate and mortality have been lowered significantly. At the present time the rate of amputation is 3% independent of the delay of admission; there was no primary mortality since 1971. Naturally the results in acute thrombosis with generalized atherosclerotic lesions are worse.

The discussion first shall be focused on the subclavian artery. Four sections of this vessel must be distinguished: The part from the aortic arch to the offspring of the internal mammary artery respectively the vertebral artery is section I, section II is the region around the offspring of the

Table 6. Number of cases I. Surgical department of the city hospital of Vienna – Lainz (1957–1977).

Acute disturbed blood supply of the upper extremities			
Embolisms	203	8% Subclavian art	-1971 Amp. rate 6% Mortality 18%
		24% axillary art. since	1971 Amp. rate 3% mortality
		19% Brachial art.	1971 0
		32% cubital art.	
		17% antebrachial-digital Aa,	
Ac. Thrombosis	34	therefrom amp. 5 (15%)	
Trauma	18	(1 replantation)	
Iatrogenic	5	(2 medicamentous)	

vertebral artery, section III lies between the offspring of the vertebral artery and the entrance to the costoclavicular space and section IV is the small part passing through the costoclavicular narrowing. Table 7 shows the localization of the arterial occlusions in chronic vascular disease of the upper extremities from which can be seen that the main localizations are

Table 7. Number of cases I. Surgical department of the city hospital of Vienna – Lainz (head: Prof. Dr. H. Denck).

Chronic disturbed blood supply of the upper extremities (1957–1977)		
Cronic subclavian art.	I	105
	II	2
	III	2
	IV	34
Art. axillaris		2
Art. brachialis		7
Art. antebrachii		13
Art. digitales anatomical		187
Art. digitales functional		29
		381

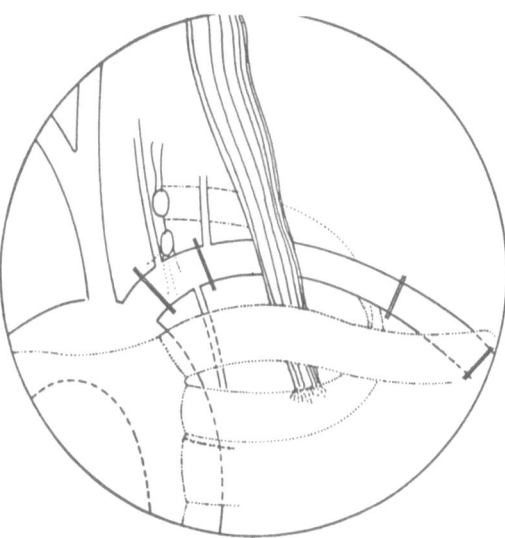

Figure 2. The four sections of the subclavian artery.

section I of the subclavian artery and the distal digital arteries; lesions of part IV in the costoclavicular narrowing are the next frequent occurrence.

Discussing now the occlusions and stenoses of the central region of the subclavian artery it must be remembered that not only the dependent arm is

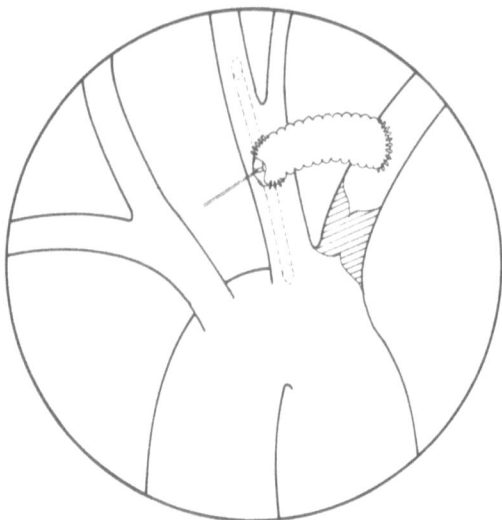

Figure 3. Schema of the carotido-subclavian bypass.

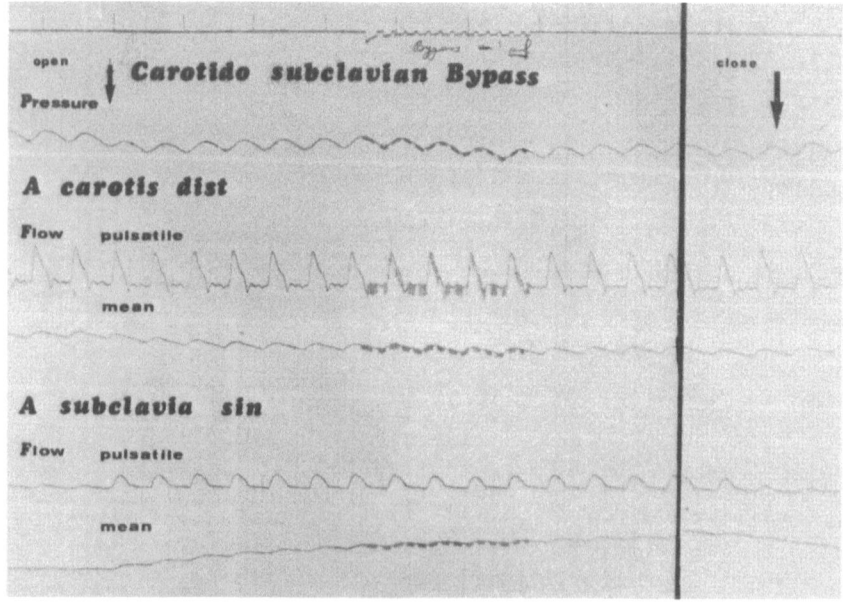

Figure 4. Hemodynamics of the carotido-subclavian bypass.

affected but also the brain by reversal of the ipsilateral vertebral artery flow, giving rise to the so-called subclavian steal syndrome with basilar artery insufficiency.

The ideal reconstruction for these occlusions still is a direct reconstruction as performed with an aortosubclavian bypass or by open desobliteration, which alone is capable of fully restoring the normal hemodynamics. Naturally a transthoracic direct operation in section I of the subclavian artery is not only a big operation but the artery itself is extremely difficult to deal with due to its extreme wall fragility. Desobliteration can not always be performed at the right layer. Therefore the extraanatomical bypass operations have been favoured and especially the carotidosubclavian bypass has been advised for the treatment of the subclavian steal syndrome. We now have examined the hemodynamics of these extraanatomical detours and could find that in spite of a considerable flow increase in the common carotid artery there is both a slight decrease of pressure in the internal carotid artery as a certain decrease of flow after opening a carotidosubclavian graft. Under normal circumstances this small pressure and flow reduction might be negligible, in cases of cerebral sclerosis however it can lead to clinical signs of carotid artery insufficiency. Another question we were interested in was how big the flow in the carotidosubclavian bypass had to be in order to reverse the vertebral flow to its normal orthograde direction. Assuming a normal subclavian artery

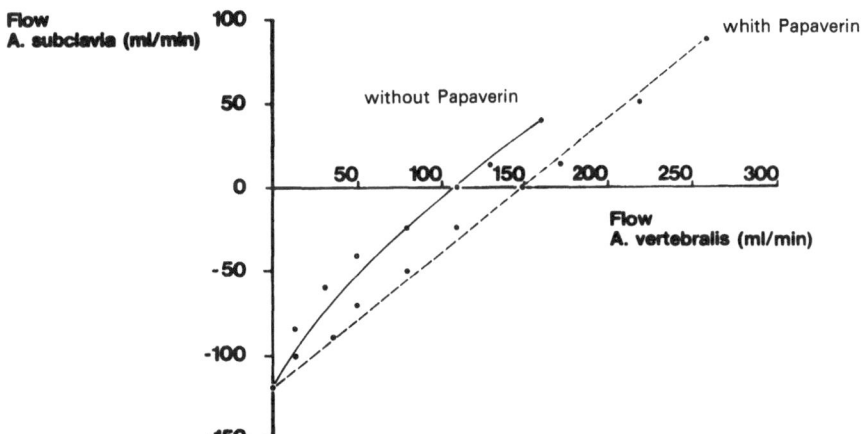

Figure 5. Hemodynamics of the subclavian steal syndrome.

Table 8. Complications following extraanatomical bypass operations for subclavian steal syndrome.

Carotidosubclavian
    Dacron graft –––––– solcograft –––––––thrombectomy ·––––– transversal dacron
               occlusion   occlusion   occlusion   graft

    Dacron graft –––––– venous graft
               occlusion
    Dacron graft –––––– stroke, death (trombosis of ipsilateral vertebral artery)
    Dacron graft –––––– stroke
    Venous graft –––––– transversal venous graft (persistent steal)
              occlusion
    Venous graft –––––– external compression ––––––– thrombembolism ipsilateral cu-
             occlusion   bital artery
Transversal grafts   0

flow of 200 to 300 ml, the critical flow in the bypass must average about 150 ml to stop the retrograde vertebral flow and should be about 200 to 250 ml to perfuse the vertebral artery sufficiently, flow values which are hardly obtained by this bypass form.

Among the complications of 52 extracranial bypass operations we find one case of persisting steal in spite of a patent graft and among the cartido subclavian grafts (table 8). A schematic drawing of these hemodynamic considerations is presented in Figure 6 suggesting that a flow of at least 150 ml/min is necessary to prevent retrograde vertebral artery flow. Such a

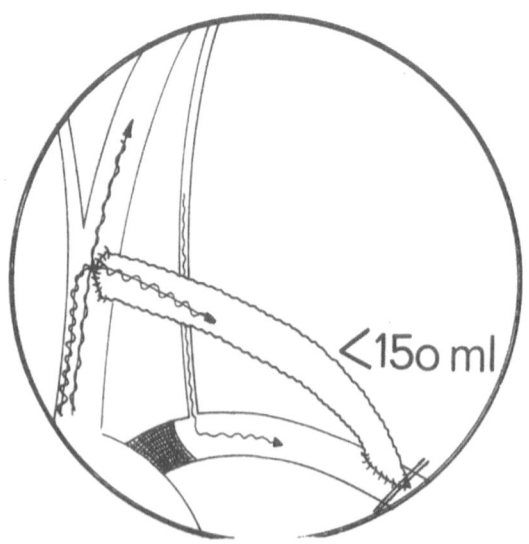

Figure 6. Minimal flow of the carotido-subclavian bypass.

borderline flow, however, can possibly lead to flow stand still in the vertebral artery with consecutive thrombosis of the vessel.

According to these facts we now prefer the subclaviosubclavian bypass as standard extracranial route for cure of subclavian steal syndrome, as here by no means reduction of the carotid artery flow occurs and the flow values generally are higher than those of a carotidosubclavian graft.

A small hint should be given to the traumatologist: In acute traumatic central subclavian artery occlusion due to a blunt shoulder trauma frequently also acute subclavian steal syndrome can be observed with possible cerebral symptoms which might suggest a contusion of the brain. Rapid angiographic diagnosis is necessary to prevent such an error and vascular reconstruction must follow immediately. In Figure 7 the angiographic features of such a case are presented.

Considering now the lesions of the subclavian artery in the costoclavicular space it has to be stated that today the standard therapy for

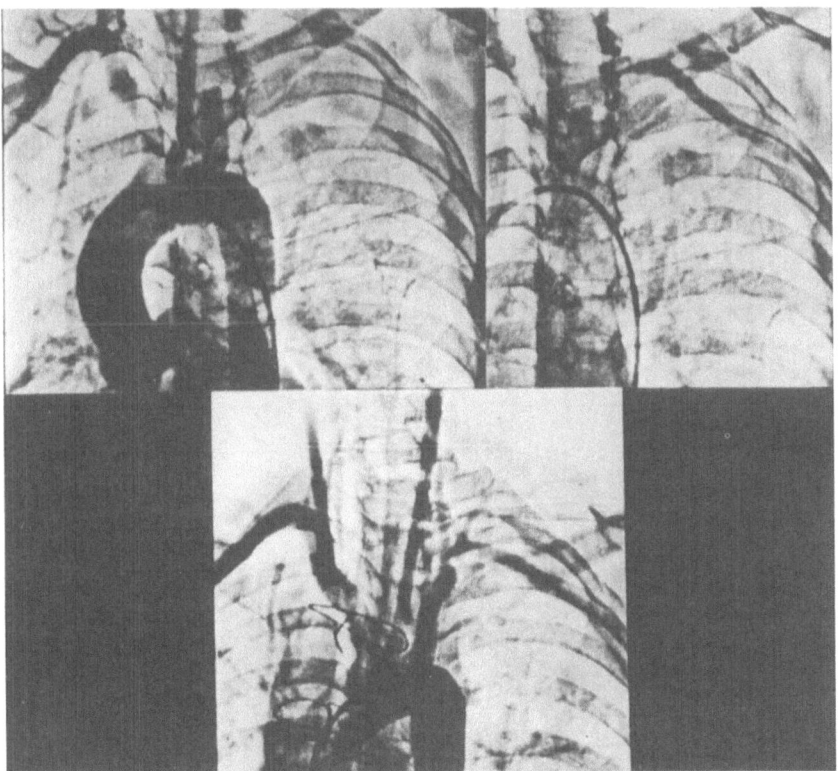

Figure 7. Post-traumatic subclavian-steal syndromes and relief by direct reconstruction.

costoclavicular compression syndrome is the transaxillary resection of the first rib from which approach also operations for poststenotic aneurysm, thrombosis of the axillary vein as well as an eventually necessary sympathectomy can be performed. For all cases of a costoclavicular narrowing proved either angiographically, hemodynamically or neurologically, we see an absolute indication for this transaxillary resection of the first rib as described by Roos. This applies also to the acute axillary vein thrombosis which primarily is best treated by fibrinolysis followed by a first rib resection either to prevent a recidivism or to improve the collateral circulation.

In case of peripheral embolies with obstruction of the peripheral circulation we perform a thoracic sympathectomy from the same incision, however first resect a small part of the third rib, which is followed by the transthoracic transpleural resection of the first four thoracic ganglia with ideal approach and accessibility. For recidivist cases this approach can, however, be difficult and even dangerous so that we try to pass this difficulty by an enlarged anterior approach or by a bypass procedure. The anterior approach with splitting of the clavicle gives good accessibility, the clavicle has to be adapted by osteosynthesis afterwards. Resection of the first rib is mandatory naturally. In four cases of recidivist occlusions we have performed extra-anatomical grafts, once from the central stump of the subclavian artery intercostally to the axilla and three times with a long

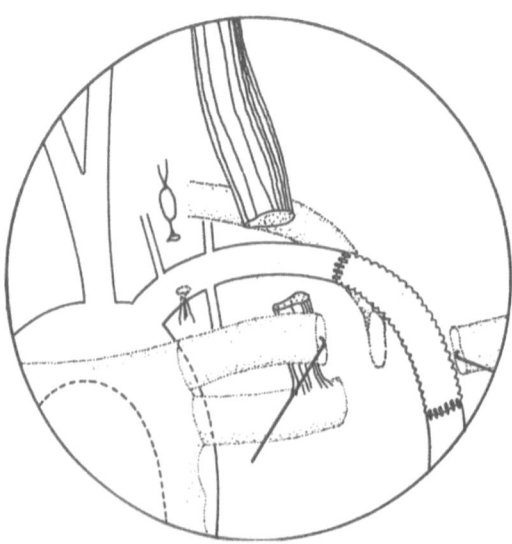

Figure 8. Anterior access at relapse-operations in the costo-clavicular area with splitting of the clavicula.

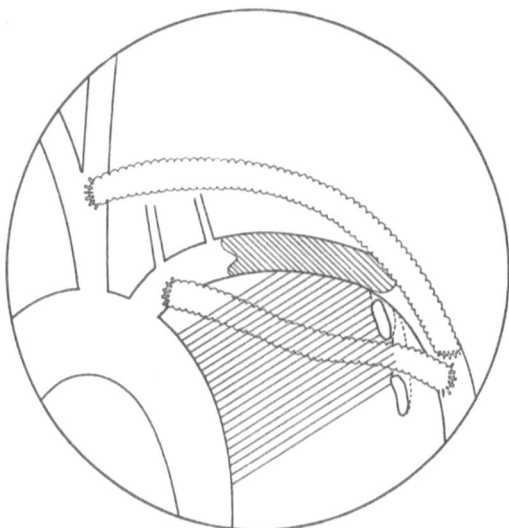

Figure 9. Exra-anatomic bypass for relapses of occlusion of the subclavian artery in section III and IV.

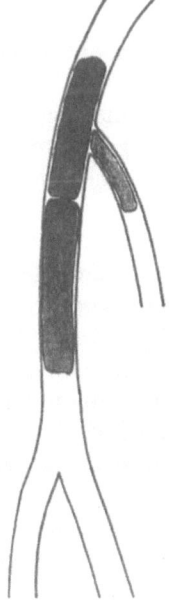

Figure 10. Chronic occlusion of the brachial artery with acute embolism of the deep brachial artery and following complete ischemia, reconstruction by embolectomy and venous bypass.

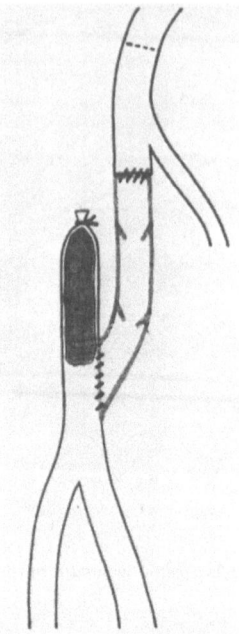

Figure 11.

subcutaneous carotidoaxillary bypass of which two are permeable for more than 8 years.

Chronic arterial occlusions in the region of the axillary, brachial and cubital artery are rare (see Table 7) and are treated according to the general principles of reconstructive vascular surgery. One special case should be pointed out:

A 78 year old man suffering from chronic occlusion of the brachial artery was admitted for additional arterial embolism into this vessel occluding all his collaterals which caused the symptoms of acute complete ischemia. The operation was performed in local anaesthesia due to the bad general condition of the patient. After embolectomy and thrombectomy from the profound brachial artery a brachiocubital bypass was performed (Figure 10 and 11), restoring the normal circulation of the arm.

The peripheral anatomical and functional arterial disorders are especially apt for the sympathetic denervation. It must be stressed that the results for Morbus Raynaud, i.e. without known underlying disease are much better than those for Raynaud Phenomenon, especially in cases of simultaneous sclerodermy. The possible operative procedures for sympathetic denervation of the upper extremity are presented in Table 9. In spite of the fact that up till now the transthoracic approach by Atkins is preferred generally, it has

Table 9. Sympathetic denervation of the upper extremity (Arnulf).

Periarterial sympathectomy (Jaboulais)
Stellectomy
Enlarged stellectomy
Rami communicantes + spinal nerves
Enlarged sympathectomy + efferent fibres of the branchial plexus (Mentha)
Preganglonic resection (White and Smithwick)
Isolated 3 Breastganglion
Monobloc 1–4 Breastganglion + spinal ganglion
                              + spinal nerve

Table 10. Thoracic sympathectomy operative access.

Ventral – supraclavicular (Ross)
Dorsal – extrapleural (Smithwick)
Transthoracic-dorsolateral (Linton)
Transthoracic-axillary (Atkins)
Dorsal-extrapleural "monobloc" (Lemmens)
Endoscopic sympathectomy (Kux)

Table 11. Thoracic sympathectomy, indication and results.

	Number of patients	Operations	Improved	**Equal**	Worse
"M. Raynaud"	69	139	115 (82%)	19 (13%)	5 (5%)
Raynaud phenomenon	8	15	12	3	
Endangitis oblit. digitus moriens	8	8	6	1	1
"Vasculitis"	2	4	2		
Crutches (embolism)	1	2	2		2
Thoracic outlet syndrome (microembolism)	17	17	12	5	
Acrocyanosis	3	6	4	2	
Hyperhydrosis	8	16	16		
M. Sudeck	2	2	2		
	118	209	171 (83%)	30 (14%)	8 (3%)

to be stated that both the transaxillary extrapleural operation of Roos and the total sympathetic denervation according to Lemmens by extrapleural dorsal monobloc resection with special consideration given to the nerve of Kuntz should be more used in the future. When the main indication is hyperhydrosis, also the endoscopic sympathectomy according to Kux can be performed (Fritsch). Our own results and complications are summarised in Tables 11 and 12 from which it can be seen that together with a low rate of complications clinical improvement can be found in 83%.

Table 12. Thoracic sympathectomy (sympathectomy).

Access		Complications		
		Horner	N. Axillaris	Pleura
Ventral supraclavicular (Ross, 16)	22	18	—	—
Dorsal extrapleural (Smithwick, 18)	4	2	—	—
Transthoracic-dorsolateral (Linton, 11)	35	7	—	2
Axillary (Atkins, 1)	132	2	4 (3%)	8 (6%)
"Dorsal monobloc" (Lemmens)	4	—	—	1 (1/4)
Endoscopic (Kux 10)	12	—	—	2
	209	29 (13%)	4 (2%)	13 (6%)
	Mortality 0			

finger roomtemperature

RP ‰

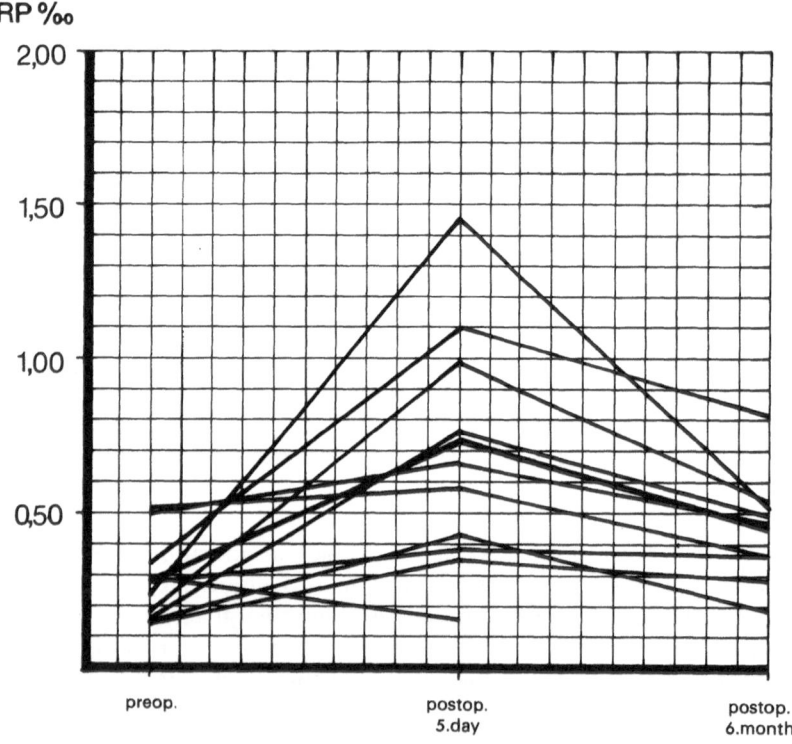

Figure 12.

The aim of the thoracic sympathectomy is depletion of the vasoconstrictoric vascular tonus, decrease of the sweat secretion and a vasodilatation. According to the experience of Walker, Lyn and Barcoff the maximum effect of the thoracic sympathectomy lasts only for two days and decreases continuously, though still the two- to threefold values as compared to the preoperative state are maintained. Also in our patients material 83% of the patients operated on subjectively claimed an improvement. We were disappointed more when we started to measure the volume pulse pre- and postoperatively. All measured values increased, as judged by the mean values, though there was a great variability. Only in one patient with endangitis and occlusions of the lower arm was a decrease seen as a paradox reaction after sympathectomy, which can also be observed in the lower extremities. Controls after six months, however, showed a clear deterioration in the average value equalling the preoperative value (Figure 12). The coldness test, with one exception, showed no improvement as

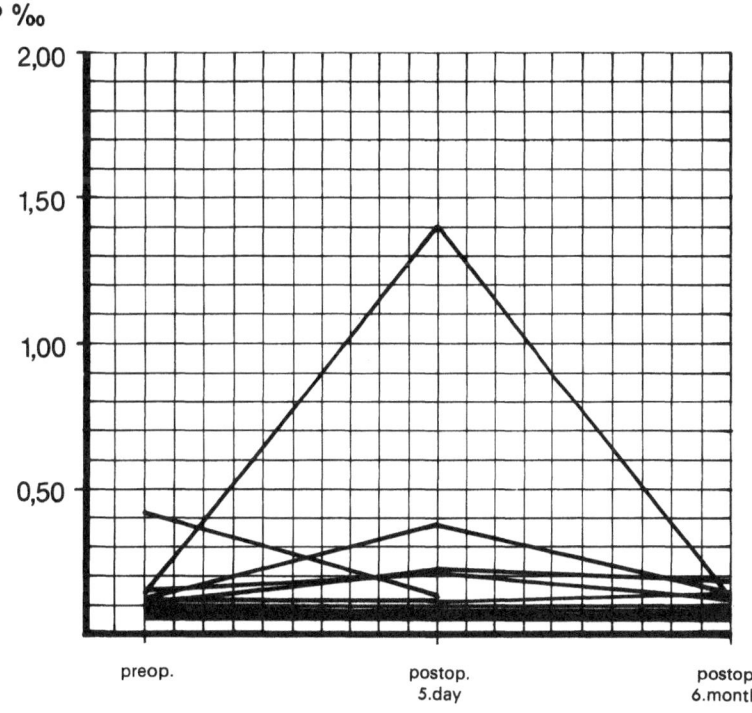

Figure 13.

148   *H. Denck, G. Kobinia, P. Weidinger*

compared to the extremely low basic situation (Figure 13). Measurement of
the influence of local heat at the fifth postoperative day again shows
improvement of the arterial volume pulse in all patients with a mean
increase of 50% except for the one case with endangitis. Similar to the
results at room temperature after 6 months a decrease of all values can be
seen, the mean value again being similar to the basic situation (Figure 14).
These results could be found in 10 patients (1 male and 9 females aged
between 30 and 70 years) by measurement before and after sympathectomy.
The arterial volume pulse was measured at 15, 22 and 40°C. Measurement
of the arterial volume pulse was done rheographically by determination of
the electrical conductivity and is standardized in pulsation per volume units
in a percentage. As the changing of the diameter of the vessel lumen is of
importance for the volume pulse the latter can be used to judge the vascular
tonus. The pathological preoperative function pattern of the arterial volume

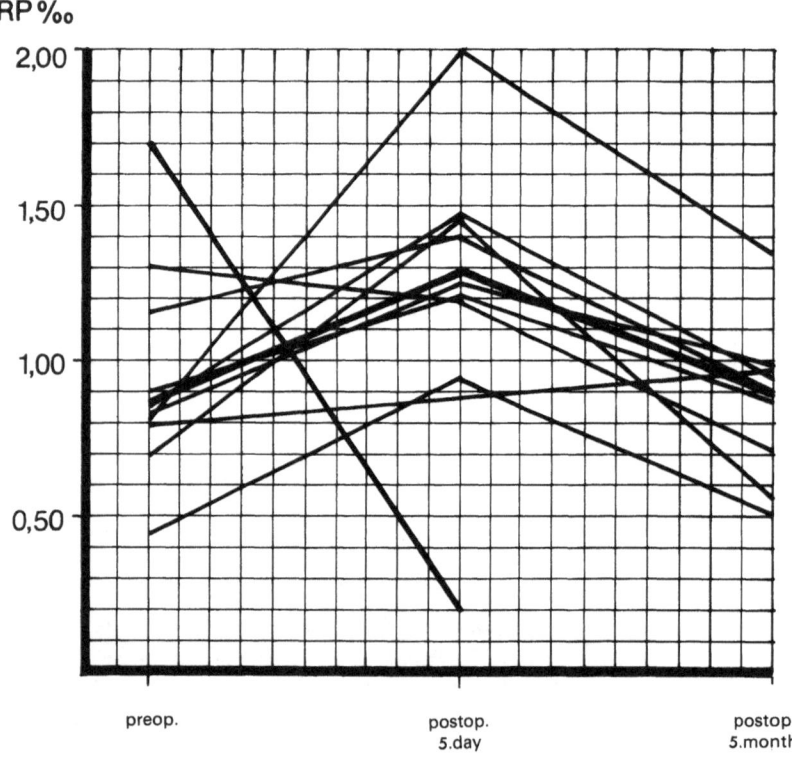

Figure 14.

pulse is explained by the angiographically proved peripheral vascular occlusions. In spite of the fact that at the fifth postoperative day a dilatation of the arterial periphery at 22 and 40°C can be found, the typical vascular spasm at coldness continues. The resection of the thoracic sympathetic nerve obviously can not break the underlying cause for the Raynaud symptoms. After the sixth postoperative month as previously stated the arterial volume pulse both at room temperature and at heat is smaller. These results can be improved by using the thoraco-dorsal monobloc resection described by Lemmens (Figure 15). Similar results also could be established by discothermographic measurements. Based on our measurements therefore it has to be stated that the optimal vasodilatatoric effect of thoracic sympathectomy is only a transient one.

Finally it can be stated that the thoracic sympathectomy nowadays is performed by resection of the first four ganglia and that the optimal vasodilatatoric effect can be measured at the fifth postoperative day, it is however transient. Results obviously can be improved by the thoracodorsal monobloc resection. Further investigations will be necessary.

In conclusion it can be said that the study of the arterial disorders of the upper extremity is one of the very fascinating fields of angiology.

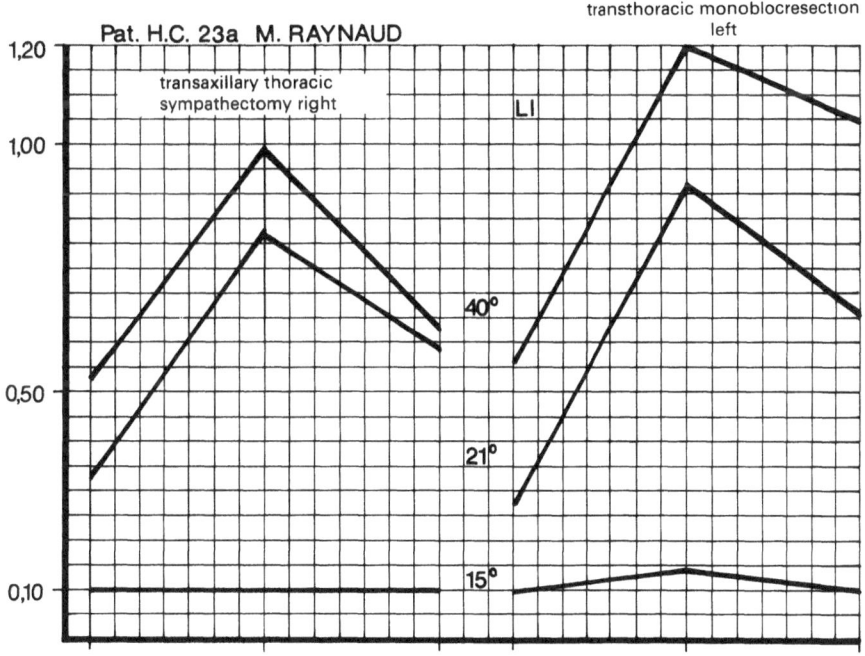

Figure 15.

Improvements have been obtained in the fields of nomenclature, research of pathogenesis and in therapy due to the improvements in diagnosis and the special therapeutic possibilities.

Part III
Thoracic outlet syndrome

13. The diagnosis of thoracic outlet syndrome

JEAN HENRI DUNANT M.D.*

ABSTRACT

It is often difficult to demonstrate that a confirmed neurovascular compression at the thoracic outlet is also the cause of the patient's complaints. A careful clinical examination must therefore be completed by objective tests to define the exact site and mechanism of compression. Such objective tests are also valuable and necessary to evaluate surgical results. The phonoangiogram is one of these simple, painless, objective and reproducible tests.

Arterial compression occurs frequently in extreme positions of the arm even in normal subjects. If, in a symptomatic patient, signs of compression are present on simple abduction, functional angiography is indicated.

Similarly, venous obstruction in extreme positions of the arm can be demonstrated by pressure measurements and phlebograms on many healthy symptom-free individuals. These two tests are nevertheless useful in the detection of intermittent, functional compression mechanisms.

A majority of the patients present neurologic symptoms. The diagnosis of TOS, especially the differentiation of normal versus pathological findings in a patient with essentially neurologic symptoms, is not easy.

Only thorough evaluation of the patient, careful clinical examination combined with objective vascular (and therefore indirect) tests, will help to make the diagnosis accurate.

It is often difficult to demonstrate that a confirmed neurovascular compression at the thoracic outlet is also the cause of the patient's symptoms. The signs of compressions are of an arterial, venous and neurologic nature and may appear separately or in combination. Chronic or intermittent compression of the nerves and blood vessels to the arm produces pain and dysfunction in various degrees. However, pain and paresthesias of the upper extremity are common symptoms and are only rarely the consequence of a confirmed vascular compression at the thoracic outlet (Table 1).

A thorough clinical examination and the standard diagnostic tests may give a lead to the mechanism of compression and its localization. Yet, if an operation is planned, we believe the clinical findings must be corroborated by objective signs in order to define the exact site and mechanism of compression. Such objective tests can also help to evaluate postoperative results.

We should like to demonstrate, how we have tried to differentiate

*Priv.-Doz. Dr. med. Jean Henri Dunant F.A.C.S., Basel, Switzerland.

Table 1. Symptoms in 92 operated patients.

Symptoms	n	%
Paresthesia/Hypesthesia	92	100
Pain	64	70
Muscular weakness	36	40
Sensation of coldness	23	25
Pallor/Sensory loss	16	18

between normal and pathological findings and to discuss briefly the advantages and disadvantages of each method.

CLINICAL EXAMINATION

The case history may yield information on symptom-inducing mechanisms and the exact localization of discomfort, intermittent or persistent symptoms, provocation, increase or relief of discomfort in various occupational postures of body or arm (Table 2). The patient is best examined from behind, while sitting.

The inspection comprises body build, posture, position and symmetry of the shoulder girdle, presence and filling of collateral veins, changes of skin color and muscular atrophy. At the distal phalanges of the fingers we may observe cracked skin, chronic paronychosis, slow-healing wounds and necrosis.

On palpation of the neck, special attention should be paid to the region of the posterior scalene triangle and the supraclavicular region. We may detect

Table 2. Symptoms.

		92 patients,	117 operations
time lag until first consultation	1 year		47
	2 years		10
	5 years		18
	>5 years		17
onset	acute		33
	slow		59
occurrence	positional		63
	paroxysmal		9
	constant		20

anomalous tenderness, a resistance or a structure (cervical rib, exostosis, callus, lymph node). Light percussion or pressure over the brachial plexus, and traction on the arm in direction of the body axis can produce symptoms.

We check muscular tonicity, strength and sensitivity of the shoulder girdle, arm and hand, and assess differences of skin temperature and sweating.

The pulses of the radial and ulnar artery are palpated. Auscultation at the thoracic outlet is done at three locations:
- in the supraclavicular region
- in the midclavicular region, below the lateral third of the clavicle.
- in the infraclavicular region, below the lateral third of the clavicle.

The standard provocative tests indicate only a positional compression of the subclavian artery and are positive in a high percentage of normal asymptomatic subjects. The radial pulse can be occluded, when the head is turned to either side, when the shoulders are braced or when the arm is elevated. Positional evaluation of the radial pulses alone is not easy, especially in extreme positions of the arms, and does not give relevant information as to the degree of compression. The observation of a supra- or infraclavicular murmur during such a provocative test does not exclude other compression mechanisms, nor does it indicate that the patient has a thoracic outlet syndrome (TOS).

We have tried to improve the results of positional tests by using phonoangiographic recordings.

Sound recordings over the subclavian artery were obtained in 80 asymptomatic persons with a normal arterial circulation of the arm. Arterial murmurs were recorded in 47 persons on hyperabduction of the arm. Our study indicates that vascular compression occurs frequently even in normal subjects in extreme positions of the arm (Table 3).

The tentative diagnosis of TOS may be made only if a murmur is present on simple abduction and if the conventional test positions produce the patient's usual symptoms. If the phonoangiogram is negative, other causes for symptoms should be looked for. The phonoangiogram is a simple,

Table 3 Positive phonoangiographic findings in asymptomatic, healthy persons.

Arm position	n = 47 persons
neutral	0/47
90° abduction	3/47
90° abduction + shoulder-bracing	16/47
150° abduction	5/47
150° abduction + shoulder-bracing	23/47

painless, objective and reproducible test, capable of combination with other routine methods, and can also be used in the follow-up of postoperative results.

An overwhelming majority of the patients complain of neurologic rather than arterial symptoms. A careful and thorough neurological examination is therefore necessary to differentiate a TOS from other diseases with similar symptoms. These neurological tests have been excellently described by Roos (10) and will not be further discussed here.

Nerve conduction velocity and electromyography provide objective measurements of a compression of nerves at the shoulder girdle and enable us to assess the results of conservative and operative treatment. Decrease of symptoms and normalization of nerve conduction velocity correlate (11). However, because of technical difficulties, these tests allow diagnostic conclusions only in particularly severe cases of nerve compression. Intermittent compression in functional position of the arms can be demonstrated only exceptionally. We believe that nerve conduction velocity measurements are useful for establishing the differential diagnosis between TOS and carpal tunnel syndrome. These syndromes are associated in approximately 5% of the cases.

DEMONSTRATION OF ARTERIAL COMPRESSION

Phonoangiography

Phonoangiography is more objective than auscultation (Figure 1). In healthy individuals a positional compression of the subclavian artery is frequent (51% in hyperabduction), a complete occlusion however is rare (3%).

Subclavian arteriography in functional positions is indicated more especially if compression can be demonstrated in 90° abduction. A further advantage of phonoangiography is that it allows reproducible postoperative controls (2, 4).

Oscillography

Oscillography has the advantage of providing reproducible, recordable, painless and simple information. (Figure 2). Stenoses and occlusions can be demonstrated with greater differentiation than by palpation of radial pulses. Pulses are recorded continuously in various arm positions. Forced positions of the arms produce tremor which falsifies the tracings. In extreme positions of the arms and during shoulder retraction, the amplitude of the tracing is often reduced; however, an interpretation of the degree of compression in intermediate positions is not possible (4).

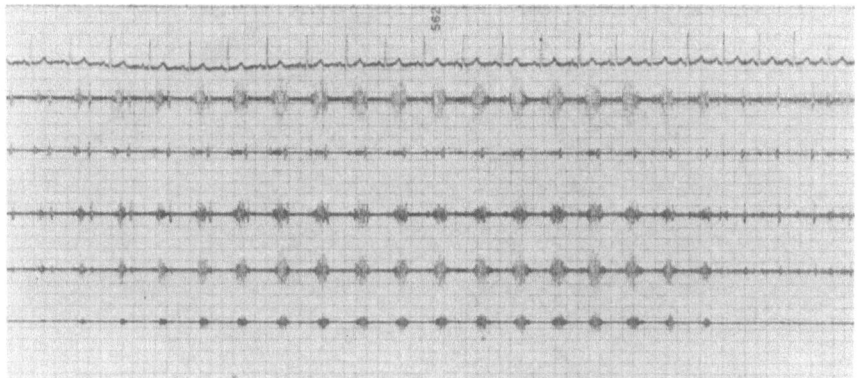

Figure 1. Phonogram of the right subclavian artery. Increase of compression under progressive abduction of the arm until maximum hyperabduction is achieved.

Neutral Position   **Costo-Clavicular Test**   **Hyperabduction**

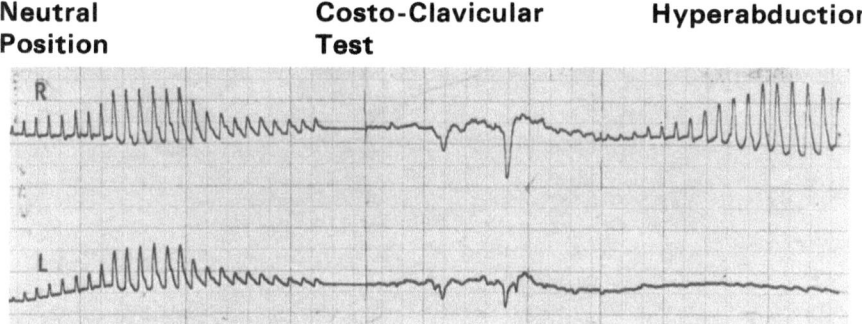

Figure 2. Oscillogram of both arms. 24 year old female with severe symptoms on the left side under hyperabduction.

Arteriography of the subclavian artery

The majority of patients with TOS have neurologic symptoms (4, 10). Nevertheless we believe that in most cases functional arteriography of the subclavian artery in provocative positions provides useful information as to the site of compression, local changes in the arterial wall and the caliber of the artery (6, 7, 8). If combined with selective brachial angiography-as has been at regular practice lately, the technique also offers information about occlusions of digital arteries (Figure 3, 4). Secondary Raynaud's phenomenon seems to be more frequently associated with TOS than generally assumed (Figure 5). Angiographic studies in patients with clinical signs of a severe TOS demonstrated ipsilateral occlusions of digital arteries in more than 50% of the cases of extreme vascular compression.

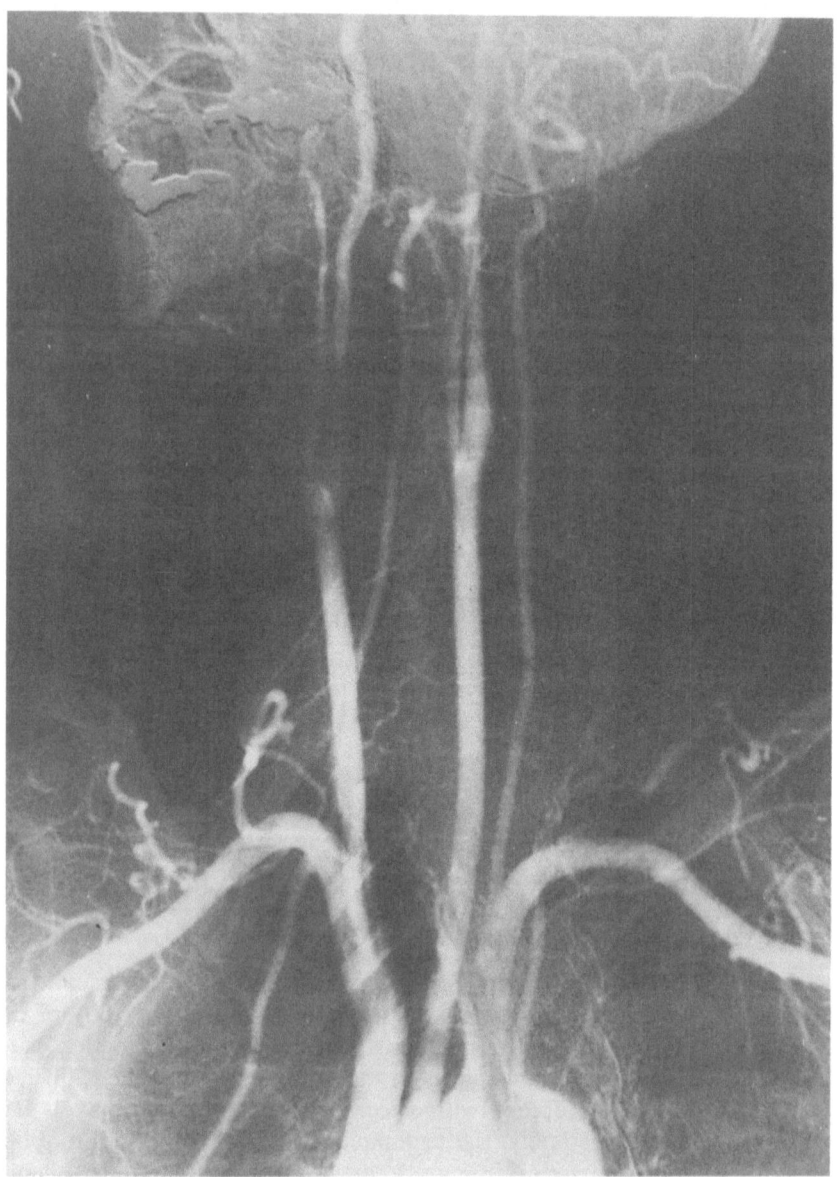

Figure 3 and 4. Bilateral thoracic outlet symptoms.
Left: neutral arm position.
Right: total occlusion under shoulder bracing.

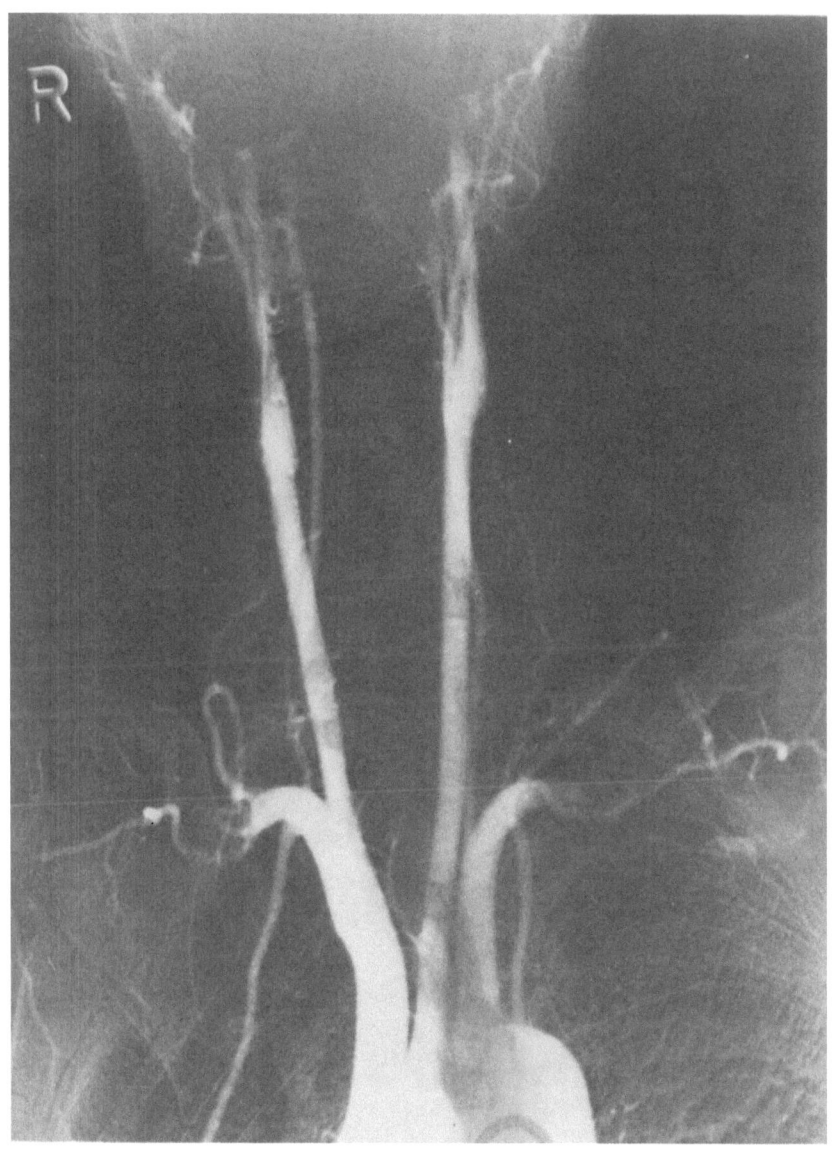

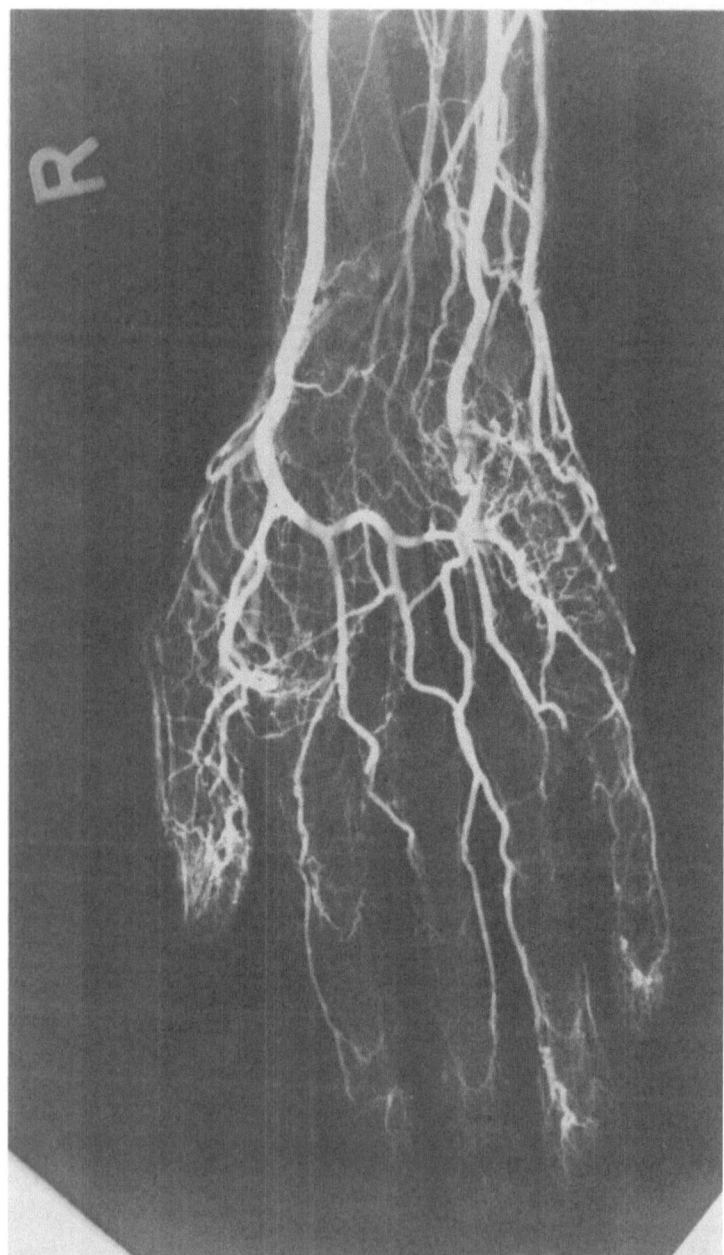

Figure 5. Same patient as Figure 3 and 4: Secondary Raynaud's phenomenon with multiple occlusions of digital arteries.

DEMONSTRATION OF VENOUS COMPRESSION

Venous pressure measurements

Compression of the subclavian vein normally occurs with backward and downward retraction of the arm, and exercise in this position leads to a further marked increase in pressure.

In 44 of 50 normal, healthy individuals (88%), the pressure in the deep venous system of the arm was markedly increased when the shoulders were hyperabducted. These observations were made on 50 asymptomatic individuals without any signs of disease at the thoracic outlet.

Phlebography

Compression of the subclavian vein in extreme positions of the arm can be demonstrated in a significant number of healthy individuals (Figure 6, 7). Narrowing of the costoclavicular space and impression by the head of the humerus seem to be the most frequent mechanism of compression.

Sixty healthy persons without clinical signs of neurovascular compression

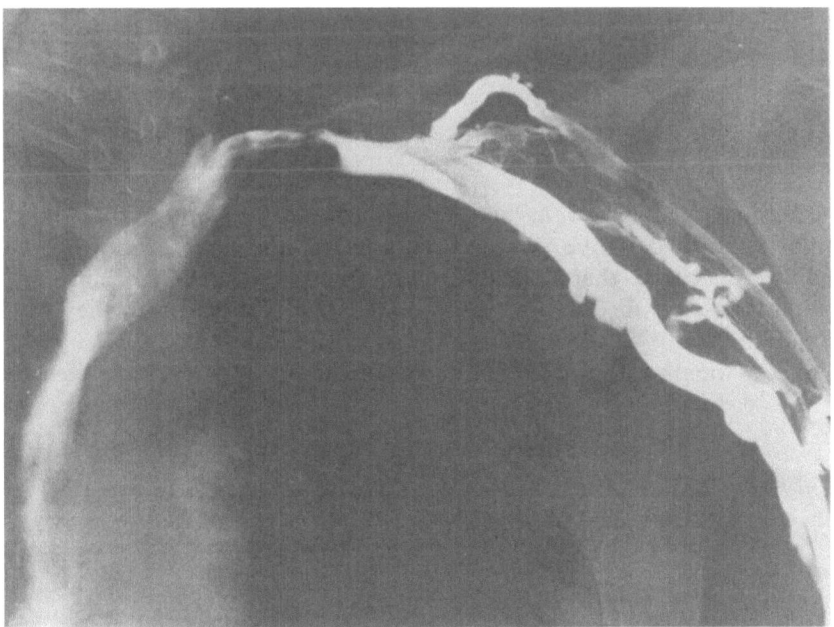

Figure 6. Functional occlusion of the left subclavian vein under shoulder retraction.

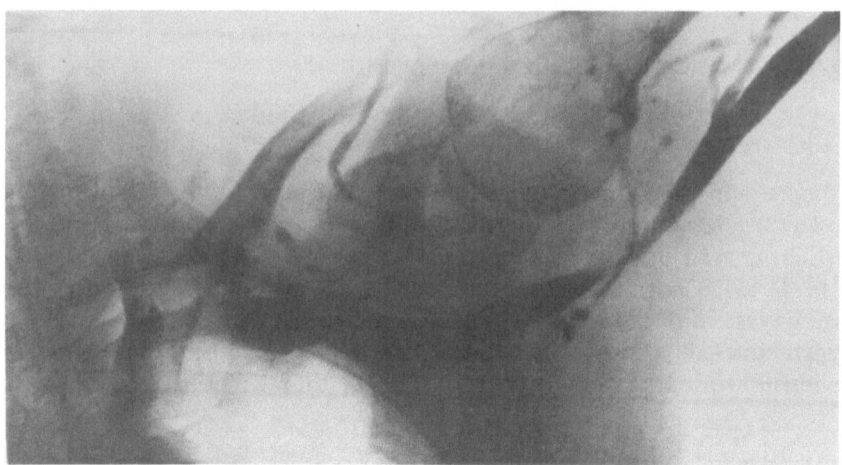

Figure 7. Significant compression of the axillary vein by the head of the humerous.

were investigated by phlebograms of the arm in various arm positions. Venous obstruction could be demonstrated in 42 of the 60 individuals (70%) under hyperabduction and shoulder retraction (Table 4).

The differential diagnosis between functional compression and constant obstruction can be facilitated by performing venous pressure measurements and phlebograms. Both of these examinations should be done in neutral and in provoking positions.

Combination of phonoangiography, phlebography and venous pressure measurements.

During our studies on asymptomatic individuals, we observed that a compression of both the vein and the artery in the same patient is rarely found. We believe, therefore, that there are two different mechanisms of compression, one for the artery and one for the vein, and that they rarely act simultaneously.

In 80 patients without disease at the shoulder girdle we made measure-

Table 4. Phlebographic findings in asymptomatic, healthy persons during hyperabduction and shoulder-bracing.

Compression	n = 60 persons	%
none	18/60	30
costo-clavicular	12/60	20
head of humerus	23/60	38
costo-clavicular + head of humerus	7/60	12

ments of venous pressure and phlebograms of the axillary/subclavian veins as well as phonoangiograms of the subclavian artery in relaxed position, in hyperabduction of the arm and with shoulders braced. The results of the same patient were compared. In extreme positions of the arm, the vein in the costo-clavicular region was more often constricted than the artery. Venous compression occurs more often at 90° of abduction of the arm than at 150°. In this latter position, arterial compression is physiological.

DEMONSTRATION OF COMPLICATIONS OF TOS

Symptoms of arterial insufficiency are not at all common (9, 10). Sometimes arterial complications, especially occlusions of digital arteries, may be the first symptoms of compression at the thoracic outlet. Elevated-arm-stress test and the Allen test may give additional information about peripheral occlusions. In cases of cervical rib marked pulsations of the subclavian artery may be palpated in the supraclavicular fossa. If there is unilateral involvement, the affected hand may be cooler, moister and look more livid than the other one, due to peripheral neuropathy.

We believe that a complete arteriographic investigation of the arm is indicated in every case of Raynaud's phenomenon in order to exclude a source of embolization at the thoracic outlet (extreme recurrent compression, aneurysm).

Symptoms of venous insufficiency are much more frequent than arterial ones. Intermittent oedematous swelling of the arm, cyanosis of the forearm and hand are typical. Enlarged venous collaterals can be seen on the medial side of the upper arm, over the pectoral muscle and on the lateral side of the neck, often with a prominent jugular vein.

Repeated compression between clavicle and first rib causes thickening of the vein wall, forced expiration (Valsalva) brings about a temporary stasis. This mechanism may be the reason for primary subclavian vein thrombosis (effort thrombosis) in otherwise healthy individuals. "Effort thrombosis" is therefore probably a venous complication of TOS (4).

It should be investigated by phlebography. The obstruction is usually located between the clavicle and the first rib. A typical collateral circulation can be demonstrated going from the cephalic/transversa colli/jugular vein system to axillary collaterals.

ESTABLISHMENT OF THE DIAGNOSIS TOS AND OUR INDICATION FOR SURGERY

The diagnosis "thoracic outlet syndrome" is a clinical diagnosis. If the patient complains of typical positional symptoms and if the physical examination, together with the standard provocative tests and phonoangio-graphy, raises a strong suspicion of TOS, a functional arteriography under local anaesthesia is carried out. If the arteriography reveals significant or total compression especially if the compression occurs on simple abduction, transaxillary first rib resection is indicated. A significant compression of the brachial plexus may, however, exist without a concomitant involvement of the artery. In these cases of essential neurologic symptomatology surgical decompression is likewise indicated if conservative treatment has failed.

Only 20% of the patients with symptoms of TOS need an operation. With a strict indication, 90% of the patients can be symptomfree after surgery. Significant arterial and venous compressions are easier to demonstrate than neurological compressions (4, 6). In the presence of an essentially neurologic symptomatology, and in the absence of signs of vascular compression, an operation is indicated only after exclusion of every other differential diagnosis.

REFERENCES

1. J.H. Dunant, H.J. Hehne, E.F. Gauer, P.P. Waibel. Venendruckmessungen im Arm zur Beurteilung von Kompressionerscheinungen beim Schultergürtelsyndrom VASA 3: 418, 1974
2. J.H. Dunant, W. Ahne, B. Heierli, H.J. Hehne, P.P. Waibel. Die Phonoangiographie als Untersuchungsmethode beim vaskulären Schultergürtelkompressionssyndrom. Dtsch. Med. Wschr. 99: Heft 7, 277, 1974
3. J.H. Dunant, H.J. Hehne, E.F. Gauer, P.P. Waibel. Phlebographische Untersuchungen über Kompressionserscheinungen beim Schultergürtelsyndrom. Thoraxchirurgie 23: 23, 1975
4. J.H. Dunant. Schultergürtelsyndrom, Hans Huber Verlag, Bern 1976
5. J.H. Dunant, P.P. Waibel. Voie transaxillaire pour la résection de la première côte dans le syndrome des défilés costo-claviculaires. Schweiz. Rundschau Med. (Praxis) 65: 1437, 1976
6. E.K. Lang. Arteriographic diagnosis of the thoracic outlet syndromes. Radiology 84: 296, 1965
7. J.W. Lord. Thoracic outlet syndromes. Current Management. Ann Surg. 173: 700, 1971
8. R.M. Nelson, R.W. Davis. Thoracic outlet compression syndrome. Ann. Thor. Surg. 8: 437, 1969
9. D.B. Roos. Transaxillary approach for first rib resection to relieve thoracic outlet syndrome. Ann. Surg. 163: 354, 1966
10. D.B. Roos. Congenital Anomalies Associated with Thoracic Outlet Syndrome. Am. J. Surg. 132: 771, 1976
11. H.C. Urschel, M.A. Razzuk, R.E. Wood, M. Parekh, D.L. Paulson. Objective diagnosis (ulnar nerve conduction velocity) and current therapy of the thoracic outlet syndrome. Ann. Thorac. Surg. 12: 608, 1971

14. The technique of measuring conduction velocity for thoracic outlet syndrome

HAROLD C. URSCHEL, JR., M.D.,*
MARUF A. RAZZUK M.D.,
EDWARD M. KRUSEN, M.D.
AND JAMES W. CALDWELL, M.D.

ABSTRACT

Nerve conduction velocity across the thoracic outlet can be performed with little discomfort to the patient and the informations so easily obtained provide objective means of diagnosis of thoracic outlet syndrome, help in the selection of therapeutic modalities, and the assessment of therapeutic results. The discrepancy in velocity values obtained by different electromyographers is technical in nature. It is realted to the methods of measuring the length of the proximal ulnar nerve segment and conduction latencies, the strength of the stimulus used and few other variables such as temperature and existing nerve disorders. The electromyographer who cannot reproduce other workers' normal velocity ranges, should establish his own values with particular observance to the basic technique of conduction study.

Nerve conduction velocity is widely employed in evaluating the parameters of nerve diseases and is used considerably in the clinical diagnosis of thoracic outlet syndrome and appraisal of therapeutic results. The test is easily performed with little discomfort to the patient. However, the information so easily obtained by different electromyographers are occasionally discrepant, leading to controversy and at times generating doubt as to the validity of this test in the diagnosis of thoracic outlet neurovascular compression.

Since most of this discrepancy is basically technical in nature, it is the aim of this communication to describe the technical details involved in the measurement of ulnar nerve conduction velocity, explain the method of calculation and outline some of the important variables that might significantly affect the results.

CLINICAL MATERIALS

Ulnar nerve conduction velocity (UNCV) was performed last year on about 8400 patients seen in consultation at the Department of Physical Medicine

*Department of thoracic surgery and physical medicine, Baylor University Medical Center, Dallas, Texas.

J.M. Greep, H.A.J. Lemmens, D.B. Roos and H.C. Urschel (eds.).
Pain in shoulder and arm: an integrated view, 165–172. All rights reserved.
Copyright © 1979 by Martinus Nijhoff Publishers, The Hague/Boston/London.

at Baylor University Medical Center for pain of the upper extremities. Seven hundred and twenty patients were found to have varying degrees of neurovascular compression at the thoracic outlet.

In analyzing the results in 247 patients, of which 172 (70%) were females (average age 37 years), and 75 (30%) were males (average age 39 years), with thoracic outlet syndrome, neurovascular compression was present in 298 extremities. Duration of symptoms in females ranged from 1 week to 15 years (average 22.2 months); and in males, it ranged from 2 weeks to 6 years (average 16.0 months). Symptoms were commonly pain and paresthesia and were distributed as follows: 36.8% in the right arm, 40.5% in the left, 20.6% in both and in 2.1% the pain was present only around the scapula or chest wall. Parascapular and chest wall pain, along with neck pain and headache were frequent symptoms in most patients. Electromyography showed no appreciable findings in 97% of patients; at least no rest denervations potentials, even in lower plexus muscles were present. The conduction velocity across the outlet averaged 59.4 m/sec on the right and 60 m/sec on the left, as compared with a normal value of 72 m/sec.

The clinical correlation between UNCV and therapeutic results was assessed in 568 patients who underwent 590 first rib resections for thoracic outlet syndrome through the transaxillary or posterior thoracoplasty approaches over a ten year period. The preoperative UNCV ranged from 32 to 65 m/sec, with the average being 55 m/sec (Table 1). Postoperative conduction values in 296 patients obtained 1 month to 5 years (average 5

Table 1. Pre and post-operative value of UNCV in patients with thoracic outlet syndrome.

Values	Velocity m/sec	
	Average	Range
Normal	72	68–75
Preoperative	55	32–65
Postoperative	68	58–75

Table 2. Clinical correlation between UNCV and therapeutic results after first rib resection for thoracic outlet syndrome.

Clinical results	Average UNCV m/sec	
	Preoperative	Postoperative
Good	55	72
Fair	60	65
Poor	63–65	65

months) after surgery ranged from 58 to 75 m/sec, (average 68 m/sec). Good results (almost complete relief of symptoms) were observed in 248 (83.8%) patients who had an average preoperative conduction velocity of 55 m/sec, fair results (improvement with residual symptoms) in 37 (12.5%) patients with average preoperative UNCV of 60 m/sec, and poor results (persistence of symptoms) in 11 (3.7%) patients with preoperative UNCV ranging from 63 to 65 m/sec (Table 2).

METHOD OF MEASURING CONDUCTION VELOCITIES

Equipment: Electromyographic examination of each upper extremity and determination of the conduction velocities was done with either the Meditron 201 AD or 312 or the TECA B-2 electromyography using coaxial cable with three needles or surface electrodes for recording muscle potentials which appear on the florescent screen.

Technique: The conduction velocity in each case was determined according to the Krusen-Caldwell technique. Each patient was placed on the examination table with the arm fully extended at the elbow and in about 20° of abduction at the shoulder to facilitate easy placement of the stimulation unit over the course of the ulnar nerve. Temperature was fairly constant at a comfortable range of 68 to 72°F for all examinations. Three needle electrodes were inserted serially in the hypothenar muscles or the first dorsal interosseous with the ground electrode placed proximally, the reference electrode distally and the recording electrode in between. If surface electrodes were to be used, the ground electrode should be placed over the palm, the reference and recording electrodes over the hypothenar eminence with the reference electrode proximal to the recording electrode. In recording the median nerve conduction velocities the electrodes are placed in the thenar muscles in the same order described for the ulnar nerve.

Sites of stimulation: The ulnar nerve was stimulated consecutively at four points.
1. at the volar aspects of the wrist at the proximal skin crease about 2 cm proximal to the base of the metacarpal bones.
2. below the elbow medially about 2.5 cm distal to the medial epicondyle of the humerus.
3. at a point over the medial aspects of the upper arm, midway between the axillary flexion line and elbow flexion line.
4. at Erb's point which is located about 2.5 cm above the clavicle and slightly anterior to the edge of trapezus muscle, which is the nearest point to the lower trunk of the brachial plexus. For stimulation of the

median nerve the stimulation unit is placed closer to the lateral head of the sternocleidomastoid or slightly more superior.

Stimulation of the ulnar nerve at the four points was affected by a special stimulation unit which imparted an electric stimulus with a strength of 350 volts with no patient's load, which is approximately equal to 300 volts with patient load with a skin resistance of 5000 ohms. Supramaximal stimulation was used at all points in order to obtain maximal response. The duration of the stimulus was 0.2 msec except for muscular individuals it was 0.5 msec. Time of stimulation, conduction delay and muscle response appear on the TECA screen with time markers occurring each millisecond on the sweep.

The conduction time or latency period of response to stimulation from the four points of stimulation to the recording electrode were obtained from the TECA digital recorder or calculated from the tracing on the screen.

Calculation of velocities

After obtaining the latencies which were expressed in milliseconds (msec), the distances in millimeters (mm) between two adjacent sites of stimulation were measured with steel tape. The velocities were calculated by subtracting the distal latency from the proximal latency and dividing the distance between the two points of stimulation by the latency difference according to

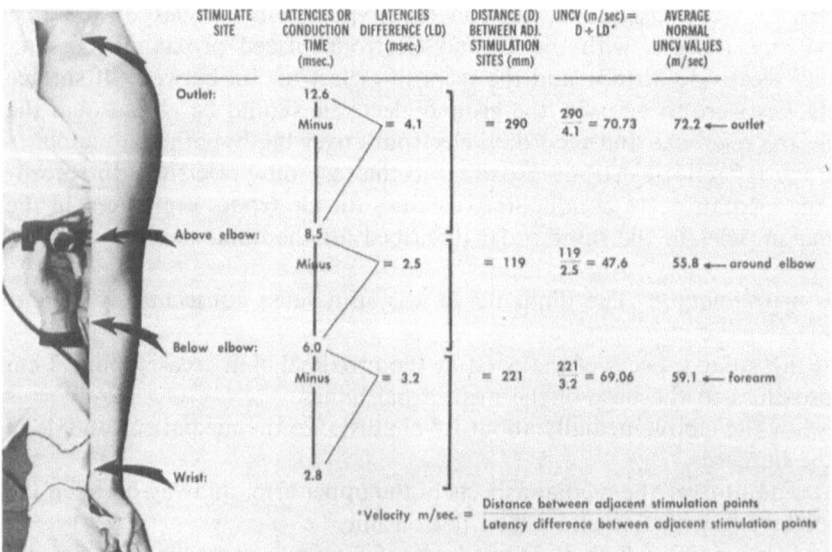

Figure 1. The method of calculating the velocity, computed by dividing the distance between two points of stimulation by the latency difference between the same two points.

the following formula:

$$\text{Velocity m/sec} = \frac{\text{Distance between two adjacent stimulation points}}{\text{Difference in latency}}$$

Consider a patient with latencies at the outlets of 12.6 msec, above elbow 8.5 msec, below elbow 6.0 msec, and wrist delay 2.8 msec; and distances between two adjacent points of stimulation of 290 mm from outlet to above elbow, 119 mm from above elbow to below elbow and 221 mm from below elbow to wrist. The velocities can be computed from the formula by dividing the distance between two adjacent points of stimulation by the difference in latencies between the same two points (Figure 1).

DISCUSSION

Since the 17th century, tremendous strides have been made towards understanding the disorder of thoracic outlet syndrome, its etiologic mechanisms, and methods of treatment (2, 6, 10, 11). However, objectivity in diagnosis remained lacking until the pioneering work of Krusen and Caldwell (1), who in 1965 performed the first conduction study of the ulnar nerve through the thoracic outlet. Ever since, this test has become widely used in the diagnosis of this syndrome, the selection of modes of treatment, and the assessment of therapeutic results (8, 9).

Although the ulnar nerve is most frequently involved in thoracic outlet compression, others such as the median nerve can also be compressed either primarily as in the high type of thoracic outlet syndrome described by Swank and Simeone (7), or secondarily by the scar of recurrent cases (11). Conduction velocities in such instances may reveal low velocities which would affirm the diagnosis of compression.

The conduction velocities of the upper extremity are of a particular value in the diagnosis of thoracic outlet syndrome in patients with predominently neural compression but without apparent motor or sensory deficit or the presence of demonstrable bony abnormalities. It is also an important asset in the work-up of the differential diagnosis of atypical chest pain in patients who have normal coronary circulation and in whom the diagnosis of thoracic outlet syndrome would otherwise be missed (10).

Whereas previously, many pain problems in the upper extremity were diagnosed as neurovascular compression on subjective clinical grounds and frequently surgical intervention was carried out as a therapeutic trial; now, by means of conduction velocity determinations, accurate assessment and precise localization of the compression and selection of patients for operation can be made on objective basis.

From the current study an incidence of thoracic outlet syndrome of 8.5%

has been observed and about 5% of those may require surgical decompression. The choice of therapy is decided on the basis of the conduction velocity. An UNCV of less than 68 m/sec across the outlet is consistent with thoracic outlet compression. If the conduction velocity is between 60–68 m/sec, most patients can be managed successfully with specific physiotherapy. If however the conduction velocity is less than 60 m/sec., the majority of patients require surgical intervention and removal of the first rib with correction of any significant bony abnormalities. Postoperative testing of ulnar nerve conduction has shown good correlation between the velocities and the clinical improvement. A significant increase in the velocities occurs following rib resection in most cases.

For normal values of UNCV across the outlet, similar means for a particular measuring technique but with different ranges have been reported by Caldwell et al. (1), London (5), and Jebsen (4) (Table 3) (5). If the steel tape is used as the measuring device the mean conduction velocity is 70.2 (5) to 72.2 m/sec (1). Whereas, if obstatrical caliper is used, the mean velocity runs at lower values of 58.9 (5) to 61.3 m/sec (4). Comparing clinical values of length of the proximal segment of the ulnar nerve across the outlet as obtained by the caliper and tape measurements with that in situ length of the same segment as measured on Cadavers (4), London (5) found the caliper measurement to be 1.18 cm shorter than the true length and the tape measurement longer by 3.32 cm. This length difference of 45 mm if divided by a normal outlet latency of 4.1 msec would account for 10.9 m/sec of difference in velocity between the two measuring techniques.

Either technique and its normal velocity ranges would be adequate to apply in clinical practice provided it is used consistently. However, if the electromyographer is unable to reproduce other workers' results, he should establish his own set of normal values by studying carefully selected normal subjects.

The anatomic landmarks for stimulation and distance measurements on the neck and upper extremities should be appropriately localized over the course of the stimulated nerve and used consistently in all cases. Wandering landmarks contribute significantly to variations in velocities noted in normal persons. For example, a 0.2 m/sec difference in calculating the time

Table 3. Studies of normal ulnar nerve conduction velocity across the thoracic outlet using caliper and steel tape measuring techniques.

Caldwell-Krusen tape (m/s)	London tape (m/s)	London caliper (m/s)	Jebsen caliper (m/s)
72.2 (68–75)	70.2 ± 5.02 (58–82.4)	58.9 ± 4.20 (50–67.7)	61.3 ± 5.4 (52–78)

delay over a 290 mm segment of nerve when the velocity is in the vicinity of 70 m/sec creates a difference of 3.2 m/sec. Likewise a 10 mm difference in determining the distance when the time delay is 4 m/sec can create a difference of 3 m/sec when the velocity is 70 m/sec.

It is also important to use supramaximal stimulation. It has been found that submaximal motor response might have a considerable delay in latency (3). Fluctuation in the magnitude of the stimulus by the same electromyographer may account for obtaining wider range of values. Krusen and Caldwell use a net potential of 300 volts with a duration of 0.2 m/sec, except in muscular individuals the duration time is increased to 0.5 m/sec. This may account for their narrow range of velocity values. The lower potentials in the range of 100–300 volts and stimulus duration of 0.05–0.2 m/sec used by London (5) may account for his wider range of normal values and velocities as low as 58 m/sec which represent compression in Krusen-Caldwell criteria. The discrepancy in the range of the two series unquestionably is technical in nature. The narrow range of 68–75 m/sec (mean 72.2) obtained by Caldwell and Krusen correlated better with the clinical picture and therapeutic results. Patients with conduction velocities below 58 m/sec get better results after rib resection than patients with velocities above 60 m/sec. Although the nerve compression is trunkal in both types of patients, nonetheless, we have observed at the time of surgery that patients with higher velocities, i.e., 60–65 m/sec have additional elements of compression which is located at the origin of the trunk. In these patients, the nerve roots C_8 and T_1 are short and converge very acutely and wrap tightly around the inner border of the neck of the rib to form the trunk. Resection of the body of the rib would relieve the compression of the trunk, however unless the neck of the rib is removed the cimpression at the origin of the trunk would continue and related symptoms persist. Resection of the neck of the rib in these cases is technically difficult without undue traction on the nerve roots and proximal trunk, which in turn may cause subsequent postoperative parasthesia. To affect complete resection of the neck of the rib and meanwhile avoid traumatization of the nerves, recently we have begun mobilizing the proximal aspects of the lower trunk and T_1 nerve root and separate them from the underlying pleura. This manoeuver exposes the remaining part of the neck and head of the rib and facilitates their total removal safely and easily. Performing such complete resection in these patients with conduction velocities 60–65 m/sec, we have noticed better clinical results.

REFERENCES

1. J.W. Caldwell, C.R. Crane, U.L. Krusen. Nerve conduction studies in the diagnosis of the thoracic outlet syndrome. South Med. J. 64: 210, 1971

2. O.T. Clagett. Presidential Address: Research and Prosearch. J. Thorac. Cardiovasc. Surg. 44: 153, 1962
3. M.M. Gassel. Sources of error in motor nerve conduction studies. Neurology 14: 825–835, 1964
4. R.H. Jebsen. Motor conduction velocities in the median and ulnar nerves. Arc. Phys. Med. 48: 185, 1967
5. G.W. London. Normal ulnar nerve conduction velocity across the thoracic outlet: comparison of two measuring techniques. J. Neurology, Neurosurgery, and Psychiatry, 38: 756–760, 1975
6. D.B. Roos, J.C. Owens. Thoracic outlet syndrome. Arch. Surg. 93: 71, 1966
7. R.L. Swank, F.A. Simeone. The scalenus anticus syndrome. Arch. Neurol. Psychiatry 51: 432, 1944.
8. H.C. Urschel Jr., M.A. Razzuk, R.E. Wood, D.L. Paulson. Objective diagnosis (ulnar nerve conduction velocity) and current therapy of the thoracic outlet syndrome. Ann. Thorac. Surg. 12: 608, 1971
9. H.C. Urschel Jr., M.A. Razzuk. Current concepts: Management of the thoracic outlet syndrome. N. Engl. J. Med. 286: 1140, 1972
10. H.C. Urschel Jr., M.A. Razzuk, J.W. Hyland, J.L. Matson, R.M. Solis, N.F. Galbraith, D.L. Paulson, R.E. Wood. Thoracic outlet syndrome masquerading as coronary artery disease. Ann. Thorac. Surg. 16: 239, 1973
11. H.C. Urschel Jr., M.A. Razzuk, J.E. Albers R.E. Albers R.E. Wood, and D.L. Paulson Reoperation for Recurrent Thoracic Outlet Syndrome. Ann. Thor. Surg. 21, 1976

15. The classical neurological syndrome associated with a cervical rib and band

R.W. GILLIATT*

ABSTRACT

Within the thoracic outlet syndrome as a whole, patients with a rudimentary cervical rib and band causing unilateral wasting of the hand form a small but clearly defined group. The interest of these cases lies in the fact that vascular features are usually lacking, and the differential diagnosis is from other causes of neurogenic hand wasting. The thenar muscles tend to be particularly severely involved and confusion with the carpal tunnel syndrome has occurred in the past. This confusion can be avoided by nerve conduction studies; in particular, the sensory action potential recorded from the ulnar nerve is likely to be small when the hand wasting is due to a cervical rib and band, whereas the median sensory action potential is normal. When sensory loss is present on the inner side of the forearm, loss of the flare normally produced by intradermal histamine provides further confirmation that the lesion is distal to the dorsal root ganglion.

It is now fashionable to use the term thoracic outlet syndrome to describe a wide spectrum of neurological or vascular symptoms and signs occurring in patients with or without radiological evidence of cervical ribs. There is, however, one group of cases, albeit a rare one, in which the clinical picture is so characteristic that it deserves separate description. This is the group in which wasting of the hand affects particularly the lateral thenar muscles; it is usually unilateral and unassociated with any vascular disturbance. Wasting of this pattern is more commonly associated with a small rudimentary rib or a prolonged C7 transverse process than with a large bony rib, and, in our experience, operation reveals a sharp fibrous band running from the tip of the bony abnormality to the first rib.

This may be called the classical neurological syndrome, and it was well described in the English literature at the beginning of the century. Why then is it not better recognized today? One reason is that the thenar wasting was, almost from the beginning, confused with that which occurs in the carpal tunnel syndrome. Partial thenar atrophy due to a cervical rib and band is a rare occurrence, whereas the carpal tunnel syndrome produces wasting in this distribution relatively frequently, and it was not until motor and sensory nerve conduction studies were widely applied in the 1960s that the two conditions could be distinguished with certainty.

*The Institute of Neurology, Queen Square, London, England.

J.M. Greep, H.A.J. Lemmens, D.B. Roos and H.C. Urschel (eds.).
Pain in shoulder and arm: an integrated view, 173–183. All rights reserved.
Copyright © 1979 by Martinus Nijhoff Publishers, The Hague/Boston/London.

Let us examine the historical development of this concept of partial thenar atrophy. In one of the earliest descriptions of hand wasting associated with cervical ribs, Howell (5) described 16 cases collected from the National Hospital, Queen Square, and from St. Bartholomew's Hospital in London. Of these, the majority showed wasting throughout the hand but particularly affecting the thenar muscles; this was usually associated with less marked wasting in the forearm and with sensory loss in the first thoracic derma-tome. In four cases, however, the thenar wasting was unaccompanied by any other motor deficit; in two of them there was sensory disturbance in a median distribution and, in retrospect, it seems likely that these were patients with the carpal tunnel syndrome who happened to have symptom-less cervical ribs in their X-rays.

Further light on these cases comes from the proceedings of a clinical meeting at the Royal Society of Medicine in London in 1913. This meeting was devoted to cervical ribs and the importance which was attached to this subject may be gauged from the fact that the proceedings of the meeting occupy eighty pages in the journal. Sir William Osler was in the chair, the anatomy was discussed by Wood-Jones, the surgery by Thorburn and by Sargent, and the medical aspects by Howell and by a Dr. Kinnier Wilson, the latter a brilliant young neurologist on the staff at Queen Square, who had recently described the condition of hepatolenticular degeneration which still bears his name. Sir Rickman Godlee, the doyen of British surgeons at this particular time, and the nephew and collaborator of Lord Lister, was unable to attend the meeting but he sent a message saying how interested Lister would have been. After sending good wishes to the meeting he wrote, "I have taken much interest in the question of cervical ribs ever since I saw Lister remove one in the days when they were called exostoses, from a middle-aged Major who had trouble in raising his rifle. He was cured by the operation."

At this meeting Wilson introduced his concept of partial thenar atrophy as the characteristic feature of the cervical rib syndrome. After showing illustrations of affected hands he commented:

"It will be seen that there is a curiously local early wasting of the thenar eminence on the right side, in which the muscles involved are the abductor pollicis and the opponens pollicis alone; all the other thenar muscles, including the flexor pollicis brevis, being intact. This definitely partial atrophy of the thenar muscles has come under my notice a large number of times, as a glance at the series of figures (Figures 2–6) will show. Sometimes the wasting is comparatively slight, sometimes it is profound, as in Figure 6, yet the other thenar muscles escape."

At a later stage of the meeting Dr. Buzzard, another physician from Queen Square, described how Wilson had first drawn his attention to this phenomenon, since when he had encountered it a number of times.

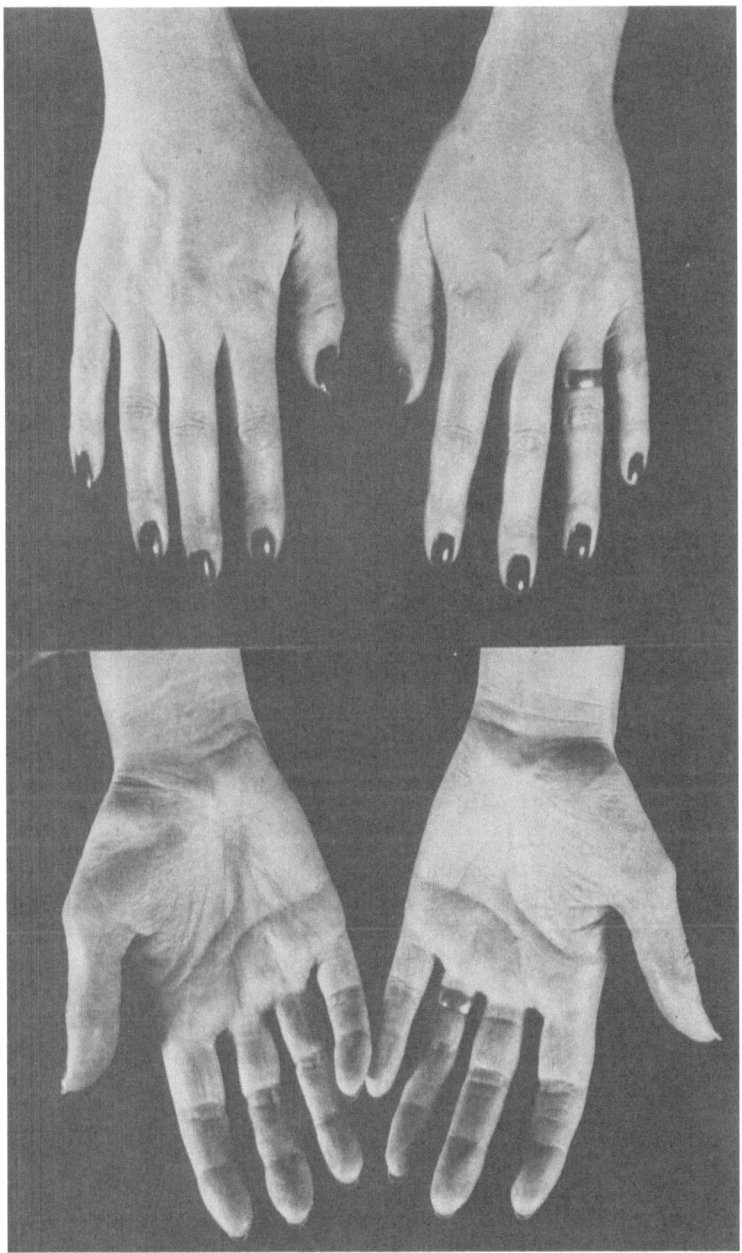

Figure 1. Mrs. A.C., aged 38 (N.H. No. A92963) An example of partial thenar atrophy in the right hand. The patient had suffered from mild intermittent pains in the right arm for many years but considered that the thenar wasting had only been present for a few months. The other hand muscles were of normal bulk except for slight thinning of the dorsal interossei on the right, with a suggestion of "guttering" between the metacarpals on the back of the hand. There was no sensory loss.

X-rays and nerve conduction studies showed typical changes, and the presence of a rudimentary cervical rib and band was confirmed at operation (Professor Valentine Logue).

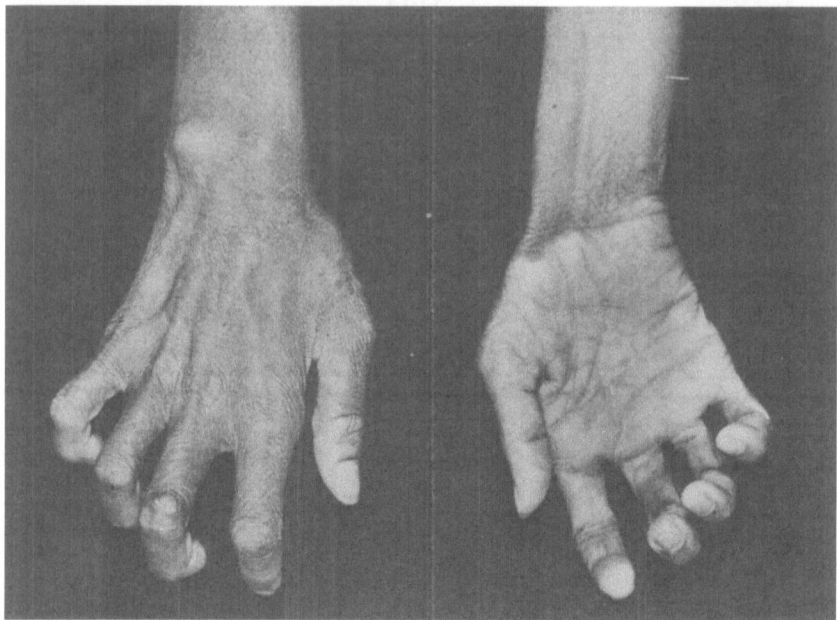

Figure 2. Miss B.M., aged 21(N.H. No. A91563) Severe generalized wasting of the right hand developing over at least five years. The forearm muscles were also affected, particularly the finger flexors. Sensory findings were variable but X-rays and nerve conduction studies showed typical changes, and the presence of a rudimentary cervical rib and band was confirmed at operation (Professor Valentine Logue).

It also transpires from the published account of the meeting that the first patient recognized by Wilson as showing this syndrome was seen in 1906, at which time he was a house physician at Queen Square. The patient was, in fact, under the care of Dr. Buzzard, who subsequently sent an account of the case to Professor Keen in Philadelphia, by whom it was published (6). The original case notes have also been traced, and from these and the published account of the case there seems little doubt that this patient had a bilateral carpal tunnel syndrome (3).

It is unfortunate that Wilson should have been mislead by this case; the result was a shift of emphasis away from the cases which Howell had described, with more generalized involvement of hand and forearm muscles and with sensory disturbance on the inner side of the forearm, towards patients with isolated thenar atrophy which we would now regard as having a different cause.

There is no doubt that Wilson's observations had a great effect on other neurologists in England. Once this pattern of wasting was accepted as part of the cervical rib syndrome, it seemed rational to assume that patients with partial thenar atrophy but without an extra rib in their X-ray had some

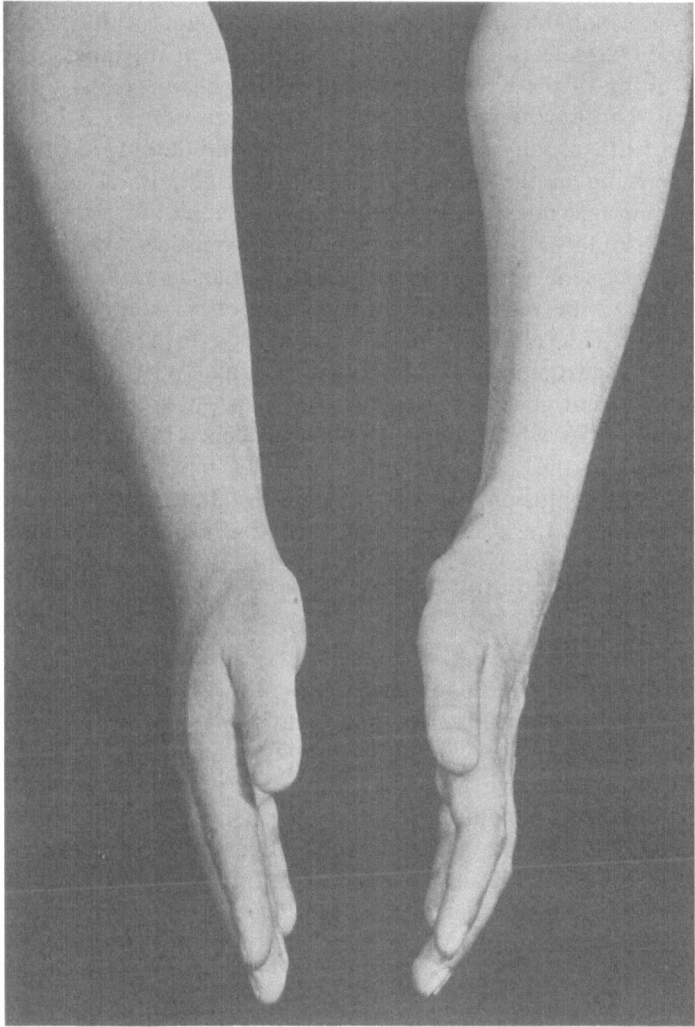

Figure 3. Mrs. S.J., aged 40 (N.H. No. A74992). Wasting of the left forearm muscles affecting particularly the thumb and finger flexors, and flexor carpi ulnaris. There was also wasting of the left hand, most marked in the thenar region. The patient had noticed pain in the arm for 18 months and weakness for 8 months. There was analgesia on the inner side of the left forearm with loss of the histamine flare.

X-rays and nerve conduction studies showed typical changes and the presence of a rudimentary cervical rib and band was confirmed at operation (Professor Valentine Logue).

disturbance at this level. Sir Francis Walshe become a strong protagonist of this view, and in his published papers referred to the clinical acumen of Wilson in picking up this important physical sign (12, 14). Once it was accepted that the syndrome could occur without a cervical rib in the X-ray, it seemed unreasonable to distinguish between patients with partial thenar atrophy and characteristic nocturnal paraesthesiae in the hands, and those without wasting of the hands but with a similar history (13).

The term "acroparaesthesia syndrome" had been used by Schultze (9) to describe patients, usually middle-aged women, who developed painful tingling and burning in the fingers and hand at night. Its association with muscle wasting had not been recognized and the condition was regarded as a form of vasomotor neurosis. As a result of Wilson's observations and Walshe's subsequent writing on this subject, the "acroparaesthesia syndrome" came to be regarded as a manifestation of some neurovascular disturbance at the level of the thoracic outlet. As a further result of this, the carpal tunnel syndrome, clearly described by Brain, Wright and Wilkinson in 1947 (2), was not generally accepted by English neurologists and neurosurgeons until 1956, when Simpson finally published the nerve conduction studies which put the diagnosis on an objective basis (10). In tracing the roots of present confusion, we can therefore conclude that the two important factors were (i) the coexistance of the carpal tunnel syndrome and (ii) the fact that many patients have cervical ribs in their X-rays which do not give rise to symptoms in the arms or hands.

From our present knowledge, what can we say about thenar as opposed to generalized wasting in the hand in patients with a cervical rib and band? The first point to be made is that both types of wasting are relatively rare. In the EMG clinics of the National Hospitals at Queen Square and Maida Vale, not more than two or three examples are seen in a year out of approximately 2000 patients referred. My personal series collected over approximately 15 years consists of only 30 cases. Some years after our initial publication on the carpal tunnel syndrome (7), my colleague Dr. Michael Kremer told me that he had seen 600 carpal-tunnel patients and, over the same period, only 12 patients with neurological deficits due to cervical ribs.

In my own 30 patients, muscle wasting restricted to the thenar region with perfectly normal bulk elsewhere was seen in approximately one fifth. Even in these cases weakness could be detected in the interossei and hypothenar muscles as well as in the thenar muscles. More commonly, wasting affected all the small hand muscles but with particular emphasis on the thenar region (Figure 1). This pattern was present in the majority of the cases. There were a few patients, however, in whom the hand was generally wasted without distinction between thenar and other muscles (Figure 2). Wasting of the forearm, visible on its anterior and inner aspect, was also present in about one third of the patients (Figure 3).

While sensory symptoms were common, a sensory deficit was less so. When present it consisted of a patch of superficial sensory loss on the inner

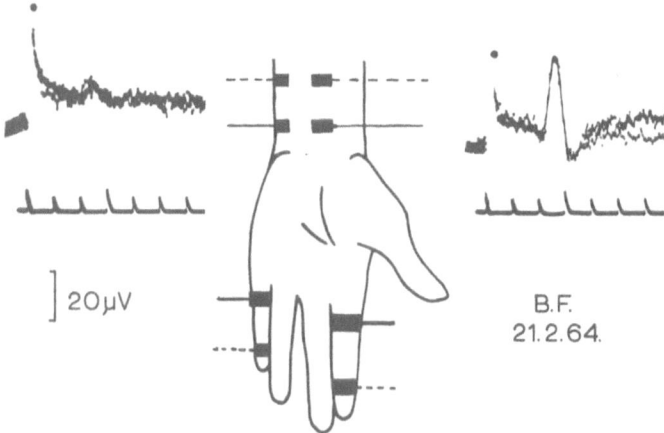

Figure 4. Mrs. B.F., aged 25 (N.H. No. A16419). Left cervical rib and band. Reduced amplitude of sensory action potentials recorded from ulnar nerve at wrist. Three successive traces superimposed. Time scale in msec.
  Source: Gilliatt et al. (3).

side of the forearm, not usually extending into the hand. Loss to pin-prick was more obvious than that to cotton-wool; appreciation of compass points was only rarely affected on the fifth finger.

These patients conspicuously lacked vascular symptoms and signs; and the differential diagnosis was from other muscle wasting diseases affecting the upper limbs, such as median and ulnar nerve lesions, brachial plexus neuropathy (so-called neuralgic amyotrophy), cervical spondylosis, syringomyelia and motor neurone disease. Clinical features which were helpful in establishing the diagnosis included the characteristic peripheral distribution of the wasting, weakness and sensory loss; and the preservation of normal deep tendon reflexes in biceps, triceps and brachioradialis.

Women appeared to be affected ten times as commonly as men but their ages ranged from the second to the eighth decade without a characteristic age incidence. The description of pain in the arm given by the patients also varied widely from one case to another and was not sufficiently constant to be diagnostically helpful. In most patients the pain was the earliest symptom, often preceding muscle wasting by several years, but it tended to be mild, diffuse and intermittent, so that patients did not seek medical help until the motor deficit in the hand was noticed. In a few patients pain in the arm was the main complaint but there were others who claimed never to have suffered pain as part of the syndrome.

The classical nocturnal paraesthesiae of the carpel tunnel syndrome, waking the patient in the early morning with numb, painful and swollen fingers, did not occur in the cervical rib patients, and this was a helpful negative point in the differential diagnosis. In spite of it, the predominantly thenar wasting commonly mislead clinicians, and carpal tunnel syndrome was the commonest mis-diagnosis in patients referred to us for further investigation.

The critical investigations were three. Of these, the nerve conduction studies were probably the most important. Not only did they exclude median or ulnar entrapment at the wrist or elbow but, in addition, the small amplitude of the ascending sensory action potential in the ulnar nerve indicated the presence of a lesion distal to the dorsal root ganglia. A typical example is shown in Figure 4. Although a low amplitude ascending action potential from the fifth finger could also result from ulnar nerve entrapment at the elbow, this is easily excluded by recording the ascending action potential above the elbow as well as at the wrist. In cervical rib patients the reduction in amplitude should be similar at the two levels and the velocity of the ascending volley in the forearm and elbow segment should be normal. In a recent group of 14 patients the ulnar sensory action potential amplitude on the wasted side was at the lower limit of the normal range in four, and below it in 10 cases. In only one of these, however, was the potential wholly absent (4).

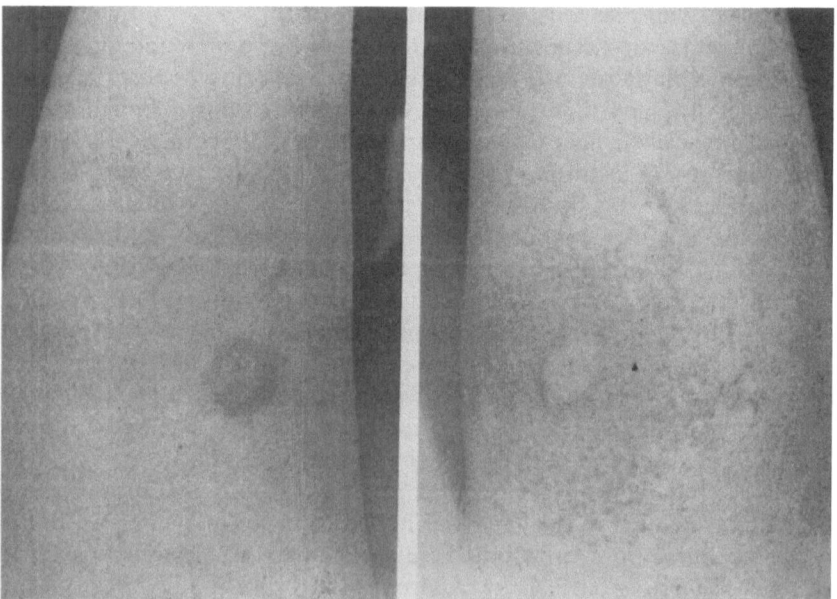

Figure 5. Miss S.M., aged 16 (N.H. No. A39707). Right cervical rib and band. Loss of flare response to intradermal histamine (0.01 ml of 1 in 1000 histamine acid phosphate) on inner side of affected forearm. Normal response on opposite forearm.
    Source: Gilliatt et al. (3).

When sensory loss has been present on the inner side of the forearm we have found the use of intradermal histamine to be valuable in demonstrating the absence of a flare (Figure 5). In three of our recent patients the response was clearly abnormal when the conduction studies showed only marginal changes.

In almost every case X-rays have shown either a rudimentary cervical rib or a long down-curving C7 transverse process on the affected side. I have referred for surgery only two patients without these changes compared with 25 patients who showed the typical radiological features. One of the two patients turned out to have a neurofibroma of the lower trunk of the branchial plexus; the other showed a typical sharp fibrous band angulating the C8 and T1 roots just before they joined. Thus a fibrous band causing thenar wasting in the absence of a rudimentary rib or long C7 transverse process in the X-ray seems to be an exceedingly rare phenomenon.

An interesting feature of the radiological abnormalities is shown in Figure 6. A wasted hand is more commonly associated with a small

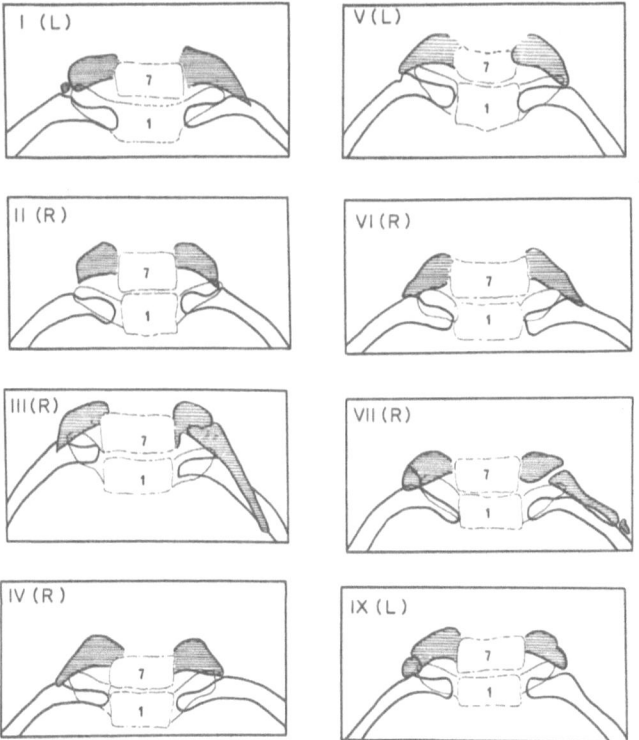

Figure 6. Tracing of radiographs of eight patients.
Source: Gilliatt et al. (3).

rudimentary rib or long down-curving C7 transverse process than with a fully formed cervical rib articulating with the first rib. This agrees with the consistent surgical finding made by my colleague, Professor Valentine Logue, that the neural damage is caused, not by the bony rib, but by the sharp-edged fibrous band which joins the tip of the bony abnormality to the first rib. In Figure 6 it can be seen that there were two patients with a fully formed cervical rib on one side and a rudimentary rib on the other; it is interesting that in both cases the wasted hand was on the side of the rudimentary rib. This was also the experience of Wilson who wrote in 1940:

"On the whole it is the small rib type that affects the plexus, and the larger, the artery, if at all; in the case of bilateral deformities the less substantial one sometimes proves more productive of symptoms than its fellow."

The presence of a sharp-edged fibrous band running in the anterior border of scalenus medius was also described by Bonney (1), and its presence seems to be critical for the development of this particular syndrome. All of us would accept that we commonly see patients with rudimentary cervical ribs or large down-curving C7 transverse processes who never develop symptoms in the hands. What is less commonly realized is that patients with unilateral wasting but with bilateral radiological abnormalities only rarely develop a similar syndrome on the opposite side. The hand wasting has been unilateral in all of the 25 operated patients I have examined personally, although the radiological abnormalities were bilateral in 24 of them. Some of these patients have now been followed for as long as 15 years, but none have so far developed wasting in the second hand. That wasting can occasionally be bilateral should not, however, be questioned. Examples were given in the recent report of Lascelles, Mohr, Neary and Bloor (8). Bilateral wasting was also present in the familial cases described by Thompson (11).

One question which I have not discussed is why the muscle wasting should particularly involve the lateral thenar muscles. As Wilson originally suggested, the abductor pollicis brevis and opponens pollicis are severely affected, whereas the flexor pollicis brevis may be spared, and indeed sometimes appears to show compensatory hypertrophy (Sunderland, personal communication). In my own cases, selective wasting of this distribution seems to have been most obvious in patients with motor deficits of relatively short duration, suggesting that it is a stage in a slowly progressive process which eventually results in wasting throughout the hand. Does this imply that the motor fibres supplying the lateral thenar muscles are already grouped together in the T1 root or lower trunk of the brachial plexus, some distance proximal to the origin of the median nerve? Basic anatomical studies on this problem are clearly required if we are to understand the cause of this interesting clinical pattern which has now been known to neurologists for 70 years.

ACKNOWLEDGEMENTS

The author wishes to thank Professor Valentine Logue for permission to quote from his operative findings. He also wishes to thank Dr. R.G. Willison for helpful discussion.

REFERENCES

1. G. Bonney. The scalenus medius band: a contribution to the study of the thoracic outlet syndrome. J. Bone Jt. Surg. 47B: 268, 1965
2. W.R. Brain, A.D. Wright, M. Wilkinson. Spontaneous compression of both median nerves in the carpal tunnel. Lancet, 1: 277, 1947
3. R.W. Gilliatt, P.M. LeQuesne, V. Logue, A.J. Sumner. Wasting of the hand associated with a cervical rib or band. J. Neurol. Neurosurg. Psychiat. 33: 615, 1970
4. R.W. Gilliatt, R.G. Willison, V. Dietz, I.R. Williams. Peripheral nerve conduction in patients with a cervical rib and band. Ann. Neurol. 4:124, 1978.
5. C.M.H. Howell. A consideration of some symptoms which may be produced by seventh cervical ribs. Lancet 1: 1702, 1907
6. W.W. Keen. The symptomatology, diagnosis and surgical treatment of cervical ribs. Amer. J. med. Sci. 133: 173, 1907
7. M. Kremer, R.W. Gilliatt, J.S.R. Golding, T.G. Wilson. Acroparaesthesiae in the carpal-tunnel syndrome. Lancet 2: 590, 1953
8. R.G. Lascelles, P.D. Mohr, D. Neary, K. Bloor. The thoracic outlet syndrome. Brain 100: 601, 1977
9. F. Schultze. Ueber Akroparasthesie. Dtsch. Z. Nervenheilk 3: 300, 1893
10. J.A. Simpson. Electrical signs in the diagnosis of carpal tunnel and related syndromes. J. Neurol. Neurosurg. Psychiat. 19: 275, 1956
11. T. Thompson. Familial atrophy of the hand muscles. Brain 31: 286, 1908
12. F.M.R. Walshe, H. Jackson, R. Wyburn-Mason. On some pressure effects associated with cervical and with rudimentary and "normal" first ribs, and the factors entering into their causation. Brain 67: 141, 1944
13. F.M.R. Walshe. On "acroparaesthesia" and so-called "neuritis" of the hands and arms in women. Brit. med. J. 2: 596, 1945
14. F.M.R. Walshe. Nervous and vascular pressure syndromes of the thoracic inlet and cervico-axillary canal. In: Modern Trends in Neurology. ed. Anthony Feiling Butterworth and Co., London, p. 542, 1951
15. S.A.K. Wilson. Some points in the symptomatology of cervical rib, with especial reference to muscular wasting. Proc. roy. Soc. Med. (Clin. Section) 6: 133, 1913
16. S.A.K. Wilson. Neurology, Vol. 2, edited A.N. Bruce, Edward Arnold: London. 1940

16. Costo-clavicular compression: a review

D.J. BAKKER. M.D.*

ABSTRACT

Costo-clavicular compression is considered as one of the thoracic outlet compression syn-dromes. The term was introduced by Falconer and Weddell (4) when they called attention to the fact that the neurovascular structures could be compressed between the clavicle and the first rib, without abnormality of the scalenus musculature. The thoracic outlet compression syndrome is a symptom complex consisting of neural, arterial and venous disorders of the upper extremity which are caused by compression of the neurovascular structures between the clavicle and the first rib (6).

DIFFERENT SYNDROMES AND THE ETIOLOGY OF THE COMPRESSION

The neuro-vascular compression syndromes or thoracic outlet compression syndromes, a term introduced by Rob and Standeven in 1958, can, dependent on the so-called level of compression, classically be divided into seven different syndromes.
1. The scalenus anticus syndrome.
2. Cervical rib syndrome.
3. Costo-clavicular compression syndrome.
4. Hyperabduction syndrome.
5. Pectoralis minor syndrome.
6. Syndrome of the narrow upper thoracic aperture.
7. Scalenus minimus syndrome.

This differentation however, is based on an interpretation of subjective complaints and doubtful results from clinical examinations and lacks clinical and experimental evidence. Many tests to confirm the diagnosis are often positive in symptom-free patients and the reverse is also true.

1. In the scalenus anticus syndrome, the compression of the neuro-vascular bundle is thought to occur between the anterior and medial scalenus muscles. This space, known as the scalenus triangle, is already small and is further narrowed by muscle contraction. This may be true, but contraction of the scalenus muscles also gives an elevation of the first rib, so

* Wilhelmina Hospital, Amsterdam, The Netherlands.

J.M. Greep, H.A.J. Lemmens, D.B. Roos and H.C. Urschel (eds.).
Pain in shoulder and arm: an integrated view, 185–200. All rights reserved.
Copyright © 1979 by Martinus Nijhoff Publishers, The Hague/Boston/London.

that the costo-clavicular compartment is narrowed and the result is a
component of costo-clavicular compression. (Figure 1.) Evidence of this
double etiology of the complaints is suggested by the poor results in
patients after single scalenotomy. (2, 8, 12, 14) (Table 3).

2. In the cervical rib syndrome we can distinguish schematically between
five different anatomic forms which a cervical rib can assume. The description was given by Roberts as early as 1908. The variations extended
from a long transverse processus of C7 to a complete cervical rib which
reaches the manubrium sterni. We must remember that an incomplete bony
cervical rib can act as complete due to its fibrous attachments to the first rib
and the manubrium sterni. The route taken by the artery through the

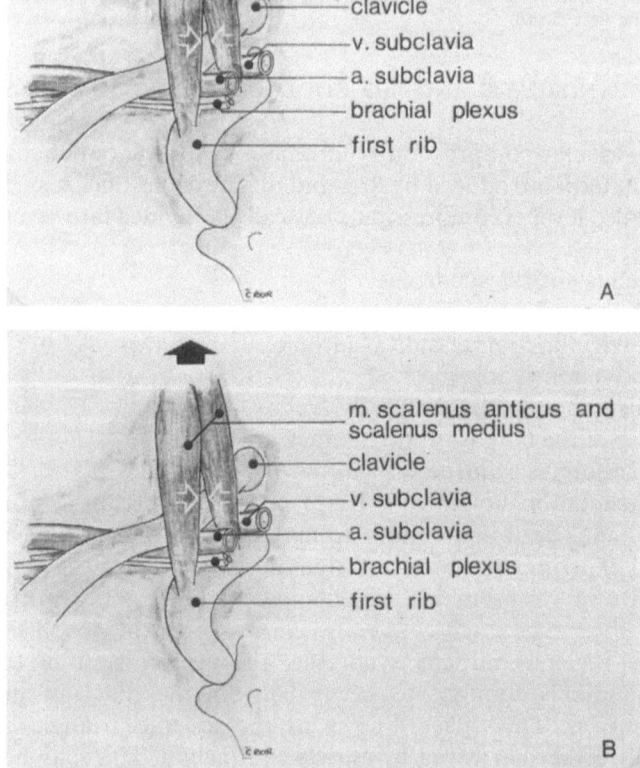

Figure 1*A* and *B*. Compression mechanism in the scalenus anticus syndrome. Narrowing of
the scalenus triangle (white arrows), and narrowing of the costo-clavicular space by muscle
contraction (black arrows).

scalenus triangle is more ventral and cranial than normal because of the cervical rib. Furthermore the artery is compressed against the tendon of the scalenus anticus muscle. A narrowing of the costo-clavicular space causes a kinking of the artery at the place where the clavicle crosses the first rib (Figure 2).

3. In the costo-clavicular syndrome there is compression of the neuro-vascular bundle between the clavicle and the first rib. To understand this we can compare the clavicle and the first rib with their fixation on the manubrium sterni, to a pair of scissors. The movable part of the scissors is the clavicle. This is very extensively described by Lo-A-Njoe (1974) in his thesis about costo-clavicular compression. Dependent on the shoulder and arm elevation, the clavicle slides posteriorly over the first rib for a distance of approximately $2\frac{1}{2}$ cm (Figure 3). During this movement there is also an endorotation of clavicle. In this way the costo-clavicular compartment is narrowed. The influence of this shoulder movement on compression and complaints is described elsewhere in this book. Normally patients do not

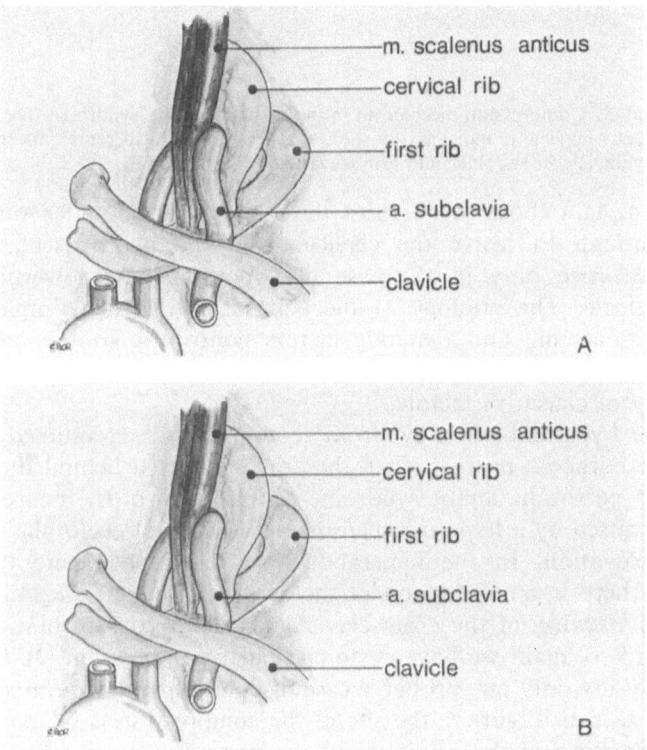

Figure 2*A* and *B*. Compression mechanism in the cervical rib syndrome.

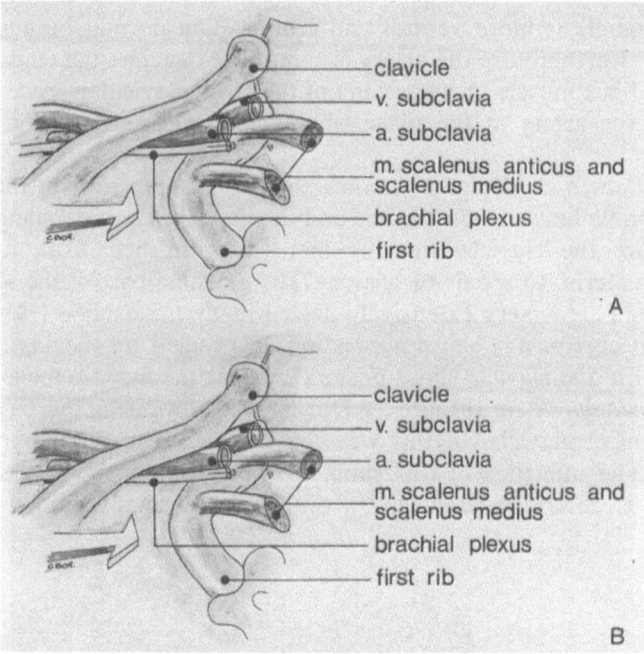

Figure 3*A* and *B*. Compression mechanism in the costo-clavicular syndrome. The scissor-like movement of the clavicle is indicated by the white arrow. This also represents the posterior sliding of the clavicle in shoulder and arm elevation.

have to complain about this because the tonus of the shoulder musculature is high enough to heave the clavicle from the neurovascular bundle. Complaints arise only in the case of hypotonus and lowering of the shoulder girdle. The etiology of the compression is not simple or monocausal. Anatomic and dynamic factors contribute to the complaints. Walsche (1944) et al. and Stammers (1950) had already emphasized the multiplicity of causative factors.

4. In the hyperabduction syndrome compression is presumed to occur against the coracoid process when the arm is elevated behind the head.

5. In the pectoralis minor syndrome compression of the neuro-vascular bundle is caused by a hypertrophied or even a normal pectoralis tendon in shoulder elevation. In the hyperabduction, as in the pectoralis minor syndrome there is an abduction of the arm and this, as we saw already, causes a narrowing of the costo-clavicular space by endo-rotation of the clavicle; and so again we have costo-clavicular compression (3). In all our patients we saw only one probable case of pure hyperabduction syndrome. As can be seen in Figure 4, the site of the compression is far more lateral than the crossing of the clavicle and the first rib, where costo-clavicular compression takes place.

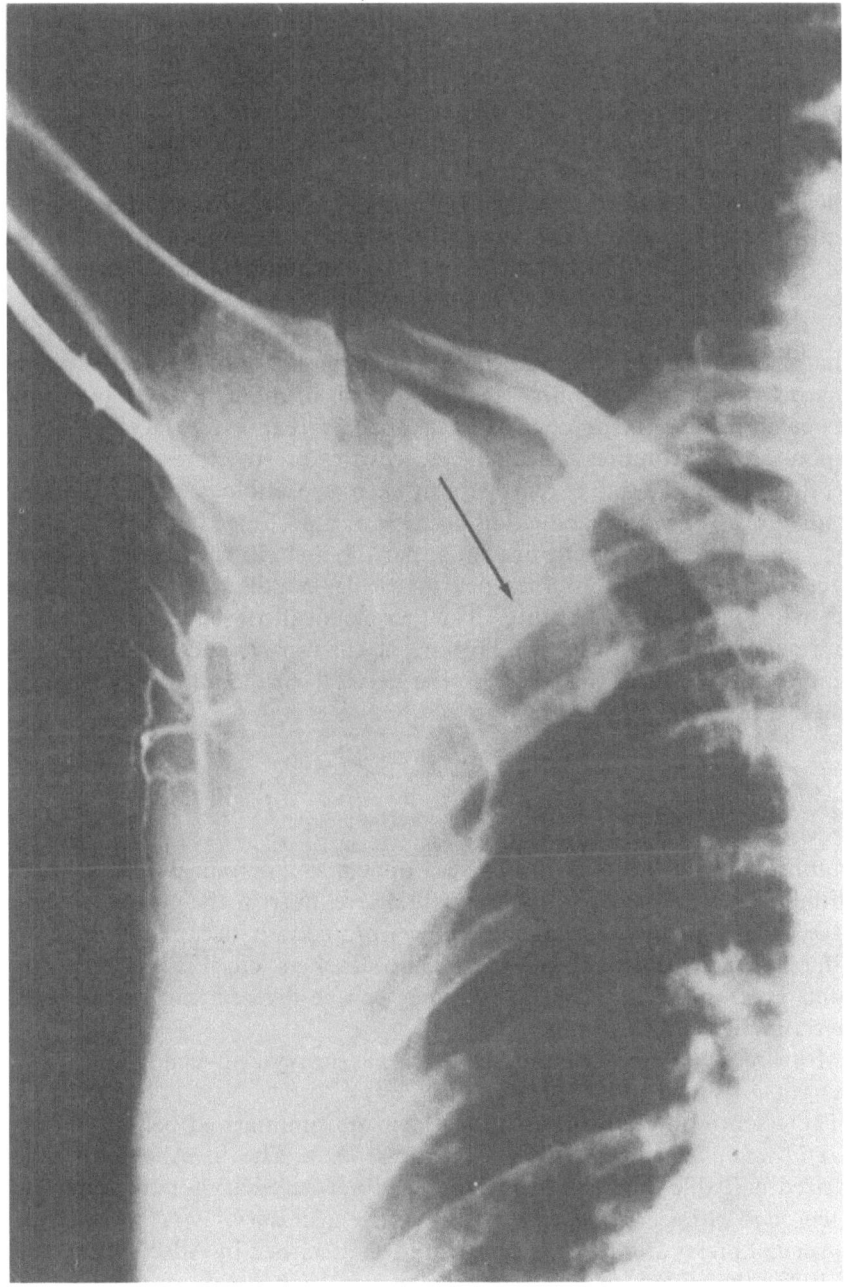

Figure 4. Hyperabduction compression. The site of artery-compression (arrow) is far more lateral than the intersection of the clavicle and the first rib.

6. The syndrome of the narrow upper thoracic aperture has no role in clinical practice.

7. The scalenus minus syndrome: This muscle varies in size. Its origin is on the transverse processes of C6 and C7; then it goes behind the scalenus anterior to its insertion on the first rib. Some of the muscle fibres are connected with the pleural tissues. Instead of a muscle there can be the so-called costopleuro-vertebral ligament. This muscle narrows the scalenus triangle and the artery can also pass through the muscle; in this case contraction gives compression. One form of the anatomic variations of this muscle or ligament belongs to the congenital bands described by Roos.

Finally, besides these different syndromes, compression in this region can be caused by a rudimentary first rib, by exostosis of the first rib or by an old clavicular fracture. Our conclusion is that a great many factors can be responsible for compression of the neurovascular structures. Lowering of the shoulder-girdle has a central position in the etiology. Other dynamic factors are a long hyperabduction position or a prolonged military attitude. The conclusion that can be drawn is that the first rib is the bottom of the space where compression of the neuro-vascular bundle takes place between this first rib and other structures. The therapeutical consequence is that first rib resection takes away the bottom of this space and terminates the compression. Besides this there is the cervical rib compression which is indeed a different syndrome.

SIGNS, SYMPTOMS AND DIAGNOSIS

Establishment of the diagnosis is very difficult. As certain movements and attitudes of the arm above the horizontal level narrow the costo-clavicular space, it is evident that patients come from certain occupations such as painters, truck drivers, housewives, school-teachers, etc. Preoperative symptoms are summarized in Table I. They can be divided into neurological, arterial and venous symptoms.

Most frequently we see pain, paraesthesias, heavy-arm-feeling and loss of strength.

The essential investigations in our view are summarized below.

Careful anamnesis is the most important point. The investigations summarized in Table 2 are supplementary and not necessary for the diagnosis.

A *thorough physical examination* is of course necessary.

Provocation tests are the classical Adson test described by Adson and Coffey in 1927, the Eden test or costo-clavicular manoeuvre or exaggerated military position, first described by Falconer and Weddell in 1943 and the Wright test of hyperabduction manoeuvre, described by Wright in 1945. In

Table 1. Thoracic outlet compression syndrome: preoperative signs and symptoms.

Neurological	Arterial	Venous
Diffuse pain	Ischemic diffuse pain	Aching
Paresthesias/hypesthesias	Numbness	Swelling
Numbness	Fatique	Bluish discoloration
Tingling	Pallor	Enlargment of the upper extremity
Loss of strength	Coolness	
Sensory loss	Sensitivity to cold	
Muscular weakness and atrophy	Intermittent claudication	
	Inability to raise the hand	

all three tests a positive result indicates a costo-clavicular compression. The value of these tests in establishing the diagnosis is doubtful. They can be positive in patients without complaints and negative in patients with a very strongly positive anamnesis.

X-ray examination is of course necessary for the diagnosis of a cervical rib or anatomical bone deformities.

We think that in uncomplicated cases, arteriography is not necessary for the diagnosis. When arterial complications have already occurred, arteriography is mandatory. If arteriography is performed it is necessary to take X-

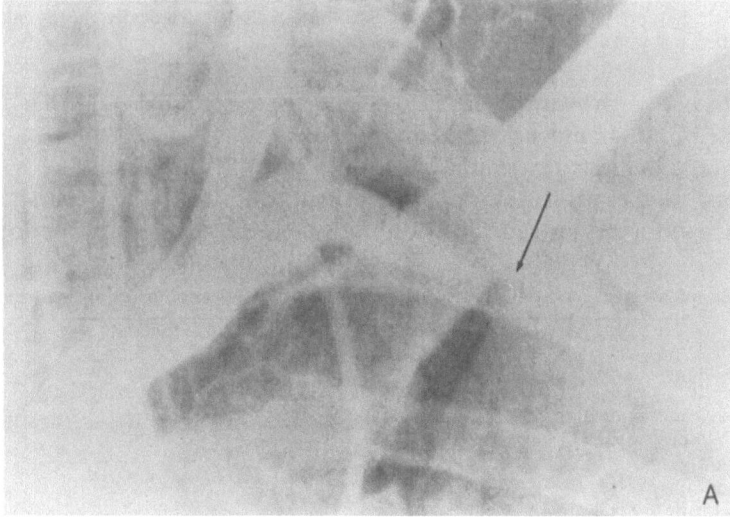

Figure 5A. Inadequate picture. The artery is totally occluded (arrow). The post-stenotic segment cannot be visualized.

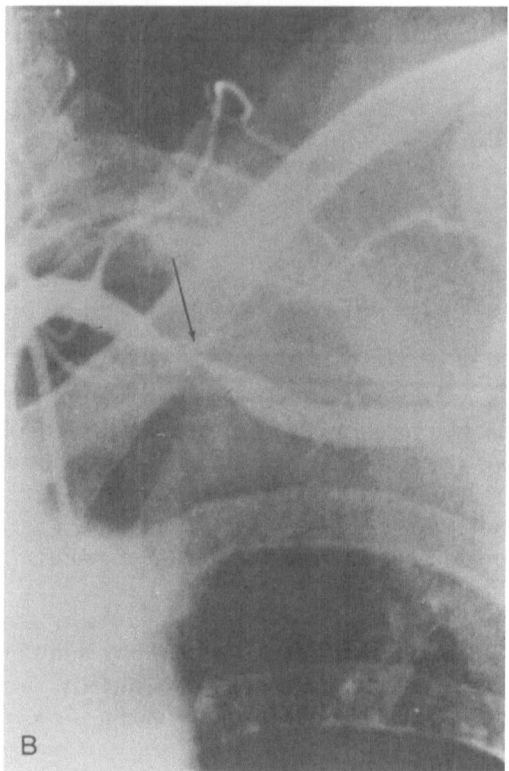

Figure 5B. Adequate picture. Artery is compressed, not occluded. Clinically the radial pulse
is diminished but not absent.

ray's during a provocation test in a positive phase. Radial pulse has to be
diminished, but should not have disappeared.

Both possibilities are demonstrated in Figure 5. In the case of a total
occlusion of the artery during the provocation test, the post-stenotic
segment cannot be judged. Secondly, arteriography has to be performed

Table 2. Supplementary methods of investigation in thoracic outlet compression syndrome.

Arteriography
Phlebography
Oscillography
Doppler-flow measurements
Plethysmography
Ultra-sound
Fonoangiography
Venous pressure measurements
Ulnar nerve conduction time
Quantitative measurement of blood flow through arm muscles by 99M technetium clearance

with the patient sitting upright under local anaesthesia. Normal functional and anatomical conditions are then present. This so-called "functional arteriography" has recently been described by Neuerer (7). The other objective methods of investigation (Table 2) are valuable perhaps for a better understanding and a better judgement of the compression syndrome; they do not have decisive significance for the diagnosis.

Urschel described the technique of measuring the ulnar nerve conduction time. He considers this helpful, noting that the average conduction velocity was reduced in patients with a costo-clavicular compression syndrome, returning to normal after operation. Phlebography has to be performed in patients with evidence of venous hypertension and stasis (see also: Complications).

DIFFERENTIAL DIAGNOSIS

Differential diagnosis covers a large field in many specialities such as neurology, rheumatology, orthopedics, pulmonology and others. Other authors in this book have dealt with this subject.

THERAPY

Therapy of costo-clavicular compression syndrome can be conservative or operative.

Conservative: In patients with moderate or minor complaints we start with physiotherapeutic treatment for 6 to 8 weeks. Principal goal is strengthening of the neck- and shouldermuscles. Good results are obtained in about 70% of the patients.

Operative therapy is indicated when:
1. Conservative therapy has failed.
2. When complications have already occurred.

We must remember that the first signs of a costo-clavicular compression syndrome can be arterial emboli (Figure 6).

Over the years we have practised the following operating techniques.

1. Cervical rib resection.
2. Resections of fibrous bands (+scalenotomy).
3. Scalenotomy alone.
4. First rib resection (+scalenotomy) via a supra- and infraclavicular approach.
5. Fixation of the 1st to the 2nd rib.
6. Versatio costae I.
7. Claviculectomy.
8. First rib resection (+scalenotomy) via a transaxillary approach.

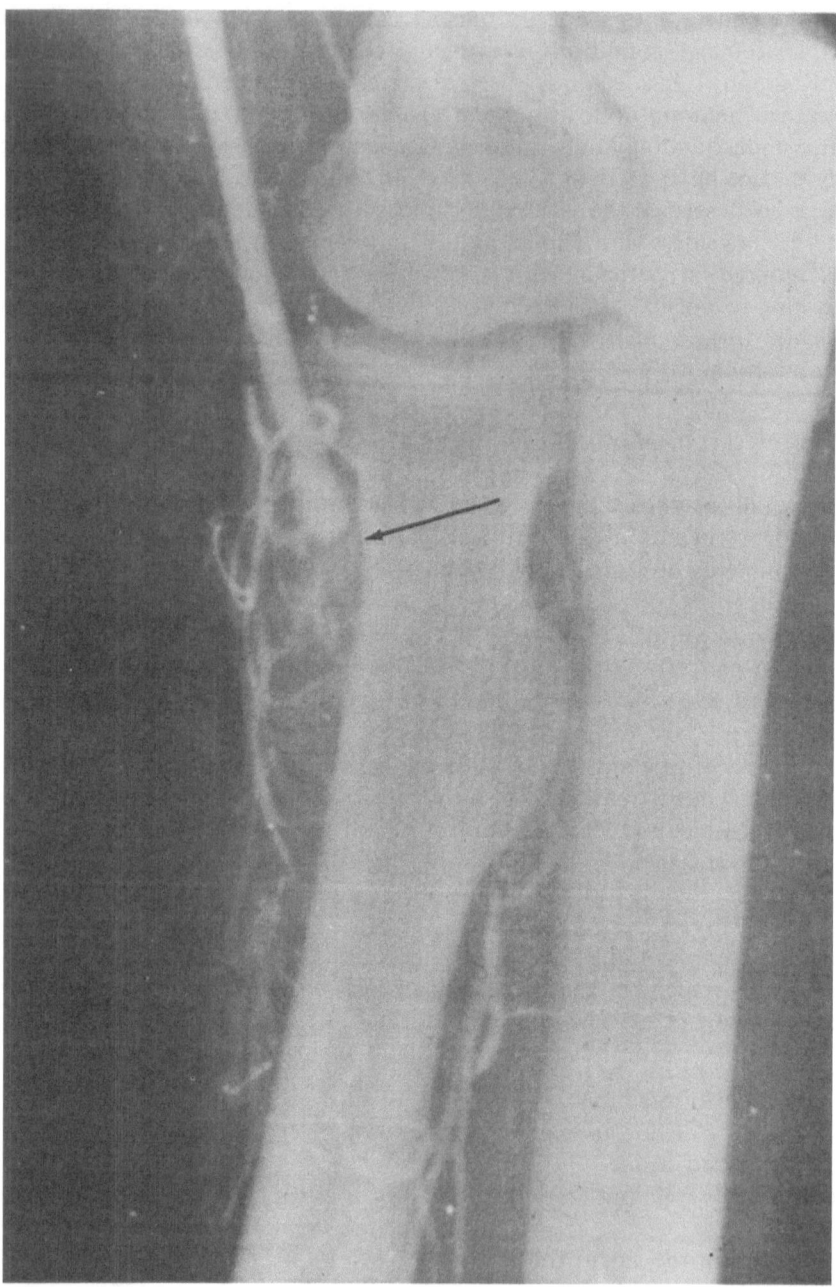

Figure 6. Embolic occlusion of the brachial artery, as the first sign of a costo-clavicular compression.

Table 3. Thoracic outlet compression syndrome: results of the operative treatment.

	N = Pat.	Without complaints after 1 year
Scalenotomy alone (until 1958)	38	$4 = 10.5\%$
Scalenotomy alone (from 1958)	22	$3 = 13.6\%$
Scalenotomy + resection of fibrous bands (scalenus minimus)	30	$21 = 70\ \%$
TOTAL:	90	$28 = 31.1\%$

From 1966, following the publications of Dr. Roos, our therapy of choice has been the transaxillary first rib resection (+scalenotomy and resection of fibrous bands). We will not discuss the different operative techniques in detail. However, some general conclusions can be drawn from the results. Table 3 shows our results with scalenotomy alone. These are as poor, as throughout the world.

Scalenotomy, is now generally accepted as a poor operation. Good results are reported in less than 30% of cases. Theoretically this operation would be sufficient in patients with an isolated form of scalenus compression. This, however, is extremely rare, if existing at all. In Table 4 the results are summarized of the operations that were intended to widen the costo-clavicular space. Although the early results were good (80%), results after one year had deteriorated (50%). This was due to technical errors. Our conclusion however, was that we were working in the right direction with these costo-clavicular space-widening techniques.

From 1966 until 1977 we did only transaxillary first rib resections with a good result in 88% of cases (table 5).

Table 4. Thoracic outlet compression syndrome: operative results of the costo-clavicular space-widening operations.

	N = Pat	N = Without complaints		
		Early	After $\frac{1}{2}$ year	After 1 year
Fixation of the 1st rib to the 2nd Rib + scalenotomy	159	128 80.5%	82	$68 = 42.8\%$
Versatio costae I	20	16 80 %	14	$14 = 70\ \%$
Partial or total claviculectomy	9	6 66.7%	6	$5 = 55.6\%$
First rib resection + scalenotomy (supra- and infraclavicular approach)	16	13 81.3%	12	$12 = 75\ \%$
Total pat.:	204	163 79.7%	114	$99 = 48.5\%$

Table 5. Thoracic outlet compression syndrome: operative results in first rib resection via a transaxillary approach from 1966–1977.

	n	Without compl. after 3 years
First rib resection	474 Pat.	417 Pat.
(Transaxillary approach)	(= 563 Extr.)	88%

Our conclusion is that there are only two operative methods left nowadays:
1. Cervical rib resection.
2. Transaxillary first rib resection.
The advantages of the transaxillary approach are:
1. It gives the best cosmetic appearance.
2. Thoracal sympathectomy can easily be performed via this approach.
3. Arterial reconstruction, if necessary, can be accomplished via this approach.
   The technique of the transaxillary first rib resection will not be described. Roos (1966) and Lo-A-Njoe (1974) have given excellent descriptions.

RECURRENT SYNDROME

During the operation the first rib must be fully resected. Incomplete resection can cause a recurrent syndrome due to regeneration of the first rib, the periosteum, or the posterior rib remnant.

Another source of recurrent complaints can be that after first rib resection the space between the clavicle and the second rib is too small and it will then also be necessary to resect approximately 8 cm from the middle part of the second rib. To avoid recurrence the patient has to be evaluated in the abduction-external rotation position before closing the incision after first rib resection. If the clavicle is extremely close to the second rib, middle part of this can also be excised.

Another question to be answered is: Do we have to operate on all patients with complaints after conservative treatment has failed? When the patient avoids certain attitudes and movements he will be able to live with

Table 6. Thoracic outlet compression syndrome: Complications.

I. Arterial:
    a. Vascular wall damage→organic stenosis
    b. Secundary thrombosis
    c. Subclavian artery aneurysm (post-stenotic)
    d. Arterial emboli
II. Venous
    e. Venous thrombosis (S.C. Paget-von Schroetter syndrome)

his disability without too serious complaints. To answer this question we must not forget that costo-clavicular compression can have serious complications that occur not too infrequently. The complications (arterial and venous) are summarized in Table 6.

COMPLICATIONS

In Figure 7 you see the X-ray of a woman with a costo-clavicular compression diagnosed in 1969. Complaints were not too serious and operation was thought unnecessary. Two years later she had far more serious acute complaints. Arteriography revealed a total occlusion of the artery. These occlusions are difficult to treat operatively. Therapy of choice in these cases is resection of the occluded artery and heterograft interposition, or a venous bypass. Van Dongen describes these techniques and possibilities elsewhere in this book. Another complication is poststenotic subclavian aneurysm.

Figure 8 demonstrates a case of such an aneurysma caused by cervical rib compression of the subclavian artery. As we saw already organic vascular wall damage can become a source of emboli with obstruction of the peripheral arteries (Figure 6).

A last complication is venous thrombosis, or the so-called Paget-von

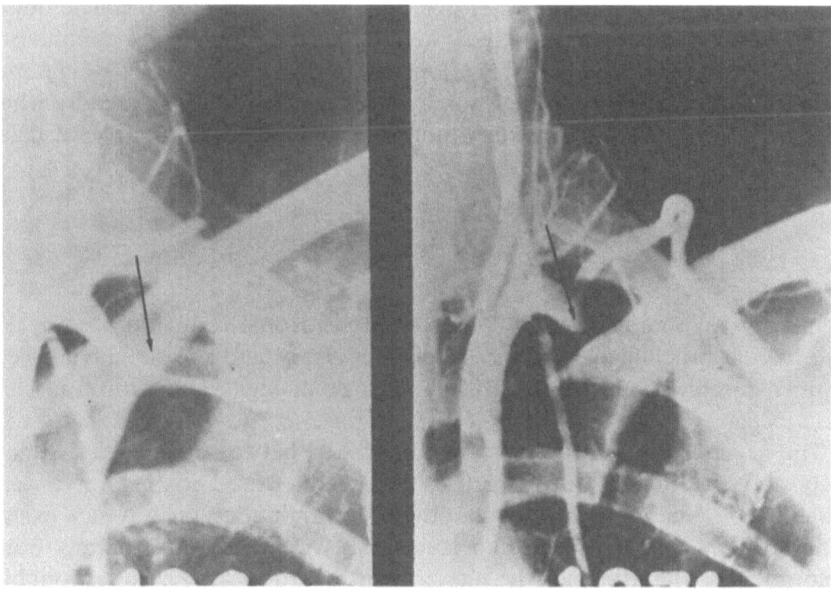

Figure 7. Costo-clavicular compression.

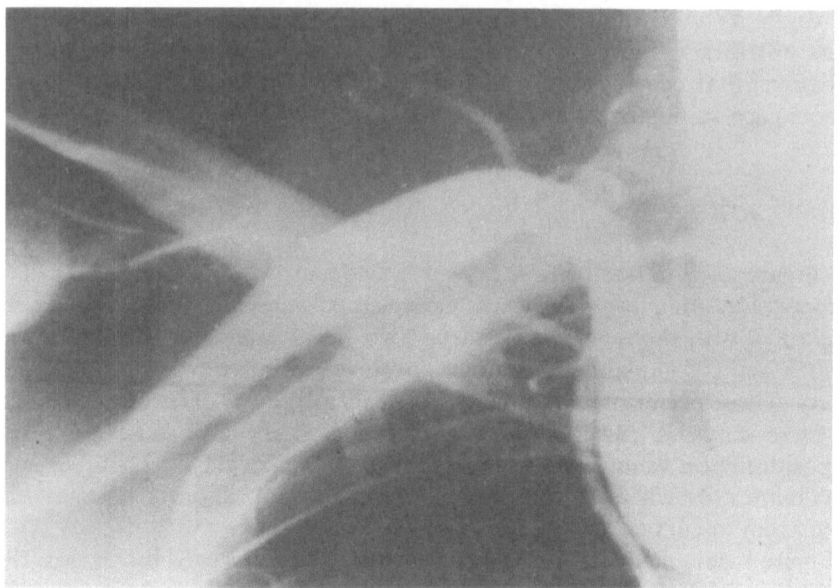

Figure 8. Aneurysm of the subclavian artery, caused by cervical rib compression.

Schroetter syndrome (Figure 9). Most of these vascular complications can be treated via the transaxillary approach.

We believe, in conclusion, that operative treatment in the thoracic outlet compression syndrome is also indicated in the case of moderate complaints. In our experience, the complications are not so rare as is sometimes thought. When they occur, the consequences can be serious, especially when they occur in a part of the artery, unfavourable for reconstructive vascular surgery.

SUMMARY

Symptoms in thoracic outlet compression syndrome result from compression of the brachial plexus, the subclavian artery and the subclavian vein or any combination of the three. The different signs and symptoms are described.

The neurovascular structures are compressed between the clavicle superiorly and the first rib posteriorly. Diagnosis is based mainly on a very careful case history, a thorough physical examination and X-ray examination of the upper thoracic aperture (to show cervical ribs or any bone deformities). The value of the classical provocation tests is questionable. Arteriography is not necessary, except when arterial complications have

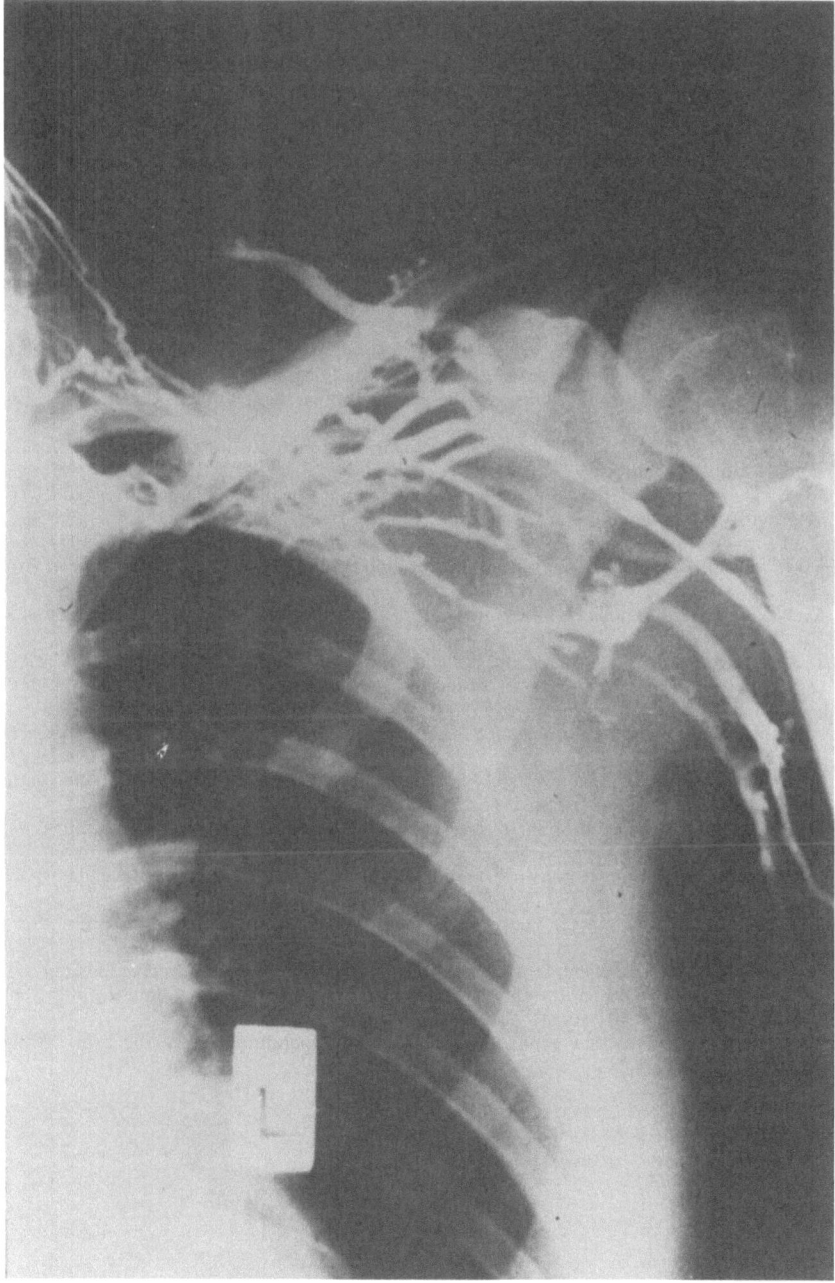

Figure 9. Thrombosis of the subclavian vein (Paget-von Schroetter syndrome).

already occurred. Therapy can be conservative or operative . The operative treatment of choice is the transaxillary first rib resection. Besides achieving the best cosmetic appearance it is possible via this approach to perform a thoracal sympathectomy or arterial reconstruction if necessary. Operative treatment is also indicated in the case of moderate complaints because of the risk of complications. These complications and their treatment are described.

REFERENCES

1. A.W. Adson, J.R. Coffey. Cervical rib: a method of anterior approach for relief of symptoms by division of the scalenus anticus. Ann. Surg. 85: 839, 1927
2. O.T. Clagett. Presidential Address: Research and Prosearch. J. Thorac. Cardiovasc. Surg. 44: 153, 1962.
3. T.R. de Bruin. Costoclavicular space enlargement; eight methods for relief of neurovascular compression. Int. Surg. 46: 340, 1966
4. M.A. Falconer, G. Weddell. Costoclavicular compression of the subclavian artery and vein: relation to the scalenus anticus syndrome. Lancet 2: 539, 1943
5. G.J.F. Lo-A-Njoe. Thoracic outlet compression syndrome. Thesis, Amsterdam 1974
6. R.M. Nelson, R.W. Davis. Thoracic outlet compression syndrome: collective review. Ann. Thor. Surg. 8: 437–451, 1969
7. G. Neuerer. Funktionelle Arteriographie bei "Thoracic outlet syndrome". Vasa, Band 6, hft. 3: 292–294, 1977
8. J. Raaf. Surgery for cervical rib and scalenus anticus syndrome. J.A.M.A. 157: 219, 1955
9. C.G. Rob, A. Standeven. Arterial occlusion complicating thoracic outlet compression syndrome. Brit. Med. Journ. 2: 709, 1958
10. J.B. Roberts. The surgical importance of cervical ribs to the general practitioner. J.A.M.A. 51: 1126, 1908
11. D.B. Roos. Transaxillary approach for first rib resection to relieve thoracic outlet syndrome. Ann. Surg. 163: 354, 1966
12. D.B. Roos. Experience with first rib resection for thoracic outlet syndrome. Ann. Surg. 173: 429, 1971
13. F.A.R. Stammers. Pain in the upperlimb from mechanisms in the costo-clavicular space. Lancet 1: 603, 1950
14. F.D. Telford, J.S.B. Stopford. The vascular complications of the cervical rib. Brit. J. Surg. 18: 559, 1937
15. F.M.R. Walsche, H. Jackson, R. Wyburn-Mason. On some pressure effects associated with cervical and with rudimentary and "normal" first ribs, and the factors entering into their causation. Brain 63: 141, 1944
16. I.S. Wright. Neurovascular syndrome produced by hyperabduction of the arms. Amer. Heart, J. 29: 1, 1945

17. New concepts in the etiology, diagnosis and surgical treatment of thoracic outlet syndrome

D. B. ROOS*

ABSTRACT

Four new concepts applied to Thoracic Outlet Syndrome (TOS) explain why certain patients are predisposed to develop symptoms, clarify the most appropriate tests for diagnosis, including the reasons positional variations of the radial pulse are of no value, and clearly explain the most effective surgical treatment for severe cases. The most valuable clinical tests for accurate diagnosis are presented in detail. The surgical treatment found to be most effective for relief is the transaxillary resection of the first rib and all anomalous muscle tissue encountered in the outlet. The anatomic advantages of this procedure, and a few technical points of special importance are discussed. Management of disease of the subclavian vein and artery, and important aspects of the postoperative care are included.

To understand thoracic outlet syndrome well, the physician must keep four basic concepts uppermost in mind. The first concept is that congenital anomalies in the thoracic outlet region cause some people to have an anatomic mechanical susceptability to develop symptoms of thoracic outlet syndrome under certain conditions.

The second important concept is that irritation or compression of the brachial plexus is the cause of symptoms in about 98% of the cases of TOS, unrelated to pressure on the subclavian artery. Symptoms arising from compression of the subclavian vein comprise only 1.5% total cases of TOS, and the subclavian artery is primarily involved in about 0.5% of all cases of outlet syndrome.

The third basic concept of TOS is that the compression of the subclavian artery does not contribute to symptoms of TOS, and therefore cannot be used logically to establish the diagnosis. The congenital anomalies, usually in the form of fibrous or muscular bands in the thoracic outlet, involve the brachial plexus primarily, and not the subclavian artery (3).

The fourth basic concept of TOS explains the most effective treatment for severe cases. As the basic cause of the symptoms is an anatomic abnormality irritating the brachial plexus, the offending structure must be removed mechanically in order to alleviate the plexus irritation causing the

*Associate clinical Professor of surgery, University of Colorado School of Medicine, Denver, Colorado, U.S.A.

J.M. Greep, H.A.J. Lemmens, D.B. Roos and H.C. Urschel (eds.).
Pain in shoulder and arm: an integrated view, 201–210. All rights reserved.

symptoms. Thus, the brachial plexus must be surgically decompressed, which presently is most effectively accomplished by removal of the first thoracic rib and all the anomalous tissue found in the thoracic outlet that may contribute to the symptoms (4, 5).

If physicians will apply these four basic concepts to patients they evaluate for neck, shoulder and arm complaints, many of the previous difficult and unexplained problems of thoracic outlet syndrome will become clear. The symptoms the patient describes in a detailed history will follow a recognizable pattern, the diagnostic tests on examination will become more appropriate and meaningful, and the management of the patient will be determined in a more logical and effective manner. If these four basic concepts are not applied, the patient with true thoracic outlet syndrome will continue to be misunderstood, misdiagnosed, and mismanaged, as they have been so frequently in the past.

SYMPTOMS

The main complaints of patients with thoracic outlet syndrome are pain, paraesthesias, and paresis. The pain is described as intermittent aching or sharp pain in the shoulder and neck, and radiating down the upper extremity. It may radiate in all directions from the focal point of brachial plexus irritation; posteriorly to the scapula, anteriorly to the infraclavicular pectoral region, medially up the side or back of the neck to the mastoid or occipital regions, and laterally down the arm. Although pain is the principle symptom that forces the patient to seek medical care, paraesthesias are usually present as well. They are felt either throughout the entire hand and upper extremity, or may be localized to a specific dermatome, most commonly the ulnar nerve area, and rarely in the radial nerve region. They are usually felt with the arm at rest, outstretched or elevated, and frequently are severe enough to awaken the patient from sleep. Paresis in the form of weakness and dyscoordination with early fatigueability of the limb is commonly present in moderate and advanced cases. Muscle atrophy is rare in the absence of a cervical rib, and limb paralysis is not seen in TOS. Headaches may frequently accompany these symptoms, and reflect referred pain from muscle tension in the paracervical muscle groups. They are occipital or hemicranial in location, may be so severe they incapacitate the patient, and are frequently refractory to medical treatment.

ONSET

Onset of symptoms may be spontaneous or post-traumatic, following a jerking type of injury to the neck, shoulder or upper extremity that results

Table 1. Neurologic symptoms of thoracic outlet syndrome.

Pain
    side of neck
    top, back and front of shoulder
    arm
Paraesthesias
    all fingers or 4 and 5 specifically
    whole arm "asleep" when elevated or in bed
Paresis
    decreased dexterity
    early limb fatigue
    weakness of arm and hand

in muscle spasm, such as cervical or shoulder sprain injury. The congenital bands are composed of muscle tissue and go into spasm as part of the regional muscle tension resulting from the sprain injury. It is the persistent muscle spasm from the injury that irritates the brachial plexus and makes the neurologic symptoms refractory to conservative treatment. In effect, trauma may make the anomalous muscle band so hard it acts functionally like a cervical rib, resulting in brachial *plexitis* as the roots of the plexus rub across the taut muscle band with head or shoulder movement. Immediately after injury, the patient may actually feel unhurt, but soon develops headache followed by neck and shoulder pain with regional muscle spasm. Only later, after the muscle spasm has caused continual irritation of the plexus, is the patient aware of the aching pain and tingling in the upper extremity. Typically, the headache, neck and shoulder pain may gradually improve with time, rest and therapy, but the brachial plexitis of the post-traumatic thoracic outlet syndrome may progress relentlessly. At operation, the anomalous muscle tissue is found frequently to be in the form of a sling from the anterior scalene to the middle scalene muscles, looping under the brachial plexus. If this muscle sling is consistantly contracted from chronic muscle spasm, it tugs the plexus upward, adding to the pressure on the nerve roots, and causing persistent discomfort to the patient in the neck and the distribution of the brachial plexus. Both the regional pain from irritation and tugging of the nerve roots by the anomalous muscle, and the emotional reaction resulting from the pain, lead to further reflex muscle tension, thereby establishing a self-perpetuating cycle that may be unresponsive to medication and physical therapy. Thus, the anomalous band may be the catalyst that perpetuates the nerve irritation (plexitis).

This sequence of events finally explains several consistent observations seen in patients with thoracic outlet syndrome. The symptoms of TOS are usually increased by an activity that causes neck or shoulder muscle contraction, such as raising the arm outward or overhead; lifting heavy objects; exposing the affected muscles to cold; vigorously exercising the neck and shoulder muscles; and emotional stress. Furthermore, it clearly explains the reasons why patients with moderate to severe outlet symptoms usually fail to respond to conservative treatment of all types, including TOS exercises, physical therapy, electrical nerve stimulators, and even acupuncture, as all these modalities fail to alter the underlying cause of the symptoms, namely the taut anomalous muscular bands found at operation (3).

DIAGNOSIS

Accurate diagnosis is of paramount importance to determine appropriate and effective treatment of thoracic outlet syndrome. This depends on a detailed history and an appropriate physical examination. All symptoms of the head, neck, shoulders, arms, hands and digits must be thoroughly evaluated to separate TOS from other considerations in the differential diagnosis, such as carpal tunnel, cervical disc and inflammatory shoulder syndromes. A complete history may take 30–45 minutes, and must be followed by a careful physical examination with appropriate tests to confirm the impression derived from the history. The physical examination must include complete evaluation of the neurologic, vascular and musculoskeletal status of the neck, shoulder and upper extremities. Careful examination of the individual muscle groups and sensory areas innervated by the ulnar, radial, and median nerves must be made in both upper extremities. Percussion and pressure tenderness of the brachial plexus, cervical and thoracic spine must be included.

The three tests that best evaluate carpal tunnel syndrome are: the Tinel percussion test over the median nerve at the wrist; the Phelan 60 second wrist flexion test, which is positive if the usual symptoms are reproduced; and the test for thenar muscle strength. The patient most certainly has carpal tunnel syndrome if any one of these tests is abnormal along with appropriate symptoms of median neuritis, as these tests will not be positive in a case of pure thoracic outlet syndrome. The carpal tunnel syndrome may coexist with thoracic outlet syndrome, however, making accurate diagnosis more difficult and challenging.

Tests to evaluate central root irritation include percussion of the cervical spine with localized pain at the sight of the root compression; tilted head test with and without cranial compression, which will cause radicular pain in the presence of root irritation; biceps and triceps reflexes; and individual muscle testing in the arm, wrist and hand. Remember, thoracic outlet syndrome affects the C8 and T1 roots most commonly, causing an ulnar neuropathy; carpal tunnel syndrome causes only pure median neuropathy; and a ruptured cervical disc most frequently occurs at the C4, 5 or C5, 6 level causing a radial neuropathy.

Table 2. Neurologic tests for thoracic outlet syndrome.

Weakness
    grip
    triceps muscle
    interosseous muscles
Pin-prick
    ulnar nerve area diminished
    radial and median nerve areas normal
Percussion tenderness
    supraclavicular fossa over plexus
    paracervical muscles
    trapezius muscle
Thumb pressure tenderness
    over brachial plexus
    reproduces usual pain and limb paraesthesias
Elevated arm stress test
    heaviness and fatigue of limb
    loss of hand coordination
    finger paraesthesias
    usual pain in trapezius and brachium
    drooping limb
    extremity drops to lap from distress before 3 minute test is completed

---

Of less importance are the tests that evaluate the vascular system of the upper extremities, as thoracic outlet syndrome rarely involves significant vascular compression or complications therefrom. Blood pressure and pulse volume in each upper extremity should be compared with the hands resting in the lap, as well as finger color, swelling, and nail bed abnormalities. The pulse changes or variations with the arm elevated or shoulders braced have been found to be of little or no significance, as the majority of normal symptom-free people may show such changes. Therefore, such tests must be considered a variation of normal.

As the symptoms of the neurologic, venous and arterial types of thoracic outlet syndrome are uniformly aggravated when the upper extremity is elevated, the most accurate test of TOS is reproduction of the patient's usual symptoms and complaints by the 3-minute timed elevated-arm-exercise test. The patient assumes the "stick-up" position with the elbows slightly braced backward, and then opens and closes his hands slowly for a full 3 minutes. A normal response is mere fatigue of the forearm flexor muscles, but an abnormal response is development of moderate to severe distress in the affected extremity, reproducing the patient's usual complaints (Figure 1). Fortunately, this test will detect the neurologic as well as the venous and arterial types of TOS, but it is generally negative in other conditions in the differential diagnosis of TOS. The old tests evaluating radial pulse changes in different elevated arm positions have been found to be totally inaccurate because they may be normal in patients with severe neurologic type of TOS, or abnormal in patients without symptoms. These

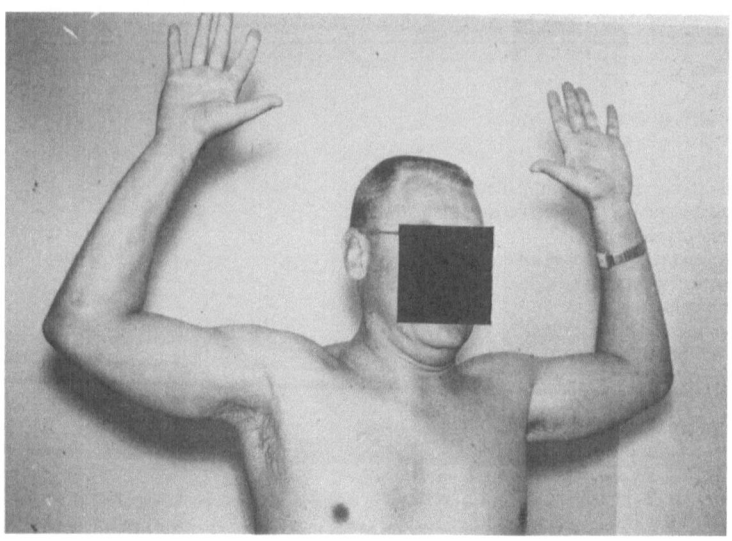

Figure 1. Photograph of patient in the "stick-up" position performing 3 minute elevated arm stress test for thoracic outlet syndrome. This is usually the most accurate test for TOS if the patient's usual symptoms are reproduced.

tests commonly lead to false conclusions and diagnoses, and ultimately incorrect and ineffective treatment of the patient. Wright found positional radial pulse diminution or occlusion in 92.6% of normal men who were symptom-free! (7, 6)

It is for the same reason that arteriography is of no benefit in the diagnosis of TOS in the majority of cases, and should never be used as a routine diagnostic measure. Arteriography is warranted only for specific indications detected on history and physical examination to evaluate possible subclavian aneurysm, plaque formation, or a source of peripheral emboli.

ANCILLARY TESTS

Cervical spine radiograms to evaluate bony anomalies, spondylosis and recent or old trauma are essential. Chest films should be evaluated routinely to avoid overlooking a superior sulcus tumor, rib anomalies, or pulmonary problems. Arteriograms are rarely necessary, as mentioned above. The neuroelectric studies (EMG and nerve conduction times) have generally proved disappointing for most of us, as the results are so variable and inconclusive that they are of little benefit in the diagnosis of thoracic outlet syndrome. Usually they are not worth the time, expense, and patient discomfort involved in obtaining inconclusive data. Also, I believe they are not beneficial in deciding which cases of TOS should be operated upon, as this is a clinical decision determined by the severity of the symptoms, the degree of incapacitation of the patient, or neurovascular complications, and not determined from a numerical print-out from a laboratory (1).

TREATMENT

After the clinical diagnosis of thoracic outlet syndrome has been carefully established by detailed history and the appropriate physical examination, treatment follows in a logical manner. If the symptoms are mild without significant distress or incapacitation, they may be readily controlled by the patient avoiding the activities known to aggravate the complaints. If aggravation is prevented, the symptoms may subside, or at least stabilize. The more the symptoms are aggravated in frequency and severity, the more likely they are to worsen. If the pressure and irritation of the brachial plexus becomes more severe and the patient develops pain that is difficult to tolerate, along with progressive weakness and dyscoordination of the hand, more aggressive treatment is required. Analgesics strong enough to keep the patient comfortable and allow adequate sleep, muscle relaxants, and light physical therapy, such as hot packs, mild exercise, massage, and ultra-sound or diathermy, may be required. Cervical traction should be avoided, as it is ineffective in TOS, and usually aggravates the pain by stretching tense cervical muscles. If these "conservative" measures control the symptoms well enough to allow the patient to lead a relatively normal life, remain productive in his job, get adequate sleep and avoid agonizing distress, they should be continued.

If the symptoms, however, do not respond to these "conservative" measures, and the patient is so miserable he sleeps poorly, has trouble at his job, or requires narcotic medication, or if he develops advanced complications of TOS, such as muscle atrophy, limb edema, or emboli, surgical relief should be offered. Currently, the most effective treatment for severe symptoms of thoracic outlet syndrome is surgical decompression of the brachial plexus by first rib, and congenital band resection (4, 5).

First rib resection offers four important benefits to the patient to help relieve TOS symptoms. First, removing the rib permanently relaxes the middle and anterior scalene muscles which are two of the cervical muscles most responsible for persistent muscle spasm, neck pain, headache and irritation of the brachial plexus. Second, removing the first rib destroys the costoclavicular scissor compressing the neurovascular bundle, especially prominent when the limb is elevated. Third, if the skeletal attachment of the anterior and middle scalene muscles is eliminated by rib resection, the muscles have nothing to reattach on to, so they retract and atrophy, leaving no functional deficit. This is of great importance, as it explains many of the failures of scalenotomy alone. On re-operation for scalenotomy failures, the anterior scalene muscle usually has been found to be reattached in its original position on the first rib by scar tissue. Fourth, the first rib resection offers clear and deep exposure of the anomalous tissue that may affect the neurovascular structures.

There are three technical points of particular importance for the surgeon performing first rib resection. First, the arm should be *gently* raised to afford adequate visual exposure for the surgeon, avoiding vigorous elevation. With the patient under general anaesthetic, it is easy for an assistant or for a brace device to pull the arm excessively, potentially causing a stretch injury of the brachial plexus. This must be evaluated carefully and avoided, and the arm should be lowered periodically during the operation to minimize this risk. Second, in dividing the muscle attachments to the first rib, the surgeon should leave the periosteum remaining *on the rib*, and not strip it off by performing a subperiosteal rib resection, as in other surgical procedures. Periosteum contains vigorous fibroblast and osteoblast cells that may reform bone and generate dense scar tissue. After the operation, when the arm is lowered, the brachial plexus lies across the bed of the old first rib. If the bed is covered by periosteal cells, the inferior trunk of the plexus may be caught in dense scar tissue, thus causing a severe nerve entrapment which may be a worse problem than the original outlet syndrome. Third, the posterior stump of the first rib should be resected or rongeured back almost to its attachment on the T1 transverse process of the vertebra to avoid leaving a posterior hook of rib. Such a hook, longer than 1 or 2 cms from the transverse process, may impinge on the lower roots of the plexus or entrap them in scar tissue formed from the tip of the rib stump.

Treatment of old thrombosis of the subclavian-axillary vein is not required if the symptoms are minimal. If significant chronic post-phlebitic syndrome of the limb results from such thrombosis, however, it can usually be relieved considerably merely by resecting the first thoracic rib. Apparently decompressing the thoracic outlet improves the collateral circulation from the arm so the previous edema and distress of the limb are alleviated.

Treatment of a fresh subclavian vein thrombosis seen within 7–10 days of onset may also be treated effectively by first rib resection after venogram confirmation that the thrombosis involves the subclavian vein. The results of this surgical approach are far better than the "conservative" treatment which leaves 65–80% of patients treated medically with a chronic post-phlebitic syndrome of the arm. I have used a more aggressive surgical approach in a few cases of fresh venous thrombosis with excellent results. This consisted of urgent first rib resection accompanied by venous thrombectomy, followed with low dose heparin. If a three day postoperative venogram shows reocclusion of the vein, which is to be expected as the intima has been damaged both by thrombosis and by surgery, then I have used a 3–4 day course of IV Thrombolysin to digest the freshly formed postoperative clot. After the enzyme treatment, the patient is kept on Coumadin for a few months. This treatment has resulted in normal venograms with asymptomatic limbs. It should not be attempted, however, without excellent surgical, radiologic and laboratory facilities available. Enzyme treatment alone has been disappointing as the etiology of the initial thrombosis remains unaltered.

Treatment of diseased subclavian artery is determined by the severity of the symptoms and selective arteriography. I have seen patients who had complete occlusion of the subclavian artery on such a gradual basis that the collateral circulation developed adequately so the patients had minimal symptoms not requiring surgical treatment. If arterial insufficiency is severe and debilitating, appropriate graft procedures may be indicated if the patient's general condition warrants an aggressive approach. If the arterial lesion lies on top of the first thoracic rib, I feel the rib should be resected through the axillary approach before a replacement graft or bypass is performed to minimize the chance of the same fate befalling the graft as the original artery. Thoracic sympathectomy may be a valuable adjunctive procedure at the same time as the first rib resection is performed. The technic of the combined first rib resection with thoracic sympathectomy is described in another paper of this meeting (5).

POSTOPERATIVE CARE

Immediately following transaxillary first rib resection or sympathectomy, no dressing, drains, slings or exercise are required. I use an absorbable suture subcuticular skin closure with a plastic spray dressing. The standard through-and-through external sutures may act as wicks to innoculate the subcutaneous tissue with axillary organisms, thus fostering wound infection. Gauze and tape dressings in the axilla are unpleasant and unnecessary.

I feel it is of paramount importance to instruct the patient carefully to keep the shoulder and brachium quiet for a month post-operatively to permit the surgical region to heal without undue motion and stress. The patient may use his hand immediately for light activities, and even bathe right away. He is permitted to raise the hand only to hair level, preferably with the elbow adducted against the trunk or raised anteriorly to minimize abduction of the brachium, which tightens the trapezius and other shoulder girdle muscles. If these muscles are strained, they may develop muscle spasm or cramp, which is painful, hard to treat and requires much more medication. I have been impressed that quiet shoulder convalescence may minimize recurrent symptoms postoperatively from scar tissue entrapment.

If physicians who may see thoracic outlet syndrome patients keep the basic new concepts of TOS in mind and take the time necessary to obtain a careful history and perform an appropriate physical examination, then follow the treatments outlined above, they will be able to offer their patients substantial relief of the previously poorly understood, inaccurately diagnosed, and ineffectively treated common medical problem of thoracic outlet syndrome.

REFERENCES

1. J.R. Daube. Nerve Conduction Studies in the Thoracic Outlet Syndrome, Neurology 25: 347, 1975
2. J. Raaf. Surgery for Cervical Rib and Scalenus Anticus Syndrome, JAMA 157: 219, 1955
3. D.B. Roos. Congenital Anomalies Associated with Thoracic Outlet Syndrome, Am. J. Surg. 132: 771, 1976
4. D.B. Roos. Experience with First Rib Resection for Thoracic Outlet Syndrome, Ann. Surg. 173: 429, 1971
5. D.B. Roos. Thoracic Sympathectomy. In Surgical Techniques Illustrated, Boston, Little, Brown & Co, Vol. 2, No. 3, 1977
6. N.L. Tillney, H.J.G. Griffiths, E.A. Edwards. Natural History of Major Venous Thrombosis of the Upper Extremity, Arch. Surg. 101: 792, 1970
7. I.S. Wright. The Neurovascular Syndrome Produced by Hyper-Abduction of the Arms, Am. Heart J. 157: 1, 1945

18. Diagnosis and management of arterial lesions in relation to the outlet compression syndrome

E. PARRY M.D.*

The incidence of neurovascular compression at the thoracic outlet is not known. If subclinical manifestations are included an incidence of about 35–40% is roughly accurate, with a sex ratio of four females to one male.

Neurological symptoms account for the vast majority of clinical presentations but, nevertheless, in a large proportion of these cases evidence of external compression on the subclavian artery and or vein can be demonstrated in the absence of significant vascular symptoms.

It is often extremely difficult to separate the neurological and vascular symptoms and decide which is predominant in a particular case. There is an overlap between neurological pain and ischaemic pain in the hand and forearm.

Rob and Standeven (1) introduced the term *thoracic outlet compression syndrome* describing a group of conditions often difficult to separate clinically.

Thoracic outlet compression syndrome includes:
Scalenus Anticus Syndrome
Cervical Rib
Costoclavicular Compression
Hyperabduction Syndrome
Pectoralis Minor Compression
Fractured Clavicle
Subclavian Vein Thrombosis
Intermittent Subclavian Vein Occlusion
C8. T1. Neurological Compression

Thoracic outlet compression syndrome simplifies the terminology, but does not simplify diagnosis or management. Clagett (2) in his Presidential Address to the American Society of Thoracic Surgeons in 1962, under the title Research and Prosearch, stressed the importance of the 1st Rib as the common denominator in all cases. He suggested that the logical treatment

*Broadgreen Hospital, Liverpool, England.

J.M. Greep, H.A.J. Lemmens, D.B. Roos and H.C. Urschel (eds.).
Pain in shoulder and arm: an integrated view, 211–215. All rights reserved.
Copyright © 1979 by Martinus Nijhoff Publishers, The Hague/Boston/London.

of the compression was not to tackle the difficult roof but to remove the floor i.e. the 1st rib as a safe and surer way of adequately decompressing the outlet.

The main anatomical factors causing compression are

1. Cervical Rib
2. Scalenus Anterior Muscle
3. Costo-Clavicular Space

External compression of the subclavian artery presents the following as two clinical groups:

I. Simple intermittent arterial compression produced by exercise and position of the arm.

II. Arterial compression with secondary arterial injury or disease.

In Group I. symptoms of ischaemic diffuse pain, numbness, fatigue, pallor, coolness aggravated by elevation of the arm, are common. Raynaud's Phenomenon in response to cold and exercise occurs and may be severe. It is doubtful if ulceration and gangrene occur in simple compression without intra-arterial disease.

Signs of arterial compression are absent when the patient is resting in the recumbent or sitting position. When the patient is sitting with the arm abducted and externally rotated 90° (AER 90°) the radial pulse may be weak or absent and bruits will be heard below the outer one-third of the clavicle. The blood pressure will fall as the arm is abducted and 20 mm Hg. is a significant change. These changes can be well shown using strain-gauge plethysmography. Exercising the hand in AER 90° is an important clinical test and pallor of the hand with fatigue of the arm occurs regularly with true compression.

In cases where the symptoms are severe enough to justify an operation, and the clinical signs confirm a degree of compression, an operation should not be planned without first having aortic arch studies carried out. Unsuspected stenoses of the brachio-cephalic, right subclavian artery or the origin of the left subclavian artery may be present, exaggerating the clinical picture and demanding different surgical management.

In Group II, secondary arterial disease is always present in the form of:

(a) Atheroma
(b) Thrombosis
(c) Fusiform or Aneurysmal Dilatation

These pathological changes can give rise to severe ischaemia to the point of gangrene of digitis or the hand, muscle infarction and intractable pain, and rarely cerebro-vascular accidents. The local stenosis or dilatation with thrombosis is, in these cases, the source of distal emboli.

The clinical picture may be dramatic with marked ischaemia of the forearm and hand, or may be transient from microemboli lodging in digital arteries. Recurring microemboli are likely, causing increasing damage to the digits with pain and/or gangrene. A microembolus may precede a larger embolus lodging in the brachial artery at its bifurcation. Although this may be compatible with a viable arm, the degree of morbidity will be high. Emergency surgery is indicated to explore the brachial bifurcation, remove the embolus and propagated thrombus from the brachial, the radial and ulnar arteries. The areteriotomy is closed with a vein patch.

CERVICAL RIB

The cervical rib needs special mention as the most important structure causing major arterial damage at the thoracic outlet. Many vascular surgeons insist that serious arterial lesions do not occur in the absence of a cervical rib and I would agree that this is true where fusiform dilatation, aneurysm formation and direct trauma to the arterial wall are concerned. Atheroma, stenosis and thrombus formation can, however, occur in the absence of a cervical rib and be associated with external compression by the scalenus anterior muscle or the costo-clavicular space. It is doubtful that the association is mere coincidence.

Complete cervical ribs are more likely to produce arterial lesions whereas incomplete ribs or fibrous bands cause neurological lesions affecting C8 and T1 roots.

Short (3) states that the point of attachment of the cervical rib to the first rib is important in deciding the type of arterial lesion. Cervical ribs are attached immediately behind or lateral to the insertion of the scalenus anterior muscle.

When the attachment is behind the scalenus anterior muscle the subclavian artery passes in one plane between the two structures and a fusiform aneurysm develops. When the cervical rib is attached lateral to the scalenus anterior muscle the subclavian becomes angulated at two points as it passes behind the scalenus anterior and then forward and laterally over the cervical rib. The angulation produces gross turbulence with weakening of the arterial wall and the formation of a true saccular aneurysm.

It is difficult to decide whether or not to advise excision of asymptomatic cervical ribs where turbulence in the form of a bruit can be demonstrated. The operation is not devoid of risk to the subclavian artery or brachial plexus in inexperienced hands. I do not believe that excision of these ribs is always necessary, but regular assessment at least annually should be carried out and the patient's family doctor alerted to possible early arterial change.

SURGICAL TREATMENT OF THORACIC OUTLET COMPRESSION

Clagett advised decompressing the outlet by removing the floor of the outlet i.e. the first rib. He advocated using a posterior approach as in a thoracop-

lasty to expose the upper ribs. This gives excellent exposure but is a major
and traumatic procedure. A similar and probably more effective method of
excising the 1st rib was described by Roos in 1968 using a transaxillary
route. This operation has made decompression in uncomplicated cases more
acceptable and gives excellent results.

Problems of outlet compression can be approached through the roof or
through the floor. My personal choice is, that where an operation is
necessary on the subclavian artery, vein, or on a cervical rib the incision
must be above the clavicle. Where the problem is that of simple intermittent
compression or pain the transaxillary excision of the 1st rib is eminently
satisfactory. I also use this route for carrying out cervico-dorsal sympathectomy for hyperhidrosis or pain in scleroderma, etc.

SUPRACLAVICULAR PROCEDURES

Exposure and decompression of the subclavian artery by scalenotomy is in
75–80% of cases inadequate. I have to add, however, that many scaleno-
tomies are incomplete because the medial tendinous fibres can be left
undivided.

The subclavian artery is the worst artery in the body to handle – its
friability is well known and terrifying. Clear exposure for absolute control is
necessary before arteriotomy or excision of a portion of the artery is
performed.

METHODS OF EXPOSURE

1. Claviculectomy
2. Dislocation sterno-clavicular joint
3. Division of the clavicle at the junction of the anterior and middle thirds
4. Supra and infra-clavicular incisions
5. Median sternotomy – partial or complete

Claviculectomy is unacceptably unsightly and unnecessary. Dislocation
of the sterno-clavicular joint does not sufficiently improve exposure at the
medial end. Dividing the clavicle between the outer and middle thirds gives
excellent exposure for dealing with post stenotic aneurysms, atheroma,
thrombus, trauma, involving the third part of the subclavian and first part
of the axillary artery. Excision of cervical ribs and partial resection of the
1st rib are similarly facilitated. Cervico-dorsal sympathectomy, if necessary,
can be carried out through the same exposure. Combined supra-clavicular
and infra-clavicular incisions allow good exposure of the brachial plexus,
subclavian artery and cervical ribs above the clavicle and below the clavicle

and are easily exposed after dividing the pectoral muscle by the combined exposure. The cervical rib and first rib can be removed at the same operation, together with any necessary procedures involving the subclavian artery or vein.

Partial or complete median sternotomy is the exposure of choice for lesions affecting the first part of the left subclavian artery and the brachio-cephalic artery.

REFERENCES

1. C.G. Rob, A. Standeven. Arterial occlusion complicating thoracic outlet compression syndrome Brit. Med. J. 2: 709, 1958
2. O.T. Clagett. Presidential Address: research and prosearch. J. Thorac. Cardiovasc. Surg. 44: 153, 1962
3. D. Short. Cervical Rib. European Journal of Cardio-Vascular Surgery, 1975

19. Costo-clavicular compression and dying digits

H.A.J. LEMMENS M.D.*

ABSTRACT

Narrowing of the cervico-axillary canal by costo-clavicular compression as well as by cervical ribs, is a potential danger for the circulation of hand and fingers, due to the possibility of microembolic showers. The lesser impairment of finger circulation, e.g. the occlusion of one digital artery, may give rise to ischaemic attacks or *asphyxia manus et digitorum*, which are to be distinguished from the Raynaud phenomenon. Progressive impairment of fingercirculation, the occlusion of both digital arteries gives rise to a ischaemic stage of the finger, the so-called digitus moriens or dying digit, which does not manifest itself in attacks, but in a permanent blueish painfull discoloration of one or more fingers and has likewise to be distinguished from the Raynaud phenomenon. On a series of 125 patients with costoclavicular compression and 15 with cervical ribs, the incidence of ischaemia of the fingers is discussed.

A costo-clavicular compression syndrome may give rise to microemboli which lodge peripherally in the smaller arteries such as the proper palmar digital arteries. The radial artery and the deep and superficial palmar arch can also become clogged due to microemboli. This induces an asphyctic condition of hand and fingers, the so called "asphyxia manus et dititorum." which is caused by a poor circulation (1,2). Collaterals, however, may guarantee sufficient circulation to avoid necrosis.

Asphyctic (ischaemic) attacks involving the fingers and hand may occur as a result of cold exposure and steal syndromes, provoked by use of the hand. These attacks can be clearly distinguished from Raynaud's phenomenon. They differ from Raynaud's phenomenon with respect to localization and natural course. They manifest themselves as a circumscript blanching of one or more fingers and are accompanied by ischaemic pain. These attacks are never symmetrical and colour changes are only temporary.

Increased activity of the hand in the presence of sufficient collateral circulation may elicit a steal syndrome causing pain in the non-affected digits. This applies especially to obstruction of the principal artery of the thumb. In this situation, the terminal artery of the superficial palmar arch, the so-called artery of Tandler, takes over the circulation of the thumb, in

*Surgical Department, Limburg University, Maastricht, The Netherlands.

J.M. Greep, H.A.J. Lemmens, D.B. Roos and H.C. Urschel (eds.).
Pain in shoulder and arm: an integrated view, 217–219. All rights reserved.
Copyright © 1979 by Martinus Nijhoff Publishers, The Hague/Boston/London.

this way withdrawing blood from the arch. Narrowing of the cervico-axillar canal may give rise to phenomena, which show much similarity with Raynaud's phenomenon, but which are still clearly distinguishable in that they are not symmetrical and show a different time course. This phenomenon disappears after removal of a cervical and/or first rib, as we could well observe.

Narrowing of the cervico-axillar canal caused by both a cervical rib and a first rib: the so-called double compression of the thoracic outlet is very dangerous for hand and finger. Even more dangerous is the recurrent cervical rib after incomplete removal of cervical rib and first rib. We have twice observed severe recurrent thromboses of radial and palmar arteries, within two years after insufficient removal of cervical and first thoracic ribs. A huge block of bone and callus formation was formed between remnants of both and severely narrowed the cervico-axillary canal, with serious compression of the subclavian artery and neural plexus. Removal of these blocks were difficult, but succesful. In a follow-up period of five years no recurrence of thrombosis and embolism were observed. Because of this condition and because of the possibility of double compression, in a case of

OPERATIONS

FOR

NARROWING OF THE CERVICO - AXILLARY CANAL

C.C.C.S.	Cervical Rib
First Rib Resections	C.R. Resections
170	21
45 bilateral	6 bilateral
80 unilateral	9 unilateral
125 patients	15 patients

ASPHYXIA MANUS ET DIGITORIUM

Hands	Hands
33 = > 19%	8 = 38%

Figure 1.

cervical rib we would advise removal of both, the cervical and the first thoracic rib.

Microemboli are a frequently occurring and serious consequence of all these conditions, and they may develop into a terminal stage of insufficient circulation of the finger: the digitus moriens or dying digit with occlusion of both digital arteries. The dying digit is a very painful, long lasting and sometimes permanent blueish, livid discolourization of one or more fingers, and can be distinguished from Raynaud's phenomenon and from asphyctic fingers in several respects. Dying digits do not occur bilaterally, nor do they present themselves in attacks. The dying digit is a progressive lesion and in case of an eventual recovery of the finger there is a clear regression. The dying digit is comparable with an infarction of the fingertips and heals by means of spontaneous or therapeutically induced collateralization, occasionally with residual necrosis of the fingertips. The fingertip becomes necrotic when the distal ends of both digital palmar arteries are and remain occluded, and when collateralization no longer occurs.

The dying digit is the end stage of any kind of progressive obstructive arterial disease in the area of the finger. Costo-clavicular compression and even more so compression by a cervical rib are the main causes for this condition with eventual loss of one or more fingers (3).

In a series of 125 patients who underwent 170 resections of the first rib, 33 instances of asphyxia of hand and fingers were observed and occlusion of digital arteries were angiografically assesed. In case of a cervical rib, the incidence of asphyxia (ischaemia) of hand and finger is even more frequent. In 21 resections of a cervical rib in 15 patients, asphyxia of hand and fingers was observed in 8 cases. Figure 1. In a total of 41 asphyctic hands, dying digits occured in 6.

In these cases removal of a cervical rib and a first rib has to be followed by a thoracic sympathectomy. Dying digits may then be transformed into asphyxia manus et digitorum. Complete healing may not be expected.

REFERENCES

1. J.M. Davis, D. Golinger. Cervical rib, subclavian artery aneurysm, axillary and cerebral emboli. Proc. Royal Society of Medicine 59: 1002, 1966
2. Thomas Lewis, G.W. Pickering. Observations upon maladies in which the blood supply to digits ceases intermittendly permanently. Clinical Science 1: 327–366, 1934
3. M.J. Raphael, Kh., Moazzez D.N. Offen. Vascular manifestations of thoracic outlet compression. Angiology 25: 237–247, 1974

Part IV

Treatment of pain in shoulder and arm

20. The treatment of shoulder pain

P. HIRSCHFELD M.D.*

ABSTRACT

The success of treatment of shoulder pain lies in a precise diagnosis. This is a clinical examination based on applied anatomy. This paper is adapted from the film "Pain at the shoulder and its treatment" as devised by Cyriax and describes some of the most common lesions and their treatment by local infiltration of steroid.

The shoulder joint enjoys more movement than any other joint in the body. Its functions therefore are manifold and many different lesions may occur. However, the tissues of the shoulder are amongst the most responsive to treatment in the whole body. Lesions which may have caused months or even years of disablement are, contrary to normal opinion, usually curable in one or two treatments, provided that an exact diagnosis is made. Unless the diagnosis is exactly made, the results from injections of steroids are disappointing, and patients may be treated for months or even years in vain. A knowledge of how to examine the shoulder is essential, and this examination is an exercise in applied anatomy.

ANATOMY

The small glenoid cavity covers only a third of the head of the humerus, the ligaments are weak and the stability therefore, is more dependent on the muscles and tendons surrounding the joint than elsewhere. This disproportion between the head and the glenoid cavity, together with the absence of bony engagement (except where the head of the humerus is roofed over by the acromion) leads to excessive rotatory and gliding movements. Such instability enhances to liability to strains. In addition the distance between the head of the humerus and the acromion becomes diminished during abduction of the arm. The soft tissues can therefore be pinched during abduction. The main muscles of the shoulder can be

*Department of clinical physiotherapy, Central Hostpial, Bremen, Germany.

J.M. Greep, H.A.J. Lemmens, D.B. Roos and H.C. Urschel (eds.).
Pain in shoulder and arm: an integrated view, 223–230. All rights reserved.
Copyright © 1979 by Martinus Nijhoff Publishers, The Hague/Boston/London.

grouped according to their function as follows.

Table 1. Shoulder muscle functions.

Function	Muscle
Abduction	Deltoid Supraspinatus
Adduction	Teres Major und Minor Latissimus Dorsi Pectoralis Major
Lateral rotation	Infraspinatus Teres Minor
Medial rotation	Subscapularis Latissimus Dorsi Pectoralis Major Teres Major

Stability is maintained during strong movements by the head of the humerus being pressed into the glenoid cavity. This is performed by the deep group of small muscles, which reinforce the capsule. These are subscapularis – inserted on the lesser tuberosity, supraspinatus – inserted anteriorly on the greater tuberosity, and infraspinatus – inserted superiorly on the greater tuberosity. Between these tendons and the acromion lies the subdeltoid bursa, which enables them to glide under the acromion on elevation of the arm. When a painful scar or calcification exists in a tendon at this area, painful pinching results, which leads to a painful arc. This is an important diagnostic sign.

Tears occur in tendons as a result of strain on degenerating tissue. The tendency to spontaneous cure in tendinitis is very slight. The reaction to injury leads to the formation of a painful scar or calcification, and movement between individual tendon fibres is impaired. In traumatic or rheumatoid lesions of the synovial membrane, the amount of synovial fluid increases and the synovial membrane becomes thickened. Movement becomes limited and adhesions finally form in the synovial folds. Much disablement results from soft tissue injuries of the shoulder, absence from work caused by these and other locomotor lesions amounting to millions of days. This is more invalidism than is caused by cardiac disease, influenza and cancer put together.

PAIN

It is interesting to note that all patients with painful shoulders point to a tender spot at the insertion of the deltoid and describe the pain as radiating down the arm to the radial side of the wrist. The reason is that pain is referred segmentally and all the structures about the shoulder are developed within the fifth cervical segment, except for the acromio-clavicular joint, which is derived from the fourth. How far the pain is referred depends on the severity of the lesion. For example, in slight arthritis or tendinitis, the pain is usually felt in the upper arm only, whereas the same lesion, should it become more intense, leads to radiation as far as the wrist. This extended reference is an error of perception occurring in the sensory cortex. A minor impulse stimulates a few cells in the appropriate part of the cerebral mosaic corresponding to the relevant dermatome; a major impulse stimulates a larger number of cells.

HISTORY

The history affords little assistance, since all lesions of the shoulder cause similar pains. However there are several questions whose answer possesses diagnostic importance, especially in deciding whether or not the pain is likely to arise from the shoulder region.

RADIOGRAPHY

A normal radiograph is not of much help as it reveals no abnormality even when clinical examination demonstrates a shoulder lesion to be present. It may also be misleading, showing areas of calcification of no diagnositc value for the presenting symptoms. Similarily, osteoarthrosis in the cervical spine is often mistakingly regarded as responsible for the shoulder pain. Arthrography may confirm certain lesions at the shoulder, but it should not replace the clinical examination.

CLINICAL EXAMINATION

The clinical examination, devised and elaborated by Cyriax, begins with a general survey to decide whether the pain arises from some other moving part or from tissues about the shoulder. To this end, the examination extends from the mid-neck to the hand, thus including all the segments from the fourth cervical to the first thoracic.

The 6 movements of the neck are examined for pain. Active scapular elevation tests the joints of the shoulder girdle.

Active elevation of the shoulder indicates range, muscle power and willingness.

Table 2.

Resisted elbow	flexion	C.5 and C.6	
	extension	C.7	
Resisted wrist	flexion	C.7	
	extension	C.6	
Resisted thumb	extension	C.8	
Resisted finger	IV/V adduction	Th. 1	

Once it is clear that the shoulder is at fault, it is examined in detail by twelve diagnostic movements:

1. Active elevation
2. Passive elevation
3. Search for painful arc
4. Passive abduction
5. Passive lateral rotation
6. Passive medial rotation
7. Resisted adduction
8. Resisted abduction
9. Resisted medial rotation
10. Resisted lateral rotation
11. Resisted extension of the elbow
12. Resisted extension of the elbow

Passive movement assesses range, and limitation and/or pain is noted. By abduction care must be taken to fix the lower angle of the scapula with the examiner's thumb. The normal range of abduction at the gleno-humeral joint is about 90°. The range of rotation, measuring from the position of the elbow by the patient's side and the forearm pointing straight forwards, is also 90°.

Resisted movements reveal pain or weakness in each muscle group. The examiner applies resistance sufficient to ensure a maximal contraction by the patient and at the same time ensures that no movement of the joint occurs.

The presence of a painful arc on active elevation of the shoulder (usually at approximately 80°–100°) indicates that a lesion is being pinched as the humerus tuberosity passes under the acromion. This is a very useful diagnostic sign, and is seen in supraspinatus tendinitis, infraspinatus tendinitis, in subscapular tendinitis (the upper part of the tendon passes under the coraco-acromial ligament) in subdeltoid bursitis and in affections of the inferior aspect of the acromio-clavicular joint.

The twelve diagnostic movements disclose a pattern of positive balanced by negative findings. In spite of the identical nature of the symptoms, the pattern identifying each lesion is different and characteristic.

A. *Limited range: capsular pattern*

Signs: Active arm elevation: painfully limited
          Passive movements: painfully limited in capsular pattern
          Resisted movements: strong and painless
Diagnosis: Arthritis
When the fibrous cuff about a joint is inflamed it is sensitive to stretch and examination reveals limitation of the passive range of movement and no pain or weakness when the muscles are tested. This limitation is in a characteristic manner and the pattern at the shoulder is: limitation of abduction, more limitation of lateral rotation and less limitation of medial rotation. CYBIAX has called this the "Capsular Pattern." Typical figures would be:
Abduction – 45° limitation
Lateral rotation – 75° limitation
Medial rotation – 15° limitation
The capsular pattern indicates that arthritis is present, and may be due to trauma, monarticular rheumatism or osteoarthrosis. Intraarticular injection of cortisone is particularly effective in traumatic and rheumatoid arthritis, the severe pain easing within the first twenty-four hours.
Technique of injection: The patient is positioned with his forearm against his abdomen. The operator identifies the posterior bony projection at the junction of the acromion and the spine of the scapula and injects at a spot 1 cm below this point aiming the needle at the corocoid process.

B. *Limited range: Non-capsular pattern*

1. Signs: Active arm elevation: painfully limited
            Passive movements: painfully limited in non-capsular pattern
            Resisted movements: strong and painless
Diagnosis: Acute subdeltoid bursitis
A common cause of limited range in the non-capsular pattern is acute subdeltoid bursitis. Sudden pain in the shoulder increases in intensity within a couple of days and spreads down as far as the hand. On examination, gross limitation of abduction is found, but, by careful movement, the range of rotation is nearly full. The bursa is tender on palpation. The pain is acute for about a week, and spontaneous cure takes from four to six weeks. Infiltration with steroid proves effective.

2. Signs: Active arm elevation: painful arc
             Passive movement: full and painless
             Resisted movements: strong and painless
Diagnosis: Chronic subdeltoid bursitis
This is a separate disorder, not the result of an acute bursitis that has failed to clear up. The outstanding sign is a painful arc accompanied by a full range of movement, with or without slight discomfort at extremes, and no pain on resisted movement. Local anaesthesia is induced diagnostically, and if the arc ceases the right part of the bursa has been reached. The anaesthesia is often of therapeutic value, but should it afford no lasting benefit, infiltration with steroid is substituted.

3. Signs: Active arm elevation: Full range
             Passive movements: Full range but painful at extreme
             Resisted movements: Strong and painless
Diagnosis: Acromio-Clavicular Strain.
The patient complains of pain felt at the point of the shoulder, a different localization from other shoulder lesions, as the acromio-clavicular joint is developed within the fourth cervical segment. Passive adduction of the arm across the front of the chest is often the most painful movement. Tenderness is usually found over the joint. One intra-articular injection of Volon A 10 brings lasting relief.

C. *Full range: One resisted movement painful*

In tendinitis, the joint is normal. Hence a full range of passive movement must be present. Occasionally, discomfort may be elicited at the extreme of range, by stretching or pinching

1. Signs: Active arm elevation: Full range with painful arc
             Passive movements: Full range
             Resisted movements: Abduction painful
Diagnosis: Supraspinatus Tendinitis
The painful arc indicates not only that the supraspinatus abductor is at fault, but also that the lesion must lie superficially at the junction of the tendon with the tuberosity. Infiltration with the steroid rapidly renders the patient painfree even if the symptoms have persisted many months.
Technique of injection: The patient sits upright with his forearm behind his back, bringing the arm into medial rotation. This bends the tendon

anteriorly as it passes to the great tuberosity making it palpable in front of the acromion. The affected part of the tendon is infiltrated.

2. Signs: Active arm elevation: Full range with painful arc
           Passive movements: Full range
           Resisted movements: Lateral rotation painful
Diagnosis: Infraspinatus Tendinitis
Resisted lateral rotation hurts. The other resisted movements do not hurt. The passive range is full. This shows the lateral rotator muscles of the shoulder to be at fault. In practice the lesion appears in the Infraspinatus tendon and not the Teres Minor. An arc shows that the lesion lies superficially at the teno-periosteal junction, and infiltration here with a crystal solution of steroid proves successful.

Technique of injection: The patient lies face downwards propped up on his elbows, his painful arm adducted and laterally rotated. This position brings the greater tuberosity outwards where it can be felt lying just behind the posterior edge of the acromion. The tendon is palpated and infiltrated with 1 ml steroid in a dozen adjacent spots to cover the lesion.

3. Signs: Active arm elevation: Full range with painful arc
           Passive movements: Full range
           Resisted movements: Medial rotation painful
Diagnosis: Subscapularis Tendinitis
Resisted medial rotation alone hurts. This indicates that the subscapularis is affected as the other medial rotators are also adductors. If a painful arc exists, the lesion lies at the uppermost part of the teno-periosteal junction. Treatment consists of one or two injections of 1 ml steroid.

Technique of injection: The patient lies face upwards, his hand resting on the front of his thigh. The bicipital groove is easily palpable and the lesser tuberosity can be felt medial to its upper end. The tendon is infiltrated at this point.

COMMENT

Local injection of steroid is most effective in the treatment of inflammation, provided it is introduced exactly in the affected area. Hence its success depends entirely on accurate diagnosis. The source must be precisely determined and adequately infiltrated.

Table 3. Analysis of 1100 cases of shoulder pain.

Pain	%
Tendinitis	52%
Bursitis	8.8%
Arthritis	27.2%
Acromio-clavicular joint	7.2%
Other pathology (Fractures, tumours)	4.8%

REFERENCES

1. J.H. Cyriax. Textbook of Orthopaedic Medicine Vol. I, 7th Ed. 1978
2. J.H. Cyriax. Textbook of Orthopaedic Medicine Vol. II, 9th Ed. 1977, Baillière Tindall, London
3. P.F. Hirschfeld. Der Schulterschmerz und seine Behandlung 2nd Ed. 1978, Schwarzeck Verlag, München

21. Prostheses and alternatives of shoulder and elbow joints

L. KINZL M.D., J. COLDEWEY M.D.
AND C. BURRI M.D.*

ABSTRACT

For different reasons there is only limited indication for the endoprosthetic treatment of the shoulder and the elbow joint at the present time.

Alternatives are resection, interposition plasty, and arthrodesis. These procedures have to be considered according to the demands of the individual cases. In the following two tables we point out schematically the treatment of choice for specific indications.

SHOULDER JOINT

In contrast to the intense discussion about alloarthroplasty of the lower extremity there has been relatively limited acceptance of the prosthetic replacement of the shoulder joint. But questions there are without any real indications.

Indications for endoprosthetic replacement

Tumors of the proximal humerus Semimalignant tumors are optimal indications for the shoulder prostheses. The same is true for isolated metastatic lesions or metastatic lesions with pathological fractures in the region of the proximal humerus.

In cases of malignant tumors, prostheses may be an alternative to disarticulation as long as the process has not infiltrated the surrounding soft tissue. If the tumor has already metastasized and amputation is too late to save the life, treatment with a prosthesis may again be indicated to preserve the arm.

Cases of benign tumors in which the joint surface has been preserved should be treated by removal of the tumor and filling of the defect with autogenous bone transplant, at least in younger patients.

Shoulder prostheses in primary chronic polyarthritis Involvement of the

*Center for Operative Medicine, University of Ulm, Germany.

J.M. Greep, H.A.J. Lemmens, D.B. Roos and H.C. Urschel (eds.).
Pain in shoulder and arm: an integrated view, 231–239. All rights reserved.
Copyright © 1979 by Martinus Nijhoff Publishers, The Hague/Boston/London.

shoulder joint in primary chronic polyarthritis is an indication for treatment with a prosthesis, if the patient has severe complaints, which cannot be controlled with medications.

Traumatic changes of the shoulder joint   In these cases all alternatives could be considered. Any decision for alloarthroplasty should be made with extreme care. This applies primarily to the proper timing of any surgical procedure for a damaged joint. No general guidelines are available for the time frame in which further improvement of the initial results after an acute injury may reasonably be expected. Not infrequently subjective and objective findings follow an undulating course. On the other hand, the final result of secondary procedures largely depends upon the basic conditions of the joint. If the shoulder is already stiff and the musculature atrophic, a less than good result must be expected with a prosthesis or a resection plasty, or even with shoulder arthrodesis.

Acute traumatic changes of the shoulder joint   Primarily, these injuries should not be treated with prostheses, but rather with early physical therapy. Prior conservative or surgical reconstruction of the joint may perhaps be attempted.

Types of prostheses

In general, two different categories of prostheses can be distinguished, simple head prostheses and total prostheses.

   The pivot point of a total prosthesis may be fixed or unfixed. In models with a fixed pivot point, head and socket are locked together with a lockring, which establishes a stable pivot point and prevents dislocation of the joint. These so-called "snap prostheses" have one advantage: Elevation of the arm does not depend upon adequate function of the rotator cuff. Normally, the rotator cuff counteracts the upward pull of the deltoid muscle during elevation and prevents superior subluxation of the humeral head. On the other hand, clinical experience has shown that these models may break or become loose because the neck of the prosthesis impinges upon the rim of the socket in the extremes of the range of motion. The functional results with "snap prostheses" are not significantly better than those with simple head or total prostheses. Apparently, a fixed pivot point does not solve the problem of mobility of artificial joints.

So far, the greatest clinical experience has been documented for the isoelastic prostheses (Figure 1). These models are preferred for several reasons:
– A wide range of different sizes of heads, different lengths of shafts, and

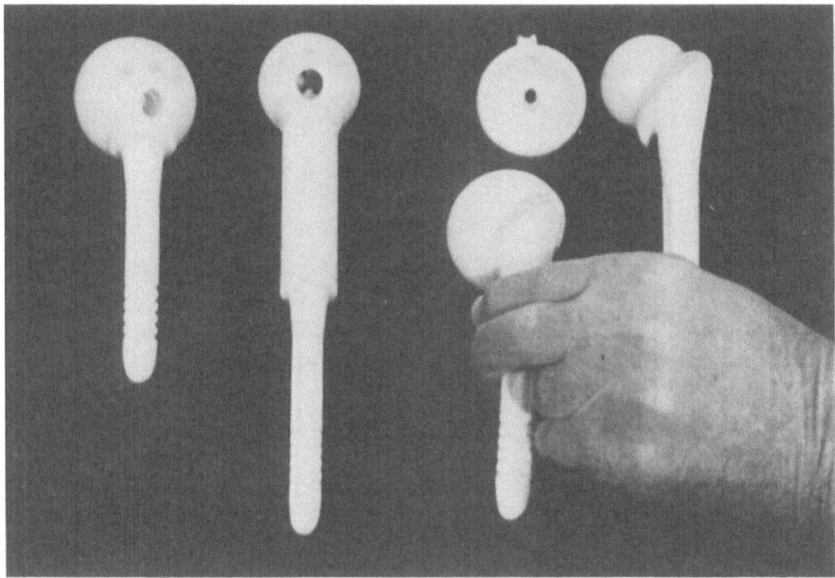

Figure 1. The different types of isoelastic shoulder prostheses from left to right: Head prosthesis, head shaft prosthesis, articular cap prosthesis and total prosthesis.

    different diameters of stems offers the proper implant for all the different individual problems.

- Fixation of the stem does not require bone cement. Numerous experiments and clinical observations confirm the implanted polyacetal resin is solidly incorporated into bone if provided with an appropriate surface contour.
- Special instruments are suitable for the particular needs of the operation. The surgical technique is relatively simple and to a large extent standardized.

Surgical technique

The surgical technique depends upon the type of prosthesis used. The isoelastic prosthesis (6), the model St. Georg (2), and the BME (BME stands for Biomechanic Eppendorf) (8), joint are implanted through an anterior approach. The Kölbel-Friedebold (5) prosthesis requires for example a posterior approach necessitated by its special fixation to the shoulder blade.

    It has not been established, if there are any advantages with respect to the postoperative mobility in using a lateral approach to the shoulder with osteotomy of the acromion when implanting a simple articular cap prosthesis. However, this approach is of interest. In cases, which only require

Table 1. Indication for the different reconstructive procedures of the shoulder joint.

		Prothesis	Osteo-synthesis	Resection-inter-position plasty	"Conservative	Arthrodesis
Severely comminuted fracture	young		+		(+)	
	old		(+)		+	
Dislocation fracture with extensive comminution	young		+		(+)	
	old	(+)	(+)		+	
Posttraumatic painful degenerative osteo-arthritis	young	+		+	(+)	
	old	+		(+)	(+)	+
Head necrosis		+			(+)	
Primary chronic poly-arthritis		+		(+)		
Tumor		+				
Infection				+		

Table 2. Indication for the different reconstructive procedures of the elbow joint.

	Prosthesis	Osteo-synthesis	Resection-inter-position plasty	Arthrodesis
Severely comminuted fracture		+		(+)
Posttraumatic painful degenerative osteo arthritis	young old		+	(+) +
Primary chronic poly-arthritis	+		(+)	
Tumor	(+)			
Infection			(+)	+

prosthetic replacement of the cap the lateral approach gives sufficient exposure, but leaves the rotator cuff more or less intact.

Reconstruction of the rotator cuff creates particular problems. In acute or old traumatic destruction, the insertions of these muscles are frequently avulsed with bone. The attached bone chips can be reattached to the humerus with screws or possibly directly to the shaft of the prosthesis, in case of an isoelastic prosthesis, for instance.

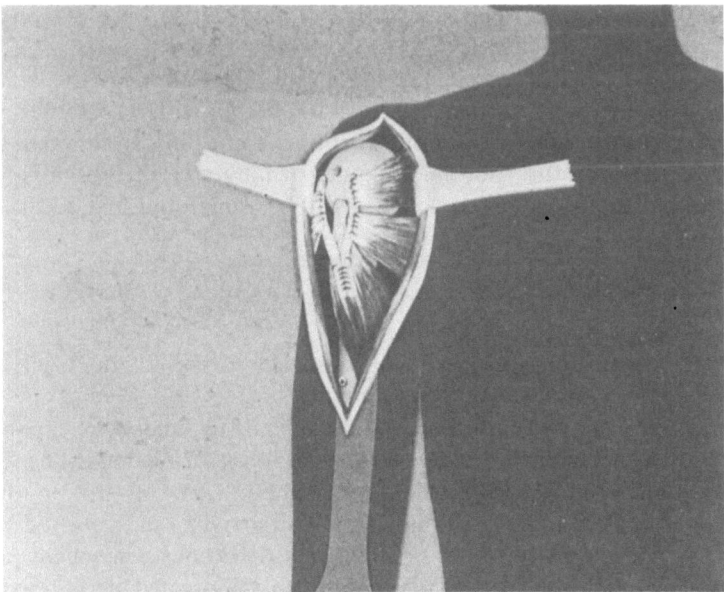

Figure 2. Attachment of the rotator insertions to the biceps tendon, which was split longitudinally, threaded through the holes of the prosthetic head and sutured to itself.

If the tubercles had to be removed it is possible to construct the tendo plate from the split tendon of the long head of the biceps for attachment of the rotators to the prosthesis (Figure 2).

Postoperative management

The postoperative treatment depends upon the condition of the rotator cuff. If the rotator cuff was not released, or if bony avulsion was repaired by stable osteosynthesis, the shoulder can be started on active assistive motion as soon as the acute postoperative pain has subsided, which is usually after the third or fourth day. Until this time the arm is immobilized in about 90°0 abduction on a pillow. If the rotator muscles were reinserted with tendon sutures, prolonged immobilization of the shoulder is necessary. This can be well accomplished with a foam rubber wedge of appropriate size. The wedge is fixed to the body with a light corset, securing the arm in abduction and allowing the patient to be out of bed and ambulate. After three weeks, the shoulder is started on free active range of motion in all directions.

Results

The subjective results are about equal for all the types of prostheses which are presented.

75 to 80% of the patients were satisfied, about 10% were disappointed with the result.

Also, objectively there were no significant differences in the achieved range of motion. Abduction is perhaps 10° better with prostheses which have a fixed pivot point. Limitation of motion is not only an inherent factor of the prostheses or the rotator cuff, but partially caused by scarring and contraction of the capsule and soft tissue. This functional loss seems to be surgically unavoidable.

Alternatives

The alternatives which still have to be considered within the spectrum of indications are pointed out in the following:
– Arthrodesis is a well established procedure and the functional capabilities have been confirmed in a large number of follow-up evaluations. Stable osteosynthesis further improved this method. Loss of motion due to surgical arthrodesis of the shoulder joint is partially compensated by the auxilliary joints and by the thoracic spine. Arthrodesis in severe painful degenerative arthritis of the shoulders is only indicated if the auxilliary joints and the opposite shoulder are free of any degenerative changes. In cases of isolated degenerative osteoarthritis of the shoulder joint, arth-

rodeses remains a worthwhile procedure, especially in patients who perform heavy physical labor (7). In paralysis of the shoulder musculature, this procedure is the treatment of choice.
- Sole resection of the humeral head proved to be a failure. However, in aggressive cases of infection, this procedure is occasionally inevitable.
- Resection-interposition plasties are quite successful in relieving pain. The mobility finally achieved is frequently equal to the mobility of a fibrous ankylosis. The stability of this type of joint plasty is questionable.

The most suitable technique appears to be Jäger's method (4) with reattachment of the articular cap of the humeral head. Then lyophilized strands of dural tissue are threaded through drill holes which are attached according to the method of Jones. If comminution of the head precludes the use of an articular cap, the surface of resection is covered with lyophilized homologous dural tissue.

ELBOW JOINT

For the endoprosthetic replacement of the elbow joint there are only a few indications:
- Primarily the elbow joint which was destroyed by polyarthritis, and secondly, posttraumatic conditions should be considered.
- Only rarely alloarthroplasty may be indicated for treatment of degenerative arthritis or of tumor disease.
- Posttraumatic and degenerative changes are also rarely indications because the disease is usually unilateral and the patient primarily uses the other extremity.

Types of prostheses

Different models of endoprostheses are available. We have personal experience only with the GSB (Gschwend-Scheier-Bähler) (3) elbow joint (Figure 3). It has the advantage of minimal resection of bone and allows revision with an interposition plasty in case of failure.

Failures are mainly due to a high number of loosening of the prosthetic shaft, especially in the area of the humerus. Gschwend (3) reported loosening within the first 18 months in 12 cases out of 39 treated with the GSB prosthesis. In spite of a positive rating of the postoperative results by 80 to 90% of the patients, the endoprosthetic treatment of the elbow joint has to be considered a failure in face of such a high rate of loosening and the long term poor mobility of the joint.

In the future the pure hinge prosthesis of the elbow joint has to be replaced with models which also replace the humero radial joint. In

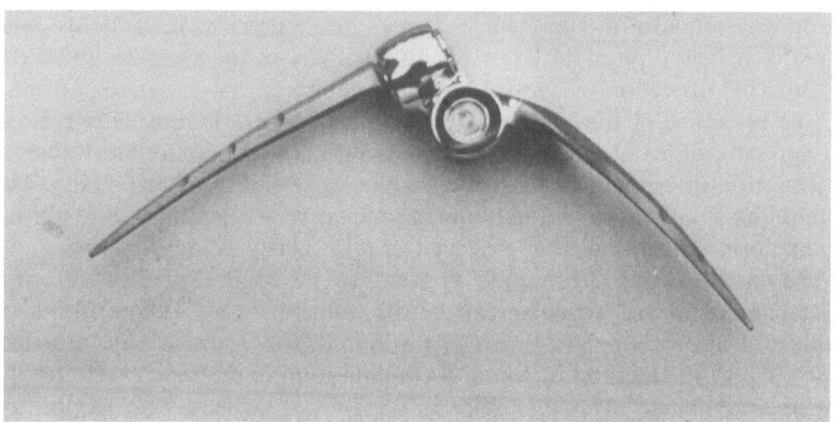

Figure 3. The GSB elbow joint.

addition the axis of the hinge should be fixed in order to absorb rotational forces. At the present time peaks of stress are transmitted to the fixation of the prosthetic shaft.

Alternatives to the endoprosthetic replacement

An indication for elbow joint plasty is found in 20 to 40 years old patients with adequate preservation of the musculature in whom severe intraarticular fractures of old non-specific infection resulted in ankylosis. Evaluation of the results after elbow plasty, often show a good strength and good mobility result. The operated patients are usually able to return to moderately strenous work and are able to engage in many sport activities. Loss of extension of 30° is usually of no great significance.

Indication for the arthrodesis is usually found in old patients with severe degenerative osteoarthritis after trauma or disease. The patient has already adapted to his disability, and arthrodesis results in permanent relieve of pain and avoids complicated plastic procedures. In addition arthrodesis is indicated in patients performing heavy manual labor, especially if great strength of the involved arm is of importance.

Arthrodeses of the elbow joint is further of benefit in a patient with paralysis of the elbow muscles or if degeneration of the elbow joint follows infection and requires resection of the subcartilaginous bone. Only the joint between humerus and ulna should be arthrodesed.

Pronation and supination should be preserved with resection of the radial head. We prefer arthrodesis of the humero-ulnar joint with help of an angled AO-Plate allowing compression of rather large cancellous bone surface. Approximation of surfaces as large as possible is felt to assure a lasting and stable arthrodesis.

REFERENCES

1. C. Burri. Isoelastische Schulterprothese (Film) Videothek 1974
2. C. Burri. Endoprostheses and Alternatives for the Arm. Hans Huber-Verlag, Bern 1977
3. G. Engelbrecht. Total Shoulder Replacement – Design St. Georg – Report. Scand. J. Traumatology 4, Suppl. 8, 1975
4. N. Gschwend. Die GSB-Ellenbogen-Endoprothese Arch.orthop.Unfall-Chir. 73: 316, 1972
5. M. Jäger. Resection – or Resection-Interposition Plastics of the Shoulde Joint. in: "Endoprostheses and Alternatives for the Arm". Huber-Verlag, Bern 1977
6. R. Kölbel et al. Shoulder Joint Replacement Kölbel – Friedebold Method. in: "Endoprostheses and Alternatives for the Arm". Huber-Verlag, Bern 1977
7. R. Mathys. Isoelastic Prostheses for the Shoulder Joint. in: "Endoprostheses and Alternatives for the Arm". Huber-Verlag, Bern 1977
8. M. Müller, M. Allgöwer, H. Willenegger. Manual der Osteosynthese Springer-Verlag, Berlin 1969
9. J. Zippel. Luxationssichere Schulterendoprothese Modell BMW. Z. Orthop. 113: 454, 1975

22. Sympathectomy for the upper extremities anatomy, indications and technics

D.B. ROOS M.D.*

ABSTRACT

Eight indications for surgical sympathectomy for the upper extremity are presented. The potential success of this procedure is easily evaluated preoperatively by the IV Tolazoline (Priscoline) test. Highlights of the surgical anatomy involved in sympathectomy, and the new technique of extrapleural thoracic sympathectomy through the axillary approach, are described. Important points of the postoperative care, and the advantages of this procedure, are included.

Sympathectomy for the upper extremity is not as commonly performed an operation currently as it was in former years. This change reflects the newer developments in vascular surgery for repair of major vessels injured by trauma or affected by obliterative disease rather than ineffectiveness of sympathectomy itself. Advances in medical treatment with newer drugs for control of vasospastic disease of the fingers also has reduced the need for upper extremity sympathectomy. As a result of these recent developments, the indications for thoracic sympathectomy have become fewer and more sharply defined.

Currently, there are eight potential indications for sympathectomy for the upper extremity. First is causalgia of the hands, consisting of medically uncontrolled burning pain with hypersensitivity to light touch of the hand that results from an injured, though not severed, nerve. Second is reflex sympathetic dystrophy, a syndrome closely associated with causalgia, consisting of pain, pallor, sweating, stiff joints and chronic edema of the hand. Both the reflex dystrophy and causalgia may be relieved by sympathectomy.

The third potential indication for sympathectomy is hand ischemia caused by arterial occlusion from disease or trauma that cannot be primarily repaired by arterial replacement or bypass graft procedures. The fourth indication is to augment or compliment an arterial repair. Some, though not all, vascular surgeons feel sympathectomy performed at the time of arterial graft increases the success rate of the primary graft procedure by dilating the peripheral arterial bed, resulting in greater flow across the new

*Associate clinical professor of surgery University of Colorado School of Medicine, Denver, Colorado, U.S.A.

J.M. Greep, H.A.J. Lemmens, D.B. Roos and H.C. Urschel (eds.).
Pain in shoulder and arm: an integrated view, 241–248. All rights reserved.
Copyright © 1979 by Martinus Nijhoff Publishers, The Hague/Boston/London.

graft and anastomoses. This might have some beneficial effect in preventing early graft failure from thrombosis, and also offers protection of the hand by increasing collateral flow if the graft should fail. A fifth indication might be severe and incapacitating vasospastic disease of the digits that has not responded to vigorous medical treatment in the absence of demonstrable collagen vascular disease. Many cases of vasospastic disease can be controlled adequately, if not cured, by medical treatment (11) (15). If collagen vascular disease is present in association with the vasospasm, surgical sympathectomy usually is doomed to failure. A sixth possible indication for surgical sympathectomy is medically uncontrollable pain of the extremity as a result of cold injury (frostbite). A seventh indication is medically refractory thromboangiitis obliterans. This apparent hypersensitivity vasculitis related to tobacco addiction is rarely seen anymore in the United States, but it is still found in other countries. The eighth possible indication for sympathectomy is disabling hyperhidrosis of the hands unresponsive to medical treatment (2).

The potential success of surgical sympathectomy may be tested in two relatively simple ways. The classic test is to perform a stellate ganglion block. This has two potential drawbacks. First, many fibers contributing to the sympathetic innervation of the upper extremity do not pass through the sympathetic ganglion itself, but arise from the second and third thoracic ganglia that may be unaffected by a block limited to the stellate ganglion. A Horner's syndrome does not necessarily indicate a complete sympathetic block of the upper extremity, as the sympathetic fibers to the eye arise from the inferior *cervical* ganglion which contributes little sympathetic innervation to the extremity itself. Second, often excessive quantities of local anesthetic are used to assure a complete block. An accurate stellate block should be performed with only 5–10 ml of 1% anesthetic solution. If greater than 10 ml is used for the block, the region may be flooded with so much local anesthetic that somatic nerve fibers of the brachial plexus may be blocked as well as the sympathetic fibers, thus giving a false impression of pain relief that may not be sympathetic in origin.

A more accurate and simpler test of the potential effect of surgical sympathectomy may be performed by intravenous injection in the opposite extremity of 1 ml (25 mg) of Tolazoline (Priscoline). After several minutes to allow full circulation of the drug, the patient is asked if he feels any relief of the burning pain and hypersensitivity of the hand, and if so, to estimate the approximate percentage of relief he feels from the injection. The result will reflect the final effect to be expected from surgical sympathectomy. If the patient feels less than 20% relief, then the surgical sympathectomy for pain relief would not be indicated, as the pain is probably mediated more through the somatic than the autonomic nervous system.

ANATOMY

The sympathetic outflow from the spinal cord generally accompanies the somatic distribution through the segmental nerves of the cord in the thoracic and lumbar levels, but this is not the case in the cervical spinal cord. In man, it has been shown that there is no sympathetic outflow from the anterior roots of the cervical spinal segments. The most superior sympathetic outflow usually begins at the T-1 spinal cord level, though in 10% of cases, there may be outflow from the C-8 level as well. The preganglionic sympathetic outflow from the spinal cord segments for the upper extremity usually arises from T-2 to as low as T-9, although again in 10% of cases, T-1 may contribute to arm innervation as well (6). Thus, for complete surgical denervation of the upper extremity, it seems wise to remove the first through the third thoracic sympathetic ganglia. This would include the nerve of Kuntz, which is a separate nerve arising from the second or third sympathetic ganglion and passing directly to the brachial plexus, bypassing the stellate ganglion (8). It is for this reason that simple stellatectomy may offer an incomplete sympathectomy for the extremity.

After surgical sympathectomy, return of apparent sympathetic vascular tone to the peripheral vessels may be a disappointing problem for the patient and the surgeon. In the past, this apparent return of sympathetic tone was attributed to "regeneration" of the sympathetic fibers themselves. Studies have shown, however, that there is no difference in regard to degeneration or regeneration between the somatic and the sympathetic nervous systems. Preganglionic fibers of the sympathetic nerves may re- generate after the rami communicantes are divided because their ganglion cells located in the anterior horn of the spinal cord, remain undisturbed. Sympathetic ganglion cells never regenerate, however, so if they are removed, the post ganglionic fibers degenerate as predicted. If the post ganglionic axis cyclinder is divided, Wallerian degeneration occurs just as in somatic nerve fibers, and new fibers will regenerate from the intact proximal ganglion cells. Goetz emphasized that the regenerated preganglionic fibers are chol- inergic, whereas the post ganglionic fibers are adrengeric. Therefore, the two different types of fibers cannot re-establish functional sympathetic neural pathways even if they should meet by chance.

Goetz (5), DeTakats (3), and Palumbo (9) each proved experimentally and clinically that cervicothoracic ganglionectomy will result in a permanent sympathectomy of the upper extremity if the procedure is performed adequately. The return of vascular muscle tone in the small vessels follow- ing surgical sympathectomy is not caused by return of sympathetic vasoc- onstrictor activity if the ganglionectomy has been complete. Although there is some difference of opinion between the authors regarding how many ganglia should be removed for "complete sympathectomy," most studies indicate that removing the first through the third, or possibly the fourth, thoracic ganglia results in as complete a sympathectomy of the upper extremity as can be obtained surgically (7). By removing the lower third of the variably shaped stellate ganglion, the first thoracic ganglion will usually be removed, but the inferior cervical ganglion will be spared, thus avoiding a Horner's syndrome of the eye (10). By removing the first three thoracic ganglia, the nerve of Kuntz will be included, so no significant sympathetic outflow to the upper extremity will bypass the interrupted chain.

TECHNIC

Over the years, several different surgical approaches for removal of the stellate ganglion or cervicothoracic ganglia have been described, and each has its strong advocates. Each has disadvantages, also. The supraclavicular approach (14) offers restricted exposure of the stellate ganglion, and no exposure of the second and third thoracic ganglia or Kuntz's nerve. The posterior paraspinous approach of Smithwick (13) involves resection of the intercostal nerves along with preganglionic fibers, but not the ganglia themselves; it offers poor exposure of the T-1 and T-4 ganglia; requires open meningotomy with some loss of spinal fluid and risk of infection; and frequently leaves a painful incision. It is performed in the prone position, thus making anesthetic or cardiovascular complications more frequent and difficult to manage.

The transthoracic approach, either anteriorly (4) or through the axilla (1), has become popular because it offers great exposure. It requires open thoracotomy with chest tube drainage, and frequently leaves a painful incision from vigorous rib spreading required for the surgeon to reach the ganglia through a small incision rather far from the sympathetic chain. The anterior transthoracic approach described by Goetz (5) and popularized by Palumbo (9) requires an incision through the pectoralis major muscle in the upper chest that is cosmetically unacceptable in women, and may be painful in men.

In 1971, this author described (12) a new extrapleural technic of approaching the stellate ganglion and thoracic sympathetic chain through the axilla after resecting the first rib. This technic affords excellent and safe exposure of the ganglia desired, requires no tube drainage, leaves a painless, inconspicuous axillary incision, and may be performed with so little postoperative morbidity that bilateral thoracic sympathectomy may be accomplished at the same time if strongly indicated. The technic of this new approach will be described, and detailed illustrations of the procedure were published recently (13).

The patient is intubated, then turned to the straight lateral position. The axilla, chest, and arm are washed with surgical soap, and draped for axillary exposure. The transverse incision is placed in the lower axilla below the hairline, in the axillomammary crease in women. An assistant elevates the elbow from the thorax, and at appropriate times, raises the arm and shoulder towards the ceiling preferably using a double wrist-lock on the patient's forearm to avoid a circumferential squeezing of the brachium. The incision should be approximately 12 cm in length in men, and 10 cm in women. The thoracoepigastric vein beneath the axillary fascia is tied and divided before dissecting the axillary tunnel to the thoracic outlet. The intercostal brachial nerve passing from the second interspace across the axillary tunnel to the arm should be preserved with accompanying fat and vein, if possible, to avoid stripping the nerve. Surgical trauma to this nerve usually causes postoperative numbness in its distribution, including the axilla and inner brachium to the elbow. The small supreme thoracic artery and vein pass from the first portion of the axillary vessels to the first intercostal space. To prevent bleeding and hematoma in the surgical field, they should be anticipated, carefully dissected, clamped, divided and tied before they are torn.

The rather tough cul-de-sac of fascia from the outer rib cage curving back to the axilla forms an anatomical barrier from the axilla to the thoracic outlet. This fascia may be tough in young people, but is thinner in older patients. It should be opened carefully by finger dissection from the sternum to the scapula, thus revealing the thoracic outlet just beyond. The subclavius muscle is carefully dissected from surrounding tissue just anterior to the subclavian vein at the costoclavicular junction. The taut yellowish ligament of the subclavius muscle is completely exposed and carefully divided under direct vision to avoid damage to the adjacent pulsating subclavian vein.

The anterior scalene muscle is then exposed by finger dissection circumferentially, hooked with a right-angled hemostat to separate it from the subclavian artery, and drawn laterally towards the axilla by the surgeon. The muscle is divided carefully at its insertion on top of the first rib, thus avoiding the phrenic nerve. By drawing the muscle laterally with the right-angled clamp, the subclavian artery is protected. The middle scalene muscle is then pushed off its attachment to the top of the first rib posteriorly with periosteal elevators. The periosteum, however, is not stripped or scraped off the bone of the rib as in a subperiosteal rib resection, but rather it is preserved intact on the bone and resected with the rib. It is important to remove all the periosteum so that no periosteal cells remain, as they may form dense scar tissue and entrap the brachial plexus which will lie across the bed of the former first rib postoperatively.

The intercostal muscle between the first and second ribs is then carefully stripped off the lateral edge of the first rib with elevators; then under the rib, the apex of the pleura is separated from the periosteum of the rib. If this is done carefully, the pleura will not be opened, and the periosteum will remain on the bone to be resected.

After the first rib is freed of all muscle attachments from the transverse process of the vertebra to the sternum, it is resected posteriorly, then anteriorly with angled rib shears, and removed. The remaining stumps of the first rib are shortened with rongeurs (Sauerbruch) leaving the posterior stump quite smooth, and only 1 cm in length from its attachment to the transverse process of the first thoracic vertebra. This length can be judged easily by finger palpation by the surgeon. No hook of remaining rib stump posteriorly should remain, as the brachial plexus may become attached to the end of such a stump, again by aggressive periosteal cells forming scar tissue. The anterior stump should be shortened to the costocartilage and left smooth so it will not tear the pleura or subclavian vein.

After the rib has been removed and the stumps shortened, the surgeon carefully strips the parietal pleura from the mediastinum by finger dissection. The upper lobe of the lung is gradually collapsed beneath his hand to second or third rib level. Finger palpation on the neck of the first rib medially will locate the large stellate ganglion that lies on the head and neck of the rib just resected. This will be found between the C-8 and T-1 roots of the brachial plexus posteriorly, and the subclavian artery anteriorly. After locating the stellate ganglion, the ganglion, and all the rami communicantes are carefully dissected from surrounding areolar tissue using long thoracic scissors. After the sympathetic chain is dissected free under direct vision beyond the third thoracic ganglion, the rami and the chain are divided sharply. The stellate ganglion is divided at its waist, which indicates the anatomic separation of the first thoracic ganglion inferiorly from the inferior cervical ganglion forming the superior half or two-thirds of the stellate ganglion. This should be done by sharp dissection with a scalpel or a very sharp scissor. No metal clips are ever applied to the ganglia, sympathetic chain or rami communicantes. The clips are totally unnecessary, and may contribute to postoperative sympathetic neuralgia by crushing afferent sympathetic nerve fibers that may stimulate sympathetic pain centrally. No bleeding ever results from dividing sympathetic nerves. If bleeding should occur, it is always from specific blood vessels, which should then be controlled with metal clips, but the clips should not be applied to the nerve tissue itself. Inferiorly, the sympathetic chain is sharply divided just below the third thoracic ganglion, which should be readily visible after careful dissection.

After removing the desired amount of sympathetic chain, the region is checked for hemastasis. The entire wound is then irrigated with sterile saline while the anesthesiologist inflates the lung to check for a possible rent in the pleura. If no pleural defect is detected, as evidenced by streaming bubbles through the saline, or a rapidly disappearing saline level as it flows into the thorax, the skin incision is closed.

If a tear in the pleura has occurred, the saline is aspirated quickly by suction to prevent all of it disappearing into the pleural cavity. The tear is then visualized, and an appropriate chest tube is placed over the second rib; the tip is passed through the rent in the pleura and part-way down alongside the mediastinum to evacuate the resulting pneumothorax postoperatively.

If no pneumothorax has occurred, the wound is filled the second time with sterile saline to the skin level as the shoulder is released by the assistant. The saline is used to fill the wound to displace the large air pocket that otherwise would remain and cause postoperative subcutaneous emphysema. By displacing most of the air in the wound with the saline, there is some fluid edema postoperatively, but only minimal subcutaneous emphysema. If a pneumothorax occurred and a chest tube is required, no saline should be instilled, as it would merely run into the pleural cavity and cause painful pleuritis postoperatively. All the remaining air will be evacuated by the chest tube anyway, so the saline displacement of the air is unnecessary.

Closure of the incision merely requires a continuous suture line to the subcutaneous fascia of the axilla, followed by a continuous absorbable subcuticular suture to close the skin surface. I avoid external through-and-through sutures in this incision, as the external sutures may act as wicks and innoculate the subcutaneous tissue with axillary organisms from the skin surface. If no chest tube is required, a plastic spray dressing is all that is necessary for the incision, thus avoiding unpleasant gauze and tape in the axilla.

If a bilateral thoracic sympathectomy is indicated, the patient is then turned on his back after skin closure, the intravenous and blood pressure cuff are changed to the arm on the side just operated upon, and the patient is turned to the lateral position on that side. The opposite axilla is then washed with surgical soap, draped for axillary exposure and the identical operation is repeated on the second side. Even if a pneumothorax has occurred on the first side operated upon, the second side may still be done safely if a proper chest tube has been inserted and attached to underwater seal drainage at the time of the original wound closure. Operative pneumothorax with this procedure is not dangerous if it is recognized prior to closure and treated properly with chest tube drainage, even if it should occur bilaterally.

Postoperatively, the patient is allowed to keep his arms in his lap, the position of most comfort, and exercise of the arms and shoulders is forbidden for one month. The patient may use his hands immediately as long as his elbows are kept adducted to the thorax to prevent much shoulder motion. It has been found that patients who move their shoulders much after first rib resection develop a lot more pain and muscle cramp than patients who keep the shoulders quiet for one month during convalescence. Quiet shoulder convalescence may reduce scar tissue formation, also.

The patient is allowed out of bed to the bathroom the night of operation, and is on a full diet the following morning. He may be discharged from the hospital in a few days when he is afebrile and feeling comfortable on oral pain medication.

With this technic of transaxillary extrapleural thoracic sympathectomy, the patients recover rapidly with less discomfort and morbidity than the older types of sympathectomy; complications are fewer; often hospitalization is shorter; the procedure may be performed bilaterally with minimum morbidity; and the results are as good as any other sympathectomy procedure, and, of course, better than stellatectomy alone. Using this technic over the past seven years, I have had no complications, failures, postoperative pain problems, or permanent Horner's syndrome from the procedure itself.

REFERENCES

1. H.J.B. Atkins. Sympathectomy by the Axillary Approach. Lancet 1: 538, 1954
2. S.I.Cullen. Management of Hyperhidrosis. Post Grad. Med. 52: 77, 1972
3. G. DeTakats. Analysis of Results Following Sympathectomy for Peripheral Vascular Disease. Am. J. Surg. 47: 78, 1940
4. T.P. Garry, A.K. Henry. Anterior Transcostal Access to Upper Parts of the Sympathetic Chain. Irish J. Med. Sci. P. 757, 1949
5. R.H. Goetz, J.A.S. Marr. The Importance of the Second Thoracic Ganglion for the Sympathetic Supply of the Upper Extremities with a Description of Two New Approaches for its Removal. Clin. Proc. (Capetown) 3: 102, 1944
6. R.H. Goetz. Sympathectomy for the Upper Extremities. Chpt 25, pg. 437 in Dale, W.A.: Management of Arterial Occlusive Disease. Year Book Medical Publishers, Inc., Chicago, 1971
7. H.A. Haxton. The Sympathetic Nerve Supply of the Upper Limb in Relation to Sympathectomy. Ann. Roy. Coll. Surg. 14: 247, 1954
8. A. Kuntz. Distribution of the Sympathetique Rami to the Brachial Plexus. Arch. Surg. 15: 871, 1927
9. L.T. Palumbo. Anterior Transthoracic Approach for Upper Thoracic Sympathectomy. Arch. Surg. 72: 659, 1956
10. L.T. Palumbo. Upper Dorsal Sympathectomy Without Horner's Syndrome. Arch. Surg. 71: 743, 1955
11. J.M. Porter, R.L. Snider, E.J. Bardana. The Diagnosis and Treatment of Raynaud's Phenomenon. Surg. 77: 11, 1975
12. D.B. Roos. Experience with First Rib Resection for Thoracic Outlet Syndrome. Ann. Surg. 173: 429, 1971
13. D.B. Roos. Transaxillary Extrapleural Thoracic Sympathectomy. Surg. Techniques Illus. Vol. 2, No. 3: 3, 1977
14. R.H. Smithwick. The Rationale and Technic of Sympathectomy for Relief of Vascular Spasm of the Extremities. New England J. Med. 22: 699, 1940
15. E.D. Telford. The Technic of Sympathectomy. Brit. J. Surg. 23: 448, 1935
16. J.T. Willerson, J.L. Decker. Raynaud's Disease and Phenomenon; A Medical Approach. Am. Heart J. 82: 572, 1971

23. Thoracodorsal sympathectomy en bloc

H.A.J. LEMMENS M.D.*

ABSTRACT

Although the numbers admittedly are still small, it is becoming evident that there is a difference between thoracic sympathectomy and thoracodorsal sympathectomy en bloc, both subjectively and objectively as demonstrated with Doppler flow-measurements and that it is necessary to resect the nerve of Kuntz.
   The best indications for the "en bloc resection" are:
-- in the first place, Raynaud's phenomenon sine scleroderma
-- secondly Sudeck's atrophy
- and finally the asphyctic finger and dying digit.
The final result however depends on the course and progression of the underlying disease.

INTRODUCTION

Results following lumbar sympathectomy for vasospastic diseases of the lower limbs, are generally satisfactory. This does not apply to sympathectomy performed for the same condition in the upper extremities. Many reports (1, 2) document recurrent sympathetic tone in a high percentage of patients treated with thoracic sympathectomy.

   The explanation for this phenomenon has to be found in the difficulty of achieving complete sympathectomy (1). Sprouting and regeneration of sympathetic fibres are thought to build up alternative pathways for the sympathetic impulse. This does not explain however, why regeneration occurs in thoracic sympathetic fibres but not in the lumbar sympathetic chain. The answer to this question may well be found in the specific anatomical differences between the thoracic and lumbar sympathetic chain, as described by A. Kuntz (5).

The success of treatment of the ischaemic hand-syndromes is dependent on the progression of the underlying disease. When an asphyctic hand is caused by arterio-sclerosis of the subclavian artery with a parietal throm-

---

*Surgical Department, Limburg University, Maastricht, The Netherlands.

J.M. Greep, H.A.J. Lemmens, D.B. Roos and H.C. Urschel (eds.).
Pain in shoulder and arm: an integrated view, 249–254. All rights reserved.
Copyright © 1979 by Martinus Nijhoff Publishers, The Hague/Boston/London.

bosis causing a shower of emboli in the small finger arteries, not only a bypass is needed to correct the steal syndrome, but also endarterectomy should be performed, and anticoagulants should be administered postoperatively to prevent recurrence of the thrombosis and consequent emboli.

When a costo-clavicular compression syndrome or a cervical rib is the cause of emboli, the cervical-axillar canal should be widened to prevent progression of the ischaemic hand-syndrome. In many cases however – therapy of the underlying disease is impossible. for instance Burger's disease, scleroderma involving the vasculature of the hand, gaint – cell angrites a.o. – therapy of the underlying disease is impossible.

Occasionally, the origin of ischaemic hand-syndromes is traumatic or functional, like "vasospastic diseases". Therefore, it is undeniable that the cause of the ischaemic hand-syndromes is of two sorts. Either the syndrome is a sequel of a systemic disease or it is a clinical nosological entity involving the hand itself. Consequently, a dual intention should be attributed to sympathectomy. In the first place, sympathectomy may achieve an additional effect during treatment of the underlying disease. For instance sympathectomy may be performed in addition to resection of the first rib in a case of costoclavicular compression causing an asphyctic hand. Another example would be adding a sympathectomy in the operative treatment of arteriosclerosis in the subclavian or axillary artery. In the second phase however, sympathectomy may constitute independent therapy.

It has become evident however, that the therapeutic effect of a thoracic sympathectomy, although very dramatic in the immediate post-operative period, is often very short-lived or incomplete (1, 3). The cause of this failure is not to be found in technical errors, but lies in the anatomy of the sympathetic nervous system supplying the upper limb. It is well known that it is not the stellate ganglion but the thoracic sympathetic ganglia No. II and III which take care of the sympathetic innervation of the hand (4, 6). The thoracic, spinal segments however provide additional preganglionar, sympathetic fibres which contribute to the sympathetic innervation of the hand and which do not always follow their course peripherally along the dorsal sympathetic chain (7).

In 1927, Alexander Kuntz described the intrathoracic nerve, a network of fine nerve fibres, that contributes significantly to the sympathetic innervation of the upper limb. This intrathoracic nerve of Kuntz is composed of several grey communicating branches. The grey communicating branches of the lower thoracic ganglia very often divide into bipartite grey communicating branches and do not follow the dorsal sympathetic chain, but bypass the thoracic sympathetic ganglia II and III, and the stellate ganglion, along spinal branches of the intercostal nerves, to supply from there the sympathetic innervation of the peripheral vasculature of the hand. This fine network of sympathetic fibres is not adequately resected in most forms of transthoracic sympathectomy and therefore is responsible for residual or recurrent sympathetic tone in the peripheral vasculature.

Any form of transthoracic sympathectomy is very often sufficient to achieve an initial beneficial effect in ischaemic hand-syndromes, but in many instances the decline of the sympathectomy effect, a decline that is always present after about a year in every form of sympathectomy, may be disastrous for the hand, when it arrives too early! To achieve a more complete and longer standing sympathectomy effect, it is necessary to resect the nerve of Kuntz. To fulfil this requirement we introduced in our hospital the "thoracodorsal sympathectomy en bloc" (Figure 1).

In this operation, a costo-transversectomy is performed through a small paravertebral incision over the second and the third rib. This approach gives easy access to the thoracic sympathetic ganglia Nos. II and III.

After meticulous dissection, the following anatomical structures are identified:

1. the intercostal nerves no. 2 and 3 over a distance of 3 cm.
2. the dorsal roots of thoracic 2 and 3 together with their spinal ganglia and the sympathetic ganglia thoracic 2 and 3.
3. an en block resection is then performed of:
- the 2nd and 3rd intercostal nerves over a distance of 3 cm.
- the dorsal roots and spinal ganglia of thoracal segments 2 and 3.
- the ventral roots of thoracal 2 and 3 and
- the sympathetic ganglia of thoracal 2 and 3 with or without resection of the lower pole of thoracal 1.
- in addition all tissue in the area of dissection between thoracal 4 and 1, comprising all intercostal musculature and all branches of the intercostal nerves.

In this way, the intrathoracic nerve of Kuntz is inevitably interrupted and the excision of the structures mentioned confines itself to the level of ganglion 2 and 3 only. This results not only in removal of all sympathetic

```
resection of :

1. ggl.sympath.th.II + III
2. intercost.nerv.II + III
3. radix post.th.II + III with ggl.spin.II + III
4. radix ant. th.II + III
5. all the tissue between int.cost.nerv.II + III
```

Figure 1. Thoraco-dorsal sympathectomy en bloc.

fibres in the grey bipartite communicating branches, but also in intersection of the so called "antidromic patchways". The significance of these antidromic pathways is difficult to understand, however their influence on vasodilatation is showed by Burn, Folkow and Uvnäs (2, 5, 8). We have the impression that the interruption of these fibres influences the increased irritability of the Raynaud hand.

Although entailing the disadvantage of the costotrans-versectomy, the operation comprises a complete sympathectomy of the hand. Compared with the transthoracic or cervical approach, it has the advantage that a Horner Syndrome was rare and, in 49 thoracodorsal sympathectomies en bloc, the phrenic nerve and thoracic duct were never severed. The disadvantages are the prone position during the operation, the paravertebral scar and the sometimes longlasting post-operative wound pain. The cardinal question however is: "Is there a difference between the results of the thoracic sympathectomy and the thoracodorsal sympathectomy en bloc?"

It is hard to answer this question, even more so because the results are

DOPPLER   L.   RAD.   ART.

M. Bürger
occl.L.uln.art.

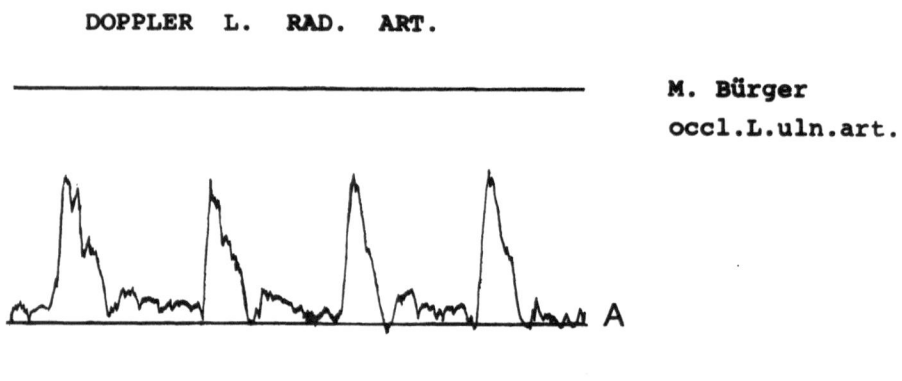

DOPPLER   R.   ULN.   ART.

M.Bürger
occl.R.rad.art.

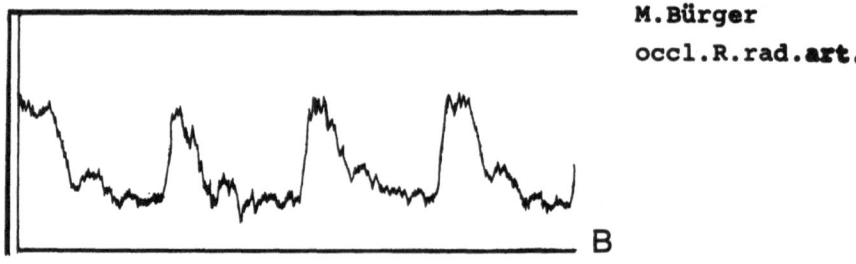

Figure 2 A Cervical sympathectomy glg. stell. + TH I-II-III.
B. Thoraco-dorsal sympathectomy en bloc TH II + III.

very much dependent on the progression of the underlying disease. In order to show a difference or even to prove that the sympathectomy en bloc gives other results, we need either a comparison between left and right sided treatment in the same patient, or an experiment. This experiment might be done clinically, when a patient initially received a thoracic sympathectomy with an unsatisfying result, later followed by completion of the thoracic sympathectomy by excision of Kuntz' nerve and the spinal ganglia, as described. Ensuing subjective and objective improvement might provide the proof that we seek.

A comparison between left and right was made twice. Objective improvement was demonstrated with Doppler flow measurements. An example is shown on Figure 2. On the left side, a cervical thoracic sympathectomy was performed, removing the stellate ganglion and thoracal 2, 3 and 4.
Post-operatively, the patient showed a Horner Syndrome, signs of a phrenic nerve lesion and a lesion of the thoracic duct. Three months later, the Doppler flow curve still showed considerable spasm of the left radial artery. The flow velocity is high, partly due to an obstructed ulnar artery. In diastole, however, flow drops to zero, which demonstrates a real periferal resistance. On the right side, a thoracodorsal sympathectomy en bloc was performed on level thoracal II and III only. Six months post-operatively a Doppler flow curve was performed showing the right ulnar artery. The flow velocity is high, higher than pre-operatively and in diastole, a continuing and even improved flow is demonstrated. Clinically, the patient experienced a better result in the right hand than in the left hand.

The experiment of the "completing procedure" was carried out six times. In all instances, the spinal ganglia, the ventral roots and Kuntz's nerve were resected after a thoracic sympathectomy was carried out in an earlier stage. In all six patients an intensified sympathectomy-effect could be demon-

	subj.improv.	obj.improv.
6 hands	6	6
M.Buerger	1	1
R.Ph.	2	2
Südeck Atr.	1	1
Asphyxia dig.	2	2

Figure 3. Excision N. Kuntz after thor. sympathectomy.

strated (Figure 3). The effect of the thoracodorsal sympathectomy was especially striking in Raynaud's phenomenon sine scleroderma, and in Sudeck's atrophy.

REFERENCES

1. R.M. Baddeley. The place of upper dorsal sympathectomy in the treatment of primary Raynaud's disease. Brit. J. Surgery 52: 426, 1965
2. J.H. Burn. Sympathetic vasodilator fibres. Phys. Rev. 18: 137, 1938
3. D.A. Felder, F.A. Simeone, R.R. Linton, C.E. Welch. Surgery 26: 1014, 1949
4. H. Foersters. Verhandl. Dtsch. Ges. Inn. Med. 253, 1939
5. B. Folkow. The nervous control of bloodvessels. In: The control of the circulation of the blood. Ed. by R.J.S. McDowall. London, Dawson, 1956.
6. R.H. Goetz, J.A.S. Marr. The importance of the second thoracic ganglion for the sympathetic supply of the upper extremities. Clin. Proc. 3: 102, 1944
7. A. Kuntz. Distribution of the sympathetic rami to the brachial plexus. Arch. Surg. 15: 871, 1927
8. B. Uvnäs. Sympathetic vasodilator outflow. Physiol. Rev. 34: 608, 1954

24. Complete reconstruction of the subclavian vein following thrombotic occlusion at the costo-clavicular level

M.A. BEAUJEAN M.D.*

ABSTRACT

Three different types of occlusion of the subclavian veins in two patients are presented. All are typical complications arising from a narrowed costo-clavicular interspace in connection with scapulo-thoracic passage pathology.

Some striking disagreement is evident between the "classical" concept of benignity of the axillo-subclavian venous occlusions and the conclusions of many reports published upon the evaluation of the respective late results of conservative and operative treatments. The high incidence of post-thrombotic sequelae advocates more selective therapeutic programmes in consideration of specific etiology in each instance. The causes of the various types of venous occlusion is discussed and it is suggested that in each case, the *constitutional, determinative* and eventually additional *temporary* factors should be systematically sought. The understanding of this pathology would be therefore clearer and the therapeutic guidelines more complete and adequate. When present, a segmental organized lesion of the subclavian vein at the costo-clavicular level-which becomes the source of additional severe thrombotic complications-, can be corrected by combination of:
- First rib resection.
- Endophlebectomy with excision of the terminal valve of the subclavian vein, included in the intraluminar fibrotic tissue.
- Occasional enlargement angioplasty of the junction of the subclavian and the brachio-cephalic veins.
- Closure of the subclavian phlebotomy with a large and rectangular autologous saphenous vein patch graft.

These procedures have been performed successfully in three instances through a combined subclavian and partial unilateral sternotomy approach permitting lateral retraction of the clavicle and the 2 first ribs. Final cosmetic aspect is very satisfactory.

Such restoration of the subclavian vein is indicated in *selected* cases in whom complete functional rehabilitation is essential. It is emphasized that the relative merits of the medical, physical and various surgical treatments – including the complete repair of the vein – should be discussed for each venous problem arising in a pathological scapulo-thoracic passage, with consideration for the general condition and capability requirements of the patient.

INTRODUCTION

Isolated or combined lesions of the nervous plexus and the main arteries and veins of the upper limb in the scapulo-thoracic passage can be due to many specific conditions. This pathology have been extensively studied in the past 50 years (60, 90), but opinions expressed in the literature, especially

* *Institut de Chirurgie* – Clinique A (Prof. D. Honoré) Universite de Liège, Clinique F.S.S. de Herstal, Belgium.

J.M. Greep, H.A.J. Lemmens, D.B. Roos and H.C. Urschel (eds.).
Pain in shoulder and arm: an integrated view, 255–279. All rights reserved.
Copyright © *1979 by Martinus Nijhoff Publishers, The Hague/Boston/London.*

about venous problems are still controverted and their conclusions remain somewhat confusing. The many denominations for the few types of occlusion of the deep veins in the upper limbs reflect the rather inaccurate understanding of the situations (5, 9, 10, 18, 19, 20, 21, 24, 37, 43, 47, 74, 80, 85, 86, 87, 88, 92):

- –"Effort," "idiopathic," "primary," "secondary," "subclavicular," "stress," "morning," "spontaneous subclavian," "iatrogenic," ... thromboses (1, 3, 16, 23, 47, 58, 61, 62, 75)
- – "Paget-Von Schrötter" syndrome (29, 31, 43, 61)
- – "Axillary," "subclavian," "axillo-subclavian" ... occlusion or thrombophlebitis (23, 32, 45, 72)
- – "Venous claudication,"
- – "Venospasm,"
- – "Intermittent venous occlusion" (2, 27, 41, 44, 45, 56, 57, 76, 77, 91)
- – Element of a "brachial plexus," "costoclavicular," "thoracic outlet," "thoracic inlet," "thoracic aperature," "scapular girdle," "shoulder girdle," "upper limb hilus," "hyperabduction," "thoracic outlet compression" "thoracic operculum," "scalenius anticus," "scapulo-thoracic passage," ... syndromes (4, 13, 25, 32, 33, 45, 49, 50, 52, 53, 57, 79, 91).
- – Etc. and many of these terms are preceded by the words "so-called"!

Discussions upon this topic should chiefly rely upon the basic etiopathologic concept: "... patients who have a 'thoracic outlet syndrome' have an underlying anatomic abnormality, not present in the general population, that predisposes them to develop symptoms under particular circumstances" (67). The latter most frequently consist of various types of injury, caused to vessels and or nerves, varying from a slight and temporary irritation or compression, to a repetitive or permanent or accidental intense squeezing (1, 12, 22, 33, 36, 38, 42, 47, 49, 63, 65, 66, 67, 68, 69, 70, 71, 80, 84, 85, 86, 88).

The pre-existing stretching or compression-producing mechanisms are usually due to the presence of:

congenital abnormal structures, such as cervical ribs or fibrous bands (4, 12, 33, 52, 67, 85, 86), unusual position of an accessory phrenic nerve (43, 44), an atypical artery (41, 43, 86), or a malpositioned subclavian vein terminal valve (17, 23, 47, 76, 77, 91).

an atypical, congenital or acquired, topographic arrangement of normal or abnormal anatomical elements.

Such conditions may lead to various pathologic symptoms which are to be accurately analyzed in order to identify precisely the original lesion(s) and the corresponding consequence(s) (18, 25, 32, 34, 41, 49, 50, 67, 74, 81, 82, 87, 91, 92). Treatment must seek to remove the cause of attrition and to restore, if possible, the integrity of the impaired organ. Gangrene due to persistent occlusion of the subclavian vein is exceptional; repermeabilization is not therefore to be considered mandatory (3, 11, 35, 36, 39, 40, 51, 74, 78).

Pulmonary embolisms are very rare (1, 3, 6, 7, 11, 28, 47, 51, 59, 74, 75, 83), but late sequelae of thrombosis are more frequent and crippling than classically assumed after conservative treatments (1, 2, 3, 13, 19, 20, 23, 43, 46, 47, 61, 66, 74, 75, 80, 86, 87, 88, 89, 91). The understanding of this pathology has changed in the past thirty years. Paradoxically, relatively few attempts have been made to re-establish a normal venous return by surgery on the lesion itself and or thrombectomy, usually associated with first rib resection (1, 3, 8, 9, 10, 12, 14, 17, 18, 19, 21, 24, 26, 28, 47, 49, 50, 54, 55, 65, 66, 67, 68, 69, 73, 74, 75, 80, 86, 87), or by-pass grafting (9, 43, 44, 48, 80, 86, 87, 91).

The surgical procedures generally advocated are mostly "indirect," such as first rib excision or claviculectomy (1, 2, 3, 10, 12, 18, 19, 20, 22, 25, 26, 33, 37, 43, 49, 50, 52, 69, 70, 74, 79, 80).

Their main purposal is to release the "first rib collateral veins" (1, 2, 3, 27, 75) and suppress the compression of the neuro-vascular structures. In a minority of cases, only pectoralis minor tenotomy (2, 13, 53), or scalenotomy (2, 4, 12, 18, 53) can be useful. The efficiency of thoracic sympathectomy alone or segmental phlebectomy is questionable (43, 47, 61). The following study reports two cases of successful direct reconstruction of formerly obstructed subclavian veins. The good physical condition of these very active patients justified a more anatomical and rehabilitative concept of treatment. Four additional cases have been successfully operated since the presentation of this paper.

RECALL OF THE "NORMAL," "SUBNORMAL" AND "PATHOLOGIC" STATES OF THE SUBCLAVIAN VEIN

The chronic, repetitive or accidental compression of the subclavian vein in the scapulo-thoracic passage is more harmful at the level of the costo-clavicular space. The squeezing of the vein between these two bones is often enhanced by the similar action of the costocoracoid ligament, the subclavius muscle or a hypertrophied root of the lower insertion of the anterior scalenius muscle lying in the same area. These structures rarely realize a significant venous occlusion respectively by themsleves only. A compression may already be evident at rest, but is more marked:
– in the hyperabduction with exorotation position ("Wright"-position),
– when the shoulder is forced backwards ("Eden"-military position) or downwards or upwards, the arm remaining along the thorax, with or without rotation-elevation of the chin and simultaneous deep inspiration ("Adson"-maneuvre).

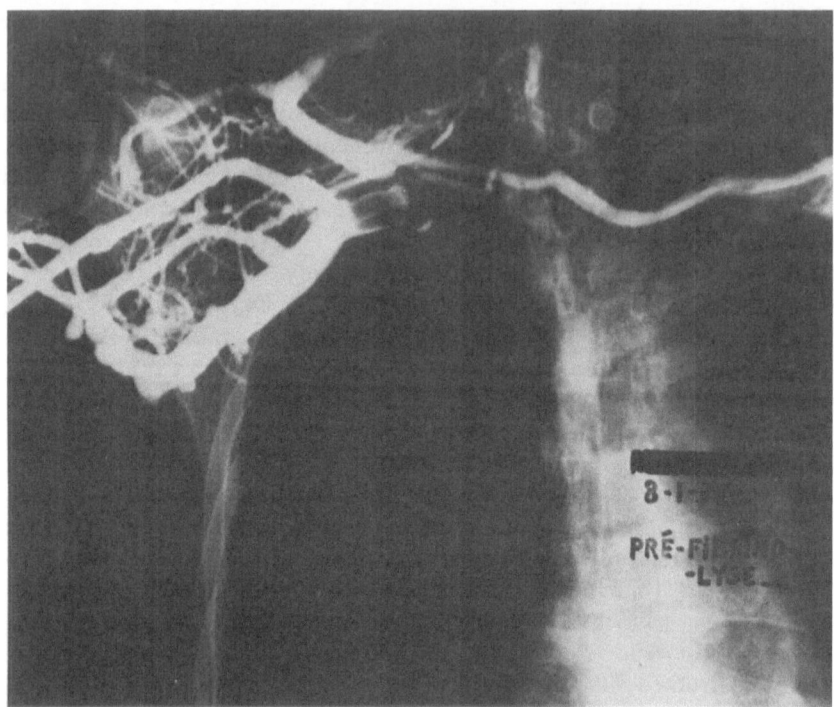

Figure 1. Case No. 1 – Phlebography at admission.

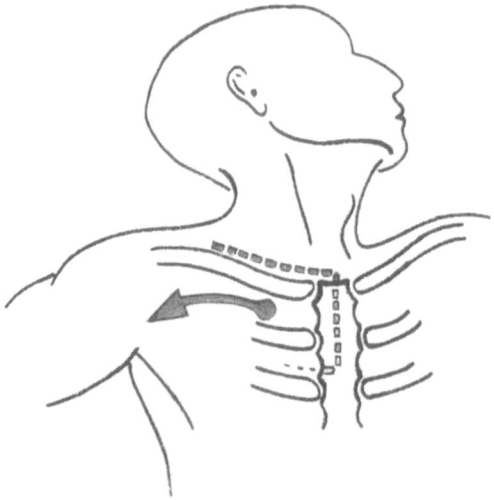

Figure 2. The "Costo-Claviculo-Sternal Flap" approach.

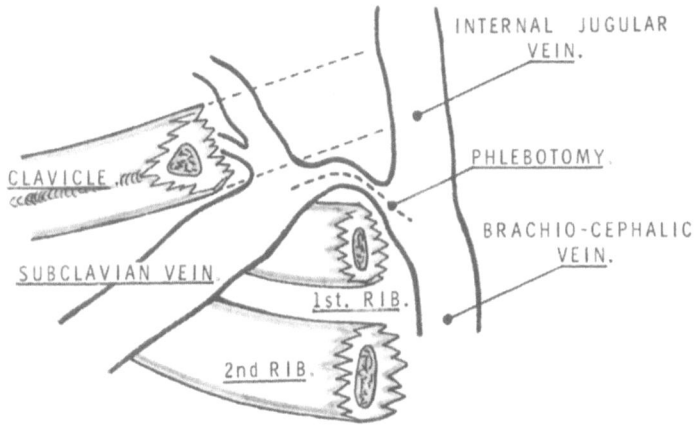

Figure 3. Approach of the costo-clavicular space and the subclavian vein.

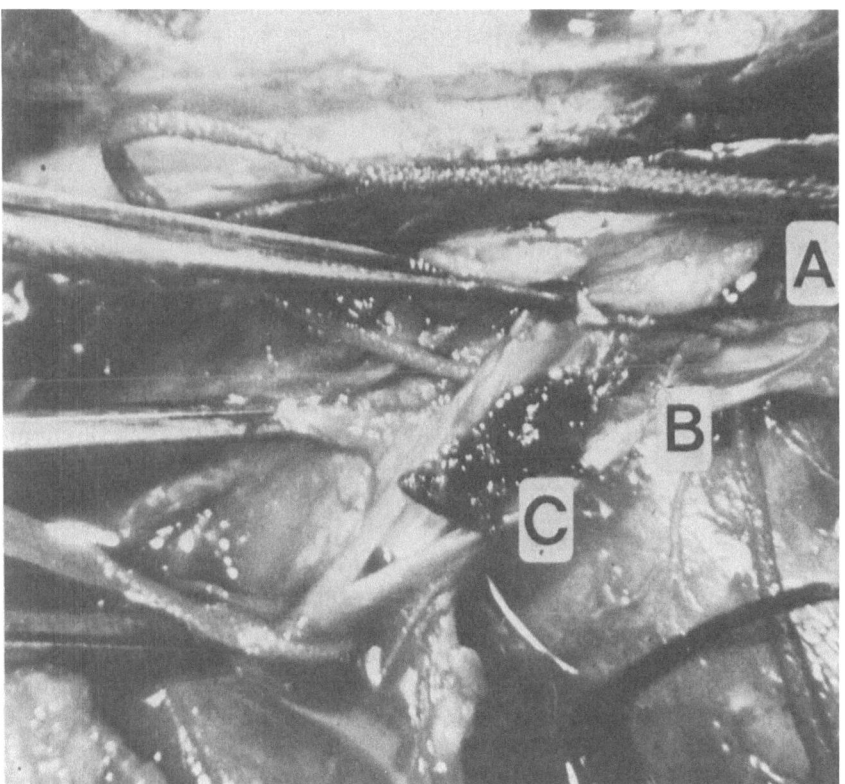

Figure 4. Aspect at phlebotomy: A. Brachio-cephalic vein; B. Organized fibrous "plug"; C. Proximal end of the recent coagulum, extending distally.

The subclavian vein may also be partially or totally occluded by the "strap" of the pectoralis minor muscle below the coracoid process or when stretched against the head of the humerus. This only happens in the hyperabduction with or without exorotation position and rarely leads to permanent lesion of the vessels.

Sixty to ninety-two percent of a normal population demonstrate partial or total occlusion of the artery adjacent to the vein in, at least, one of these attitudes. In a large percentage of active people, some degree of sub-occlusion of the subclavian vein, at rest or in the positions mentioned above may be present but completely asymptomatic. Temporary total occlusion may even occur and remain ignored, if these unusual, but potentially hazardous, positions of the limb, are assumed only for short times.

These compression mechanisms may however result in two main types of local alterations:

Type I   Extrinsic compression without significant lesion of the vein wall (2, 17, 23, 27, 29, 30, 31, 41, 43, 44, 45, 56, 57, 76, 77, 86, 91)
The narrowing of the lumen of the vessel varies widely with the anatomical arrangements in each individual, and the position of the arm and shoulder with regard to the thorax.

Type II   Segmental stenosis or occlusion with a localized and short in-traluminar thrombosis, occuring at the point where repeated crushing of the vein wall by a narrowed costo-clavicular claw, induces a perivenous and parietal fibrous reaction. (3, 9, 13, 17, 19, 20, 21, 27, 28, 29, 30, 31, 74, 75, 80, 85, 86, 87, 91).
In addition, the terminal valve of the subclavian vein is frequently found to be implanted precisely in this chronically injured segment, thus completing obstruction of the vessel. (9, 17, 74, 76, 77, 91). This combination of factors may finally lead to the formation of a connective tissue plug, not or partially recanalized (72, 75), in the proximal part of the subclavian vein. Consistent collateral venous network is usually developed; the clinical symptoms, at this stage, may be quite absent or more or less disabling, in relation to the efficiency to compensate for the blood return.

Either of these two types of lesions mentioned above may be complicated by an acute, rapidly extending, venous thrombosis if the previously "stabi-lized situation" is disrupted by a particular circumstance:
- Intense muscular work of the arm which suddenly exagerates the injury to the vein walls (e.g. effort thrombosis).
- Prolonged hyperabduction – with or without exorotation – of the arm.
- Squeezing of the shoulder against the thoracic wall (e.g. during sleep: "morning thrombosis").

From the site of compression, the thrombosis always progresses peripherally, occluding the ostia of collateral veins and therefore produces a sudden distal swelling of the limb (Paget-Von Schrötter syndrome). In rare cases, the clot also progresses proximally, causing a slight risk of pulmonary embolism. The degree and duration of the peripheral congestion depends on the capacity of the collateral veins still patent, to compensate again for the thrombosed deep ones during the early and late periods, and in all conditions of physical activity.

The main actual notions in the management of the treatment are:

1. It is classically assumed that spontaneous lysis and recanalization of the clot, assisted by *anticoagulant therapy*, along with the developement of a collateral network, very often lead to an almost complete recovery. However, it has been more recently demonstrated that 60 to 75% of the patients who were treated conservatively after extensive acute thrombosis sustain moderate to serious "postthrombotic" sequelae with increased distal venous pressure worsened by muscular activity.

2. Venous thrombectomy (preferably through the axillary approach) or fibrinolysis performed less than 5 to 8 days after institution of the acute thrombosis can completely eliminate the fresh coagulum. The veins can thus be restored to normal, if their structure has not been previously modified by the traumatic injuries (Type I).

3. Any significant organic cause of extrinsic compression should be removed: excision of the first rib, also through the axillary route, is usually preferred to claviculectomy.

4. If a previous segmental organized intraluminar thrombosis is present (Type II), classical thrombectomy or fibrinolysis would only evacuate the recent clots from the main deep veins and the orifices of the collaterals, but will not have any action on the chronic short fibrotic lesion which is permanent and may lead to recurrence of the acute thrombosis (1, 2, 3, 10, 12, 17, 19, 20, 21, 25, 26, 49, 61, 66, 74, 75, 80). In such cases, removal of the costo-clavicular "bottle-neck" by costectomy or claviculectomy only decompresses the "first rib collateral veins" therefore facilitating the venous blood flow, but do not reestablish a normal venous pathway nor suppress the "conjunctive plug". Satisfactory improvement depends on the previous existence and patency of this particular venous network in the costoclavicular slit, which should be, therefore, evidenced preoperatively, by phlebogram.

The direct reconstruction of the altered segment of the subclavian vein associated with resection of the first rib appears to be the logical solution in severely handicapped patients. Simple removal of the obstacle followed by direct suture of the phlebotomy is impossible in almost all cases, due to the atrophy of the vein walls in the chronically injured portion. Till now, segmental replacement or by-pass of the lesion using an autologous saphenous vein graft have only been rarely performed.

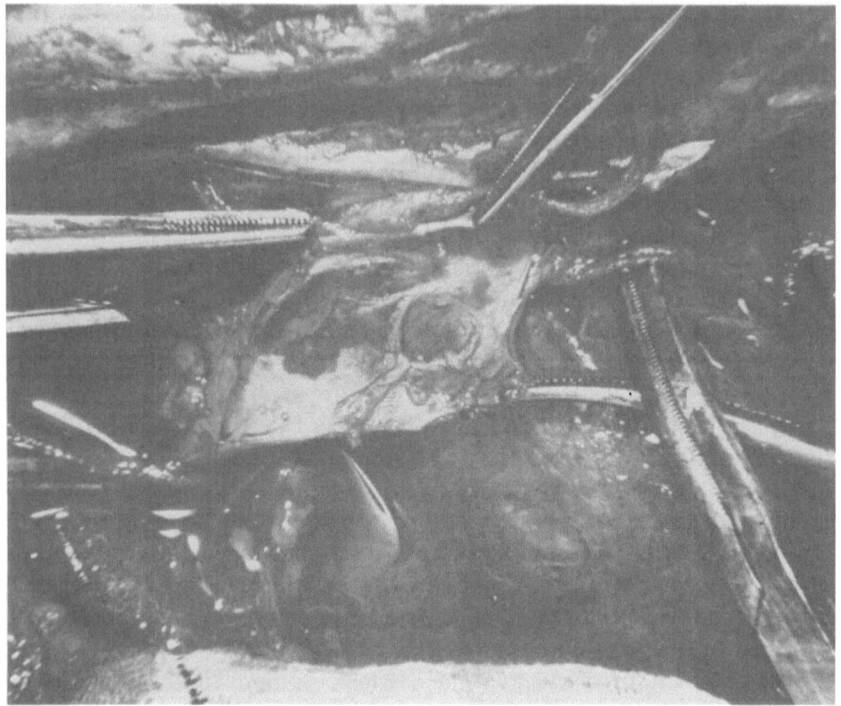

Figure 5. Remains of the terminal valve of the subclavian vein wedged in the "fibrous plug" (Case No. 1).

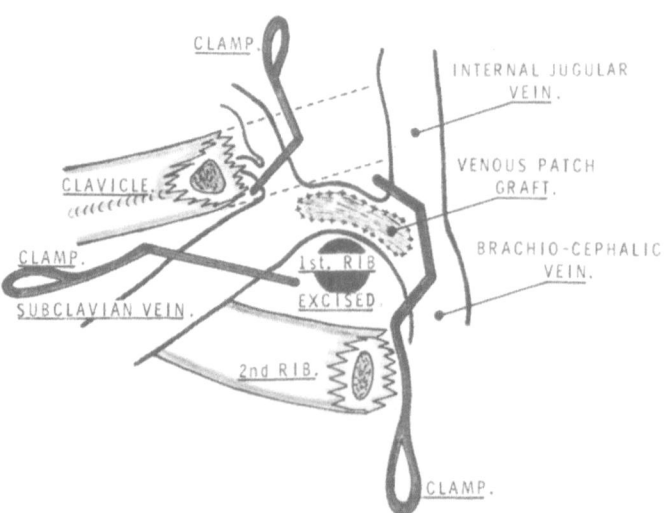

Figure 6. Restoration of the subclavian vein completed (Technical principles applied in all cases).

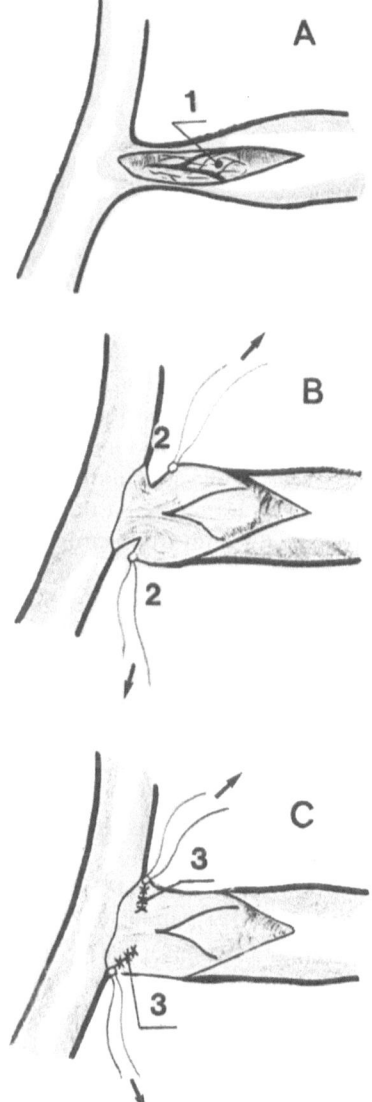

Figure 7. Angioplasty of the junction of the subclavian and brachio-cephalic veins (Case No. 2).

A. Incision of the subclavian vein.

1. remains of the terminal valve and fibrous plug, in the atrophied portion of the vein walls. B and C. Enlargement of the junction of the subclavian and the brachiocephalic veins, by a "pyloroplasty-like" angioplasty.

2. traction on the rims of the longitudinal phlebotomy.

3. transverse suture of the subclavian vein rims on the rims of the inlet of the brachio-cephalic vein, using separated (7–0) stitches.

CASE REPORT

Case No. 1

This 25 years old right-handed man does not mention any previous important illness or trauma. He works as an electrician, and therefore, frequently handles tools with elevated forearms or hyperabducted arms. Moreover, each day, he carries all his equipment, which weights 20 to 25 kg, in a particular leather satchel, traditionally used in his occupation. This bag has a single shoulder belt. He always hangs this heavy load on his right shoulder, which is therefore, forced downwards. All the muscles of the shoulder girdle and the arm are isometrically contracted in order to maintain the stability in this support for few hours every day. Upon waking, on January 8th 1977, he observed an important oedema of the right upper limb with a marked distension of the subcutaneous veins of the forearm along with a cold hand. The pressure in the basilic vein was 39 cm of water at rest, horizontally, in bed. At clinical examination, the radial pulse early disappeared when the arm was abducted. The diagnosis of combined venous and arterial compression within the scapulo-thoracic channel was evident. A phlebography demonstrated a subclavian vein thrombosis at the level of the slit between the first rib and the clavicle. The patient was considered to be a good candidate for fibrinolysis which was performed 12 hours after the onset of the symptoms. When the streptokinase perfusion was completed, the clinical state was only partially improved: a mild edema of the hand and the forearm persisted with some distension of the superficial veins. Peripheral venous pressure was 16 to 20 cm of water. Anticoagulant therapy was started by intravenous perfusion of heparin and simultaneous oral intake of anti-vitamin K. drug. A right control phlebogram disclosed a persistent clot almost completely occluding the lumen just at the site of the costo-clavicular interspace. The collateral venous network appeared, however, "satisfactory" (Figure 1). On the left, a similar examination showed only a slight compression of the vein at the same level but without hemodynamic disturbance. The arteriogram showed normal vessels when both limbs were in "indifferent" position. When the right arm was hyperabducted, the subclavian artery was totally occluded by the costo-clavicular claw. Moreover, the axillary artery was almost squeezed shut below the pectoralis minor muscle. On the left side, the same manoeuvre did not produce any significant compression. Eight hours after fibrinolysis was ended, all symptoms of acute venous occlusion recurred despite continuous perfusion of heparin. A direct surgical approach of the right subclavian vein was therefore attempted through a supra clavicular incision prolonged by a vertical partial unilateral and upper sternotomy down to the second right intercostal space (Figure 2). The sternocleidomastoid muscle was transected in its fibrous root, for further easy repair. The proximal 5 cm of the subclavian vein appeared atrophic (approximatively 6 to 8 mm of external diameter), and was occluded by a firm plug. Just distally, the vein was blueish and dilated (up to 15 mm in diameter), and also occluded, but by a soft fresh clot which penetrates into the terminal part of the cephalic vein. The first rib was then resected. Afterwards, under general heparinization (1.5 mg/kg of body weight), a phlebotomy was performed on the 5 last cm of the proximal segment of the subclavian vein (Figure 3).

It was extended onto the anterior aspect of the brachio-cephalic vein, which was clamped laterally, in front of its junction with the latter. A distal and quite recent, 12 cm long, thrombus was easily removed from the subclavian and cephalic veins using a thrombectomy balloon catheter (Figure 4). This fresh material was not present at the time of the post-fibrinolysis control phlebogram. A much older cellular and fibrotic intraluminar thrombus was resected from the 3 cm long segment formerly crushed in the costo-clavicular slit. This thromboendophlebectomy disclosed the remains of the terminal valve of the subclavian vein, which were wedged in the organized thrombus (Figure 5). These altered elements were resected. The vein wall corresponding to the site of the costo-clavicular claw appeared critically atrophied and retracted although of still good "mechanical" quality. After excision of a small sample for microscopic control, the phlebotomy was closed by means of an angioplasty rectangular venous patch taken from the saphenous vein at the ankle. This enlargement was prolonged on the anterior aspect of the brachiocephalic trunk, over its junction with the subclavian vein (Figure 6). Within four hours, all symptoms of venous hypertension disappeared and, two months later, the patient was working normally. Thirty months later, the subclavian vein remains patent and asymptomatic.

No anticoagulant therapy was given postoperatively.

Case No. 2

This 40 year old woman complained of bilateral early weakness of both upper limbs upon physical exercise for almost 20 years. This sensation is associated in the last 6 years with progressive swelling from the hands to the forearms followed by hypoesthesis swarming, and coldness of the fingers. These symptoms slowly developed and were more intense at the left whereas the patient is right handed. The "arm claudication test" is tolerated less than 40 seconds at the left and 90 seconds at the right. She also suffered from intermittent headaches with visual troubles of the left eye. At examination, the left external jugular vein was dilated. Phlebograms disclosed a chronic localized occlusion of the left subclavian vein in the costo-clavicular

claw. Significant external compression of the right vein at a comparable
location, but without mural alteration was also present. Through a "costo-
claviculo-sternal flap" approach, identical to the one used Case No. 1, a
similar procedure was performed on 16 June 1977:

Operative findings and the appearance of the lesions were similar to those
of the operation in Case No. 1, except for the absence of the fresh clot distal
to the chronic venous lesion.

The first rib was excised.

After intravenous heparinization (1.5 mg/kg of body weight), a longitudinal phlebotomy, incision – 5 cm long – was performed on the anterior
aspect of the terminal segment of the subclavian vein and was prolonged
onto the wall of the brachiocephalic vein. This latter was cross-clamped,
separately above and below its junction with the subclavian vein. Endophlebectomy with resection of the remains of the terminal valve was performed.

An enlargement by plasty of the ostium of the subclavian vein was
constructed as the vein wall was markedly retracted and atrophied at its
junction with the brachiocephalic vein (Figure 7A, B and C). The phlebotomy was then closed with a large rectangular saphenous vein patch
taken from the upper segment of the saphenous vein. The diameter of the
lumen was finally restored to normal size (Figure 8).

All symptoms, including headaches, promptly receded in the early postoperative period. No anticoagulant therapy was given. Six months postoperatively, no vascular symptoms recurred but nervous alterations partially persist, with some peripheral conduction velocity impairment. The
right first rib was excised a few weeks later through the classical transaxillary approach.

COMMENTS AND DISCUSSION

*I. The operative findings corroborate the diagnosis in both cases and
clearly explain the main symptoms.*

The passage for the subclavian veins between the first ribs and the clavicles
are 3 to 7 mm in size at the particular place where their anatomic
impairments are observed. Their external walls closely fit these bones and
are surrounded by unexpected fibrous tissue beside the insertions of the
subclavius and costo-coracoid ligaments.

The roots of the scalenius anticus muscles do not appear to be involved
in this compression mechanism. Alterations of the vein walls are obviously
due to chronic injuries without any evidence of spastic participation. It
results in a fibrotic indwelling within their histological structures leading to
retraction and atrophy of the last 5 cm of the veins, even involving their

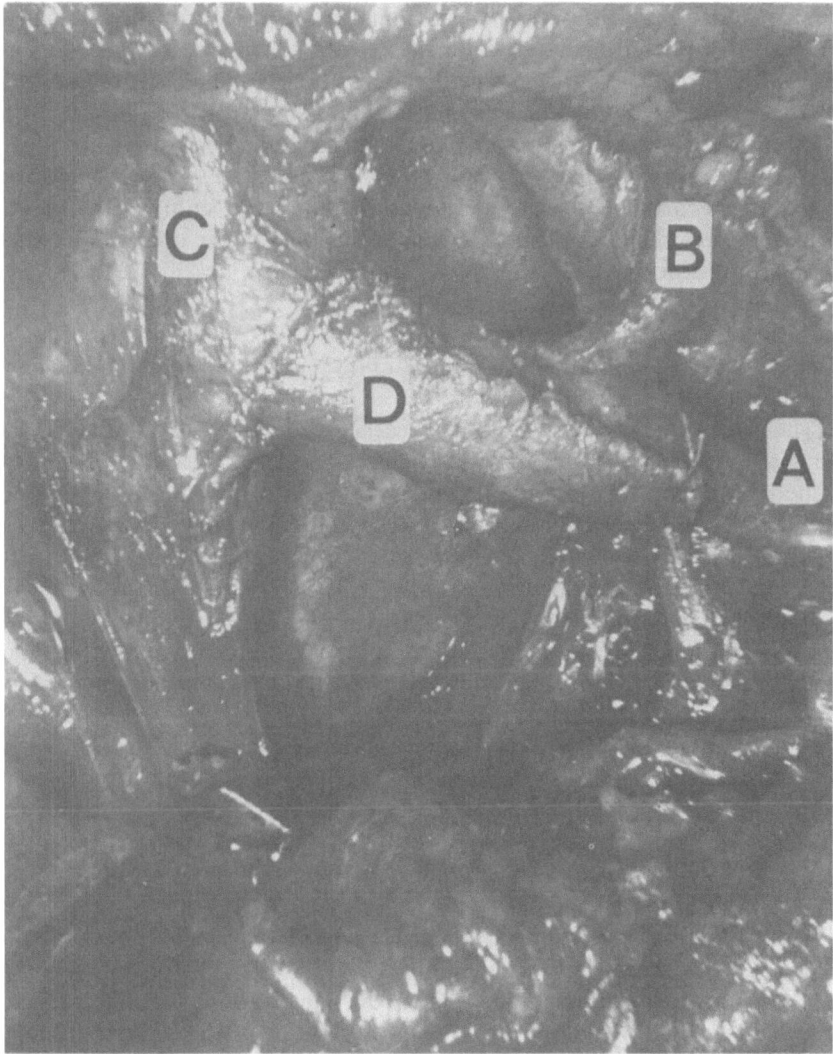

Figure 8. Final view of the subclavian vein restored after closure of the phlebotomy using a large saphenous vein rectangular patch.

A. subclavian vein.

B. main "extra-costoclavicular collateral vein", running outside of the slit, visualized on the phlebography in Figure 9.

C. brachio-cephalic vein.

D. transplanted patch venoplasty.

openings at the junction with the brachiocephalic trunks. Distally no similar modification of the vein is observed.

– In addition, in both cases, the terminal valve of the subclavian vein is found to be inserted exactly at the site of attrition in the costo-clavicular claw. Therefore, this structure cannot function normally, aggravates the obstruction of the venous lumen, and facilitates the local thrombosis, from which the short occlusive fibrous plug is formed. Furthermore, Case No. 1 developed a rapidly extensive venous thrombosis distally from this chronic lesion. Its recurrence within a few hours after the completion of the fibrinolytic treatment, confirms the role of this plug in the initiation of such acute complications.

Analysis of these factors, combined with elements from former clinical observations, and opinions in the literature, suggest the following concepts of their pathogenesis:

A. The *chronic venous lesions* in the scapulo-thoracic passage are located mostly at the level of the costo-clavicular space. They usually result from the combination of two main factors

   1. *Constitutional Factor*:   A narrowed costo-clavicular claw may exert an external "scissor-like" significant flattening of the vein associated – or not – with compression of other elements. (12, 16, 18, 32, 49, 50, 65, 67, 68, 75, 81, 82, 85, 86, 87)

     – The insufficient opening between the two bones could be from *congenital* origin(s) affecting one or both sides, eventually, at various grades and by different mechanisms.

     – In most instances, these atypical anatomical and topographical aspects recognize an *acquired* origin:

      a. Specific frequent movements or static situations inducing retraction of the muscles of the scapular girdle,

      b. Consequences of unique or repeated action of various "traumatic" factors.

      c. Excessive and progressive descent of the shoulders occurring incidentally around the thirties, ...

      ... may modify the reciprocal localizations of normal elements, leading to compression of the neurovascular structures.

     Such latter situation is more likely to be *unilateral* in case of: Traumatisms,

     "Specific movements or attitudes" after which the upper limb usually preponderant is more frequently involved.

    – At early stages, physical therapy alone can correct many of the forementioned situations (12, 13, 15, 18, 22, 37, 49, 50, 64, 66, 67, 70, 74)

- The occasional presence of the *terminal valve* of the subclavian vein etween the clavicle and the first rib may be a further
  occlusive "CONSTITUTIONAL" factor.
- Other circumstances, such as secondary consequences of a
  trauma (e.g.: fracture of the clavicle,...), or an intrathoracic
  tumor, etc., may also become a "CONSTITUTIONAL factor".

2. *Determinative Factor*: Repeated mechanical crushings of the vein by
an "abnormal" costo-clavicular claw, may be produced by normal physical
activity outside the awareness of the patient. The vein walls can eventually
be more or less modified by this attrition. However, the clinical symptoms
do not always correspond closely to the severity of the anatomic and
histologic modifications found in the localized chronic lesion.

A very short thrombus may develop at this particular site and this
intraluminar materiel further becomes fibrous and sometimes partially recanalized.

Despite the development of plugs of similar constitution the patient
No. 2 becomes heavily handicapped by the lowering of the venous
return whereas patient No. 1 is quite asymptomatic.

Microscopic examinations of the remains of the vein wall at the site
of the organized thromboses show a persistence of the tunica elastica
in both cases. The intima is replaced by a thin and adherent fibrous
layer which was easily cleared from the outer layers and amazingly
permitted "endophlebectomy". The external layers appear thickened
and muscular elements are still present but are separated by diffuse
fibrotic tissue.

One definite "determinative factor" may simultaneously produce
alterations in other structures located beside the vein. (Case No.
2).

Other circumstances may be also regarded as "determinative factors" including a rapidly extending tumor ("Pancoast-Tobraz Syndrome").

B. The development of an *acute extensive venous thrombosis* (which induces the most impressive symptoms and difficulties) seems to require an
additional "TEMPORARY FACTOR" (such as prolonged compression
of the shoulder during sleep – morning thrombosis – (Case No. 1) – or by
strongly intensified venous attrition and contusion due to scapular girdle
muscle contraction after unusual effort – effort thrombosis- ...) These
occasional circumstances may further decrease the venous flow already
impaired by a pre-existing topographical narrowing of the scapulo-
thoracic passage (Type I alteration) or an occlusive or stenotic intrinsic
lesion of the axillary or subclavian veins (Type II alterations). The Case No.
1 is demonstrative of this concept.

II. The treatment, in each case, is individually guided by the latter etiologic concepts

Pathogenic modifications of the topographical distribution of the constitutive anatomical elements, should be first treated, when disclosed in the absense of an acute extensive thrombosis, by physical therapy. If clinically unsuccessful, surgery is to be considered: first rib resection (preferred to claviculectomy), may achieve a decompression of the "first rib collateral veins", around a Type I or Type II occlusion of the subclavian vein, in

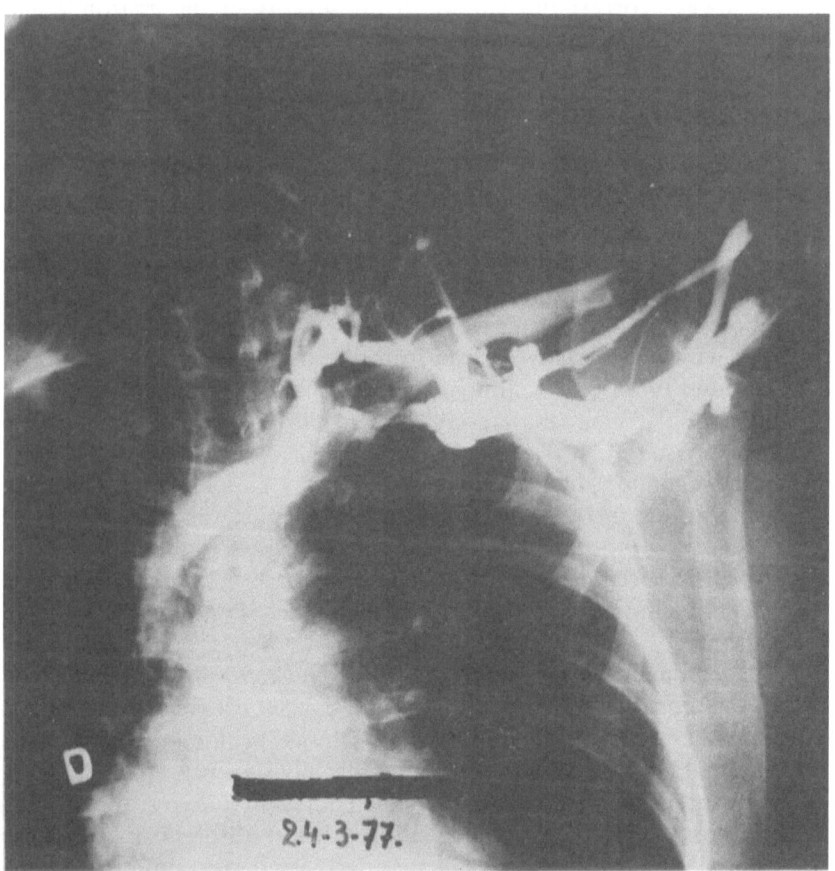

Figure 9. Phlebography of Case No. 2 at admission. The "first collateral rib venous network" was very poor in any position of the arm. Almost all the compensating collaterals run outside of the costoclavicular slit. The study of the venous drainage includes comparison of aspects in the "indifferent", "Wright," "Eden" and "Adson" attitudes.

case where some impairment of their drainage is demonstrated by phlebography. The flow of the venous return can be, therefore, improved, allowing a better effort tolerance and lowering the risk of further acute thrombosis. If few compensating collaterals are not- or poorly-visualized within the costoclavicular interspace, it is likely that no significant improvement will be achieved by excision of the clavicle or first rib only. [Case No. 1 – right side (Figure 1) and case No. 2 – left side (Figure 9)].

In addition, it must be remembered that the collateral network around a limited chronic venous lesion may appear "satisfactory" on the phlebographic pictures despite the presence of a clinical impairement and physical disability. (Case No. 1 – Right – , and case No. 2 – Left –). (Figure 1–Figure 9.), due to some dysfunction of the venous muscular "pumping".

In the presence of extended acute peripheral thrombosis, medical treatment based upon intravenous heparin must be started at once, almost in all cases. Fibrinolysis is indicated in some others (Case No. 1.). Afterwards, the attitude is eventually reviewed in favor of a surgical procedure, preferabily before the fifth to eighth day following the onset of the sudden venous stasis, according to:
- the clinical status of the venous return,
- the controls of the venous pressure with phlebodynamometric tests (12, 37, 74, 75,
- the controls of the venous pressure with phlebodynamometric tests (12, 37, 74, 75, 80, 88, 89).
- the type, length and situation of the coagulum demonstrated by phlebograms, with special consideration for the patency of the central outlets of the cephalic and "first rib collateral" veins (3, 27, 29, 30, 31, 61, 74, 76, 85, 86, 87).
- the general condition, age, and physical requirements of the patient.

Old and fibrotic connective tissue forming the *localized intravenous plug* cannot be eliminated by fibrinolysis nor balloon-catheter thrombectomy alone. It may even be the source of a new extensive thrombosis after these types of treatment (Case No. 1). These arguments support the opinion that removal of the first rib (or clavicle) should be followed in *selected cases*, by direct *surgical repermeabilization of the subclavian vein*. Such a therapeutic programme is the one most likely to restore normal venous return and avoid the risks of pulmonary embolism, crippling post-thrombotic sequelae or recurrence of acute extensive thrombosis. Excision of this thrombogenic structure by phlebectomy does not combine the prevention of recurrent thrombosis with the needs for an anatomical restoration, to provide management for the most complete physical rehabilitation.

Logical indications for sympathectomy in venous occlusion remain questionable, except in cases presenting a risk of peripheral gangrene.

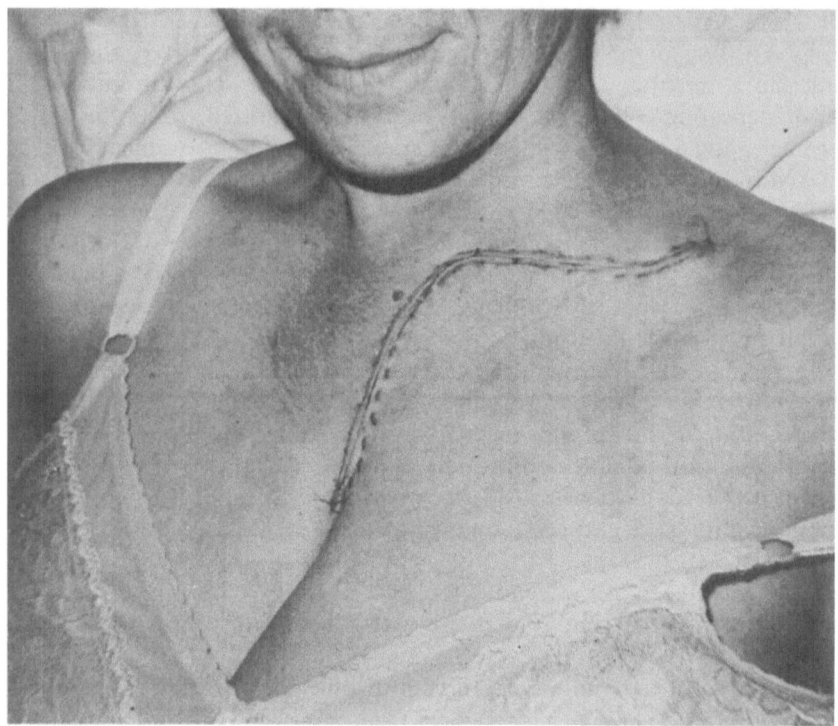

Figure 10. Skin incision for completion of the "Cleido-Sterno-Costal flap (Case No. 2).

III. Indications for the complete surgical restoration of the subclavian vein must be appraised with regard to its technical requirements

The transaxillary approach is recommended when simple balloon-catheter venous thrombectomy can achieve the desobstruction, in addition to the excision of the first rib. This method is obviously incomplete when a costo-clavicular "chronic plug" is present. The suggested operative procedure requires the completion of a "cleido-sterno-costal flap" with a partial sternotomy which is remarkably well tolerated, cosmetically acceptable, and even less damaging than claviculectomy (Figure 10). After removal of the first rib, a "thromboendophlebectomy" can be achieved, using a "thromboendarterectomy-like" dissection technique. The repermeabilization of the subclavian vein (Cases Nos. 1 and 2), is completed by excision of the remains of the terminal valve encased in the fibrotic material (Figure 5). Patients in good condition for whom functional rehabilitation is essential, may be considered as candidates for this operative treatment. The classical and more conservative procedures might prove to be sufficient in the elderly and those in delicate health or without marked impairment of the venous return.

IV. Reconstruction of the chronic venous lesions involves specific technical procedure

The external circumferences of the altered terminal parts of the subclavian vein are roughly 50% (Case No. 1) and 75% (Case No. 2) smaller than those just distal to the lesion. Axial phlebotomy along the atrophied segments is performed and prolonged 4 mm (Case No. 1) and 8 mm (Case No. 2) onto the anterior aspects of the brachio-cephalic veins. In case No. 1, distal thrombectomy is first performed. In both cases, the vein walls, when cleared from the conjunctive "plug" by endophlebectomy, appear unextensible, slightly thickened, and retracted, due to their fibrotic infiltration. The areas of junction of the subclavian and the brachio-cephalic veins are similarly stiffened. In Case No. 2, the lumen, at this level, is reduced to less than 10% of the normal size. A direct suture of the phlebotomies would obviously lead to unacceptable stenoses, and therefore angioplastic enlargement is mandatory. In Case No. 1, a 12 mm large rectangular vein patch removed from the lower saphenous vein achieves a very satisfactory result.

In Case No. 2, a larger – 16 mm – rectangular patch is obtained from fragments of the upper saphenous vein which is unfolded to use its full circumference. This material appears suitable for restoration of a normal diameter in the 6 last centimeters of the subclavian vein but is insufficient in width at the level of its junction with the brachiocephalic trunk. Enlargement of this ostium is therefore performed, using "pyloroplasty-like," transverse, separate stitches sutures to approximate the rims of both axial incisions of the confluent veins (Figure 7.A, B, and C). The combination of these two procedures restores the venous outflow in the upper limb to an almost normal size (Figure 8).

The analysis of the clinical histories emphasizes the need to investigate systematically all causes of neurovascular compression and attrition in both scapulo-thoracic-passages, even in patients demonstrating only one type of unilateral lesion

a) In case No. 1, the sole clinical picture is a right axillo-subclavian acute venous thrombosis.

Angiograms with the right arm hyperabducted demonstrate a compression of the artery and vein within the costo-clavicular claw and below the pectoralis minor muscle. The left scapulo-thoracic passage is considered within "normal range."

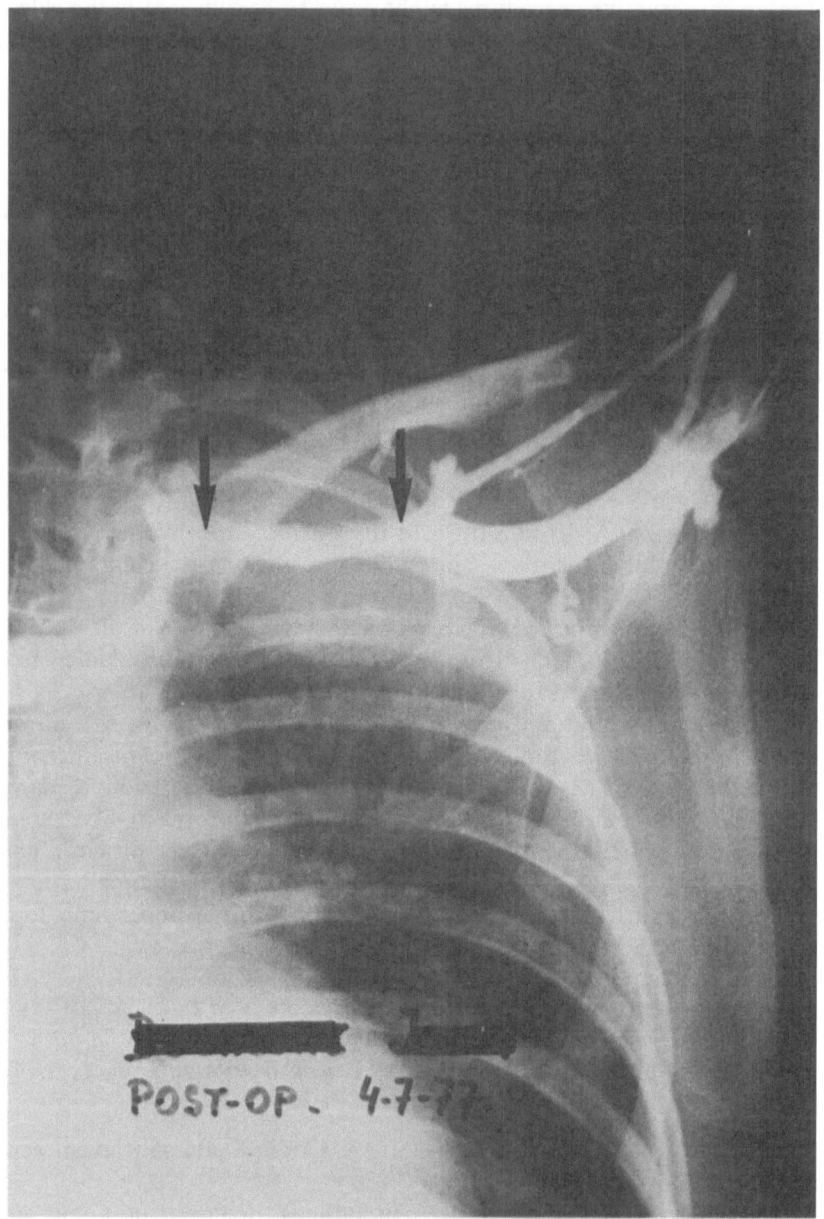

Figure 11. Post-operative phlebography of Case No. 2. The collateral venous network no longer appears very significantly as the venous return is almost completely drained through the restored subclavian vein.

Arrows indicate the location of the venous patch graft.

The "*constitutional factor*" contributing to this pathology has *no* obvious congenital origin; the specific occupational activity led in the past two years, to a narrowing of the costo-clavicular space and a chronic retraction of the pectoralis minor muscle at the right side. Topographical modifications of normal anatomical elements proceed from an acquired etiology and induce the "hyperabduction syndrome." Repetitive subsequent venous attritions are the "determinative factor" which finally produces the localized thrombotic plug at the costo-clavicular level. This occlusion remained asymptomatic until the "*temporary factor*" (long lasting shoulder compression during sleep) initiated the acute peripherally extensive thrombosis of the deep veins. No evidence of nervous alteration was present. A complete correction of the lesion at the level of the right costo-clavicular slit was indicated but physical therapy for this arm is likely to release the retraction of the muscles of the right scapular girdle particularly of the pectoralis minor.

b) The clinical history of Case No. 2 discloses essentially headaches and symptoms of compression of arteries and nerves - and perhaps the "vasa nervorum" of the brachial plexus (50) – in both scapulo-thoracic passages, for 20 years. Slowing of the venous return is evident in the past few years: it is produced, on the right side, by an intermittent occlusion of the vein when the arm is abducted and on the left side by a poorly recanalized chronic occlusion of the terminal segment of the subclavian vein. First rib excision is indicated on both sides. Left venous reconstruction is recommended as the collateral venous network is clinically insufficient, despite a "satisfactory" appearance of the phlebogram, while being not mainly dependent of the "first rib collateral veins". The "constitutional factor" is probably a descent of both shoulders which is not infrequent after the third decade of life due to some elongation of elevator muscles of the scapular girdles. The situation produces repeated pinchings of the subclavian veins in the costo-clavicular spaces which are the "determinative factors" leading to the intermittent occlusion at right and to the alteration of the vein wall at the left with subsequent formation of localized intraluminar thrombosis. No "temporary factor" had yet produced any acute phenomenon in this case.

c) The role of the terminal valves of the subclavian veins as an additional "constitutional factor" contributing to thrombosis is evident in both cases.

It appears from reviews of the literature that etiologic details of each particular case of venous occlusion has not always been completely disclosed and understood. The striking disagreement between opinions from various authors on the evaluations of the late results of conservative and surgical treatments reflects this situation. The infrequency of clinically significant upper limb venous lesions among the pathological problems of the scapulo-thoracic passage limits the possibility of extensive and systematic experience in their management. Subsequently, treatment may often have been insufficient or inadequate and this accounts for the relatively high incidence of additional further recurrence of thrombosis and of post-thrombotic sequelae in conservatively treated patients.

The specific symptoms of venous obstruction are sometimes associated with others from nervous and/or arterial origins, due to the same etiologic factors. These clinical elements must be separately identified. They contribute to the choice of the specific therapeutic guidelines for each affected scapular-thoracic passage, even in the same patient.

REFERENCES

1. J.T. Adams, J.A. De Weese. "Effort" thrombosis of the axillary and subclavian veins. J. Trauma. II: 923, 1971
2. J.T. Adams, J.A. de Wesse, E.B. Mahonet, C.G. Rob. Intermittent subclavian vein obstruction without thrombosis. Surgery. 63: 147, 1968
3. J.T. Adams, R.K. Mac Evoy, J.A. de Weese. Primary deep venous thrombosis of upper extremity. Arch. Surg. 91: 29, 1965 + Discussion by A. Haller.
4. A.W. Adson, M.D. Coffey. Cervical rib. A method of anterior approach for relief of symptoms by division of the scalenus anticus. Ann. Surg. I: 839, 1927.
5. E.V. Allen, N.W. Barker, E.A. Hines Jr. Peripheral vascular diseases. Ed. Saunders Cy., Philadelphia. 1972
6. A.H. Aufses Jr. Venous thrombosis of the upper extremity complicated by pulmonary embolus. Surgery. 35: 957, 1954
7. T. Barnett, and L.M. Levitt. "Effort" thrombosis of the axillary vein with pulmonary embolism. J.A.M.A. 146: 1412, 1951
8. L. Bazy. Thrombose de la veine axillaire droite. Bull. Mem. Soc. Nat. de Chir. 52: 529, 1926
9. M.A. Beaujean. La reconstruction chirurgicale de la veine sous-clavière obstruée ou thrombosée. In preparation
10. H.J.P. Beerstecher. La thrombose primitive des veines profondes du bras. Phlébologie Fr 23: 69, 1970
11. J.K. Berman. Discussion of the communication of Coon and Willis. Arch. Surg. 94: 662, 1967
12. S. Bertelsen. Neurovascular compression syndromes of the neck and shoulder. A survey based on a clinical series. Acta. Chir. Scand. 135: 137, 1969
13. J.A. Beyer, I.S. Wright. The hyperabduction syndrome with special reference to its relationship to Raynaud's syndrome. Circulation 4: 161, 1951
14. M. Biebl. Thrombektomie bei Blender Thrombose der Vena axillaris und Subclavia. Zbl Chir. 66: 1560, 1939
15. L.P. Britt. Nonoperative treatment of the thoracic outlet syndrome symptoms. In Urist, M.R. ed.: J.B. Lippincott (Philadelphia). Clinical Orthopaedics and Related Research. 51: 45, 1967
16. U. Brunner. "Thrombose par effort" des sportlers. Z. Unfallmed. Berufskrh. 61: 42, 1968
17. U. Brunner. Aspects chirurgicaux de la thrombose axillaire d'effort aigüe. Phlébologie 30: 51, 1977
18. O.T. Clagett. Research and prosearch. Presidential address. J. Thorac. Cardiovasc. Surg. 44: 153, 1962
19. W.W. Coon, P.W. Willis III. Thrombosis of axillary and subclavian veins. Arch Surg. 94: 657, 1967
20. W.W. Coon, and P.W. Willis. Thrombosis of deep veins of the arm. Surgery. 64: 990, 1968
21. J.M. Cormier, J. Sautot, C. Frileux, G. Arnulf. In noveau traité de technique chirurgicale. Tome V. Artères, Veines, Lymphatiques. Masson. Paris 1973

22. J.J. Cranley. Vascular Surgery. Chap 10. Neurovascular compression syndromes. Harper and Row. 1972
23. D.L. Crowell. Effort thrombosis of the subclavian and axillary veins: review of the literature and case report with two-year follow up with venography. Ann. Intern. Med. 52: 1337, 1960
24. W.A. Dale, T.R. Allen. Unusual problems of venous thrombosis. Surgery. 78: 707, 1975
25. W.A. Dale, M.R. Lawis. Management of thoracic outlet syndrome. Ann. Surg. 181: 578, 1975
26. J.A. de Weese, J.T. Adams, D.L. Caiser. Subclavian venous thrombectomy. Circulation. Suppl. 41: 158, 1970
27. J.A. de Weese, S.M. Rogoff. Phlebography of upper extremity. Vascular Roentgenology, New York. MacMillan Co., 482, 1964
28. T. Drapanas, W.L. Curran. Thrombectomy in the treatment of "effort" thrombosis of axillary and subclavian veins. J. Trauma. 6: 107, 1966
29. J. Drewes. Bemerkungen zur Etiologie des Paget-Von Schrötter-Syndroms. Fortschr. Röntgenstr. 105: 865, 1966
30. J. Drewes. Die Phlebographie der Oberen Körperhälfte. Springer. Verlag. Berlin. Göttingen. Heidelberg, 1963
31. J. Drewes. Phlebographische befunde bei der Venensperre der oberen Extremität (Paget-Von Schrötter Syndrom), Fortschr. Röntgenstr. 80: 341, 1954
32. M.A. Falconer, G. Weddeli. Costo-clavicular Compression of Subclavian artery and vein: Relation to the scalenus anticus syndrome. Lancet. 2: 539, 1943
33. T.B. Fergusson, T.H. Burford, C.L. Roper. Neurovascular compression at the superior thoracic aperture: Surgical management. Ann. Surg. 167: 573, 1968
34. J.N. Fiessinger, E. Housset. Thromboses veineuses des membres. Aspects cliniques et étiologiques. Rev. Prat. 27: 1305, 1977
35. R. Fontaine, R. Kieny, L. Tuchmann, A. Suhler, M. Kuhlman. Les gangrènes des membres d'origine veineuse. A propos de quatre nouvelles observations. Lyon Chir. 61: 52, 1965
36. J.A. Gravel. Direct thrombectomy and repair of traumatic occlusion of axillary vein. Arch. Surg. 101: 796, 1970
    Discussion of the communication of Tilney and Coll.
37. S.M. Greenstone, T.B. Massell, E.C. Herringman, H.A. Raphael. The thoracic outlet compression syndrome. A reappraisal. Vasc. Surg. 5: 121, 1971
38. P.H. Guilfoil, T. Christiansen. An unusual vascular complication of fractured clavicle. J.A.M.A. 200: 72, 1967.
39. H. Haimovici. The ischemic forms of venous thrombosis. VII Congress of the International Cardiovascular Society. Philadelphie. Minerva. Medica. 164
40. H. Haimovici. Ischemic forms of thrombophlebitis. Charles C. Thomas 1965
41. O. Horwitz, H.F. Zinsser Jr. Subclavian vein obstruction: Report of case studied by venography and relieved by surgery. J.A.M.A. 151: 997, 1953
42. F.M. Howard, S.J. Shafer. Injuries to the clavicula with neurovascular complications. J. Bone and Joint Surg. 47: 1335, 1965
43. E.S.R. Hughes. Venous obstruction in upper extremity (Paget-Von Schrötter's Syndrome). (Review of 320 cases). Surg. Gyn. Obstet. Int Abst. Surg. 88: 127, 1949
44. N.J. Jackson, E.M. Nanson. Intermittent subclavian vein obstruction. Brit. J. Surg. 49: 303, 1961
45. J.A. Kirtlex, R. Kesterson, MacCleery. Subclavian and anterior scalene muscle compression as a cause of intermittent obstruction of the subclavian vein. Ann. of Thorac Surg. 133: 588, 1951
46. S. Kleinberg, M.A. Levine. Headache as a symptom of cervical rib. Ann. Surg. 105: 299, 1937
47. L.J. Kleinsasser. "Effort" thrombosis of axillary and subclavian veins: Analysis of 16 personal cases and 56 cases collected from literature. Arch. Surg. 59: 258, 1949
48. G. Kobinia, H. Denck, F. Olbert, R. Passl, O.J. Russe, S. Szalay, P. Weidinger. Das Paget-Schrötter Syndrom prä- und posttherapeutische befunde. Kongressband "Angiographie International," Baden-Baden. 1976. Personnal communication

49. G.J.E. Lo-A-Njoe. Thoracic outlet compression syndrome. Academisch Proefschrift. Universiteit van Amsterdam. 1974
50. M. Lopes Cardozo. De Behandeling van het Costoclavicular compressie Syndroom door resectie van de eerste rib. Verkrijging van het doctoraat in de geneeskunde aan de Rijksuniversiteit te Groningen (Nederland – 1976)
51. J.W. Lord Jr. "Complications of treatment outlet system." In G.J.B. Beebe, "Complications in Vascular Surg." Lippincott. Company, 1973
52. J.W. Lord, L.M. Rosati, F. Netter. Thoracic outlet syndromes. Clinical symposia. Ciba-Geigy. Corp. R.H. Roberts 23: 3, 1971
53. J.W. Lord Jr., P.W. Stone. Pectoralis minor tenotomy and anterior scalenomy with special reference to hyperabduction syndrome and "effort thrombosis" of subclavian vein. Circulation 13: 537, 1956
54. H. Mahorner. Technique of thrombectomy for massive venous thrombosis Surg. 60: 773, 1966
55. H. Mahorner, J.W. Castleberry, W.O. Coleman. Attempts to restore function in major veins which are site of massive thrombosis. Ann. Surg. 146: 510, 1957
56. C.W. McLaughlin Jr., A.M. Popma. Intermittent obstruction of the subclavian vein. J.A.M.A. 113: 1939, 1960–1963
57. R.S. McCleery, J.E. Kesterson, J.A. Kirtley, R.B. Love. Subclavius and anterior scalene muscle compression as a cause of intermittent obstruction of the subclavian vein. Ann. Surg 133: 588, 1951
58. M.D. McDonough, M.D. Altemeir. Subclavian venous thrombosis secondary to indwelling catheters Surg. Gyn. Obstet. 133: 397, 1971
59. A. Ochsner, M.E. DeBakey, P.T. Decamp, E. Darocha. Thromboembolism analysis of cases at Charity Hospital in New Orleans over a 12 years period. Ann. Surg. 134: 405, 1951
60. J. Paget. Clinical lectures and essays. London. Longmans, Green & Co, 1875
61. J.R. Parienty Michel. Syndrome de Paget-Von Schrötter-Phlébite du membre supérieur dite "d'effort". Ann. Radiol. 8: 331, 1965
62. L. Pedinielli, A. Quilichini, H. Ravelojoana. Les thrombophlébites dites d'"effort" du membre supérieur. A propos de 2 observations. Marseille Med. 105: 365, 1968
63. I. Penn. The vascular complications of fractures of the clavicle. J. Trauma. 4: 819, 1964.
64. R.M. Peet, J.D. Hendricksen, T.P. Anderson, G.M. Martin. Thoracic outlet syndrome: Evaluation of a therapeutic exercise program. Proc. Staff Meet. Mayo Clin. 31: 281, 1956
65. D.B. Roos. Transaxillary approach for first rib resection for relief thoracic outlet syndrome. Ann. Surg. 163: 354, 1966
66. D.B. Roos. Experience with first rib resection for thoracic outlet syndrome. Ann Surg. 173: 429, 1971
67. D.B. Roos, Congenital anomalies associated with thoracic outlet syndrome. Anatomy, Symptoms, Diagnosis, and treatment. Am. J. Surg. 132: 771, 1976
68. D.B. Roos. Transaxillary extrapleural thoracic Sympathectomy. Surgical Techniques Illustrated. 2: 3, 1977
69. D.B. Roos, J.C. Owens. Thoracic outlet syndrome. Arch. Surg. 93: 71, 1966
70. L.M. Rosati, J.W. Lord. Neurovascular compression syndromes of the shoulder girdle. Grune & Stratton. New York. 1961
71. J.J. Sampson, J.B. Sanders, C.S. Capp. Compression of subclavian vein by first rib and clavicle. Am Heart J. 19: 292, 1940
72. H. Schäffer, H.A. Thies. Thrombotischer verschluß der Vena axillaris. Fortschr. Röntgenstr. 86: 268, 1957
73. E. Schepelmann. Demonstration eines Patienten mit Thrombose der linken Vena Subclavia Seltener Aetiologie. Munchen. Med. Wschr. 57: 2444, 1910
74. A. Serradimigni, C. Mercier. Les thromboses veineuses profondes des membres. Masson et Cie., Paris. 146, 1973
75. N.W. Swinton, J.W. Edgett, R.J. Hall. Primary subclavian axillary vein thrombosis. Circulation 38: 737, 1968
76. P. Tagariello. Value of phlebography in the diagnosis of intermittent obstruction of the subclavian vein. J. Int. Coll. Surg. 17: 789, 1952

77. P. Tagariello. L'Ostruzione intermittente della vena subclavia. Omnia. Med. (Pisa). 30: 215, 1952
78. P. Tagariello. Pathogenisis of venous gangrene. J. Cardiovas. Surg. 7: 510, 1966
79. S.A. Taheri. Present status of surgical treatment of thoracic outlet syndrom. Vasc. Surg. 4: 217, 1970
80. N.L. Tilney, H.J.G. Griffiths, E.A. Edwards. Natural history of major venous thrombosis of the upper extremity. Arch. Surg. 101: 792, 1970
81. T.W. Todd. The thoracic operculum; Factors controlling its presence and its size; its bearing on the morphology of the shoulder, with four cases. J. Anat. & Physiol. 46: 244, 1912
82. T.W. Todd. The descent of the shoulder after birth. Its significance in the production of pressure symptoms on the lowest brachial trunk. Anat. Anzeiger. 41: 385, 1913
83. C.E. Tomlin. Pulmonary infarction complicating thrombophlebitis of upper extremity. Amer. J. Med. 12: 411, 1952
84. H.C. Urschel, M.A. Razzuk. Management of the thoracic outlet syndrome. New. Eng. Med. J. 286: 1140, 1972
85. J. Van der Stricht, L. Jeanmart. Les thromboses veineuses du membre superieur. J. Belge Radiol. 48: 539, 1965
86. J. Van der Stricht, M. Goldstein, L. Garcia, M. Ectors. Thrombose veineuse du membre supérieur. Phléologie. 18: 57, 1965
87. J. Van der Stricht, M. Golstein, P. Vanderhoeft. Etiologie et traitement de la thrombose de la veine cave supérieure et de ses branches. Acta Chir. Belg. 68: 564, 1969
88. J.R. Veal, N.J. Cotsonas Jr. Diseases of the superior vena caval systems with special considerations of pathology and diagnosis. Surgery. 31: I, 1952
89. J.R. Veal, H.H. Hussey. Use of "exercise tests" in connection with venous pressure measurements for detection of venous obstruction in upper and lower extremities. Amer. Heart J. 20: 308, 1940
90 L. Von Schrotter. "Erkrankungen der Gefässe" in Nothnagel Handbuch der Pathologie und therapie. Holder, Wien 1884
91. J.R. Wilder, E.T. Habermann, R.L. Nach. Subclavian vein obstruction secondary to hypertrophy of terminal valve. Surgery. 55: 214, 1964
92. I.S. Wright. The neurovascular syndrome produced by hyperabduction of the arms. Am. Heart J. 29: 1, 1945

25. Lesions of the subclavian artery: reconstructive procedures

R.J.A.M. VAN DONGEN M.D.*

ABSTRACT

Only a few lesions of the subclavian artery require a sternotomy, a thoracotomy or another comprehensive approach. In most cases reconstructive surgery is possible by means of an extra-thoracic bypass procedure or by transaxillary approach. The advantages are clear. The operation takes less time and is less comprehensive. The blood loss is small. Muscle cutting and repairing is not required. Closure of the wound is done quickly. There is less postoperative morbidity and the cosmetical results are acceptable.

Pain is a common symptom of vascular insufficiency. The nature and the location of pain may be indicative of the underlying disease (Table 1). In Raynaud's disease it is an intermittent pain largely dependent on temperature. Thoracic outlet compression syndrome is suggested by pain or paresthesia which occurs during activities reaching the arms above the head. The pain caused by arterial occlusion is an ischaemic pain, which always indicates an inadequate supply of arterial blood to contracting muscles. It is an intermittent pain dependent on excercise.

To establish the diagnosis an exact clinical evaluation is important (Table 2). In most cases the diagnosis can be made by careful questioning, palpation of pulses, measurement of blood pressure, auscultation, performance of the different outlet manoeuvers and neurological examination.

Table 1. Common vascular causes of a painful arm.

Spastic	– Raynaud's disease
	Ergot intoxication
Compressive	– Thoracic outlet syndrome
Occlusive	– Arteriosclerosis
	Buerger's disease
	Takayasu's disease

*Wilhelmina Hospital, Amsterdam, the Netherlands.

J.M. Greep, H.A.J. Lemmens, D.B. Roos and H.C. Urschel (eds.).
Pain in shoulder and arm: an integrated view, 281–291. All rights reserved.
Copyright © 1979 by Martinus Nijhoff Publishers, The Hague/Boston/London.

Table 2. Signs of vascular insufficiency.

Pallor
Cyanosis
Gangrene or pre-gangrene
Atrophy of skin, subcutaneous tissue or muscles
Pulse differences
Blood pressure differences
Bruits
Adson, hyperextension and hyperabduction maneuvers

The cause of vascular insufficiency may be elucidated by special procedures as shown in Table 3. Arteriography is indicated, because in many
cases it will be the only manner to find out or to verify the exact diagnosis
and especially to be acquainted with the site and extension of the arterial
obstruction or compression. This applies also to the lesions of the subclavian artery.

Table 3. Procedures to elucidate the
cause of vascular insufficiency.

Cold stimulation
Oscillography
Plethysmography
Phonoangiography
Measurement of venous pressure
Plan x-ray study
Angiography
Electromyography
Nerve conduction study

ANATOMIC CONSIDERATIONS

With a view to the application of the different reconstructive procedures
some anatomical considerations are important. We divide the subclavian
artery into four segments (Figure 1):

The first part extends from the origin of the subclavian artery to a point
just proximal to the origins of the vertebral and internal thoracic arteries.

The second segment is the portion of the artery where the vertebral and
internal thoracic arteries arise.

The third portion is the segment between the origin of the thyrocervical
trunc and the costoclavicular space. This is the supraclavicular segment.

The fourth part is the costoclavicular segment; it is located in the space
between the clavicle and the first rib.

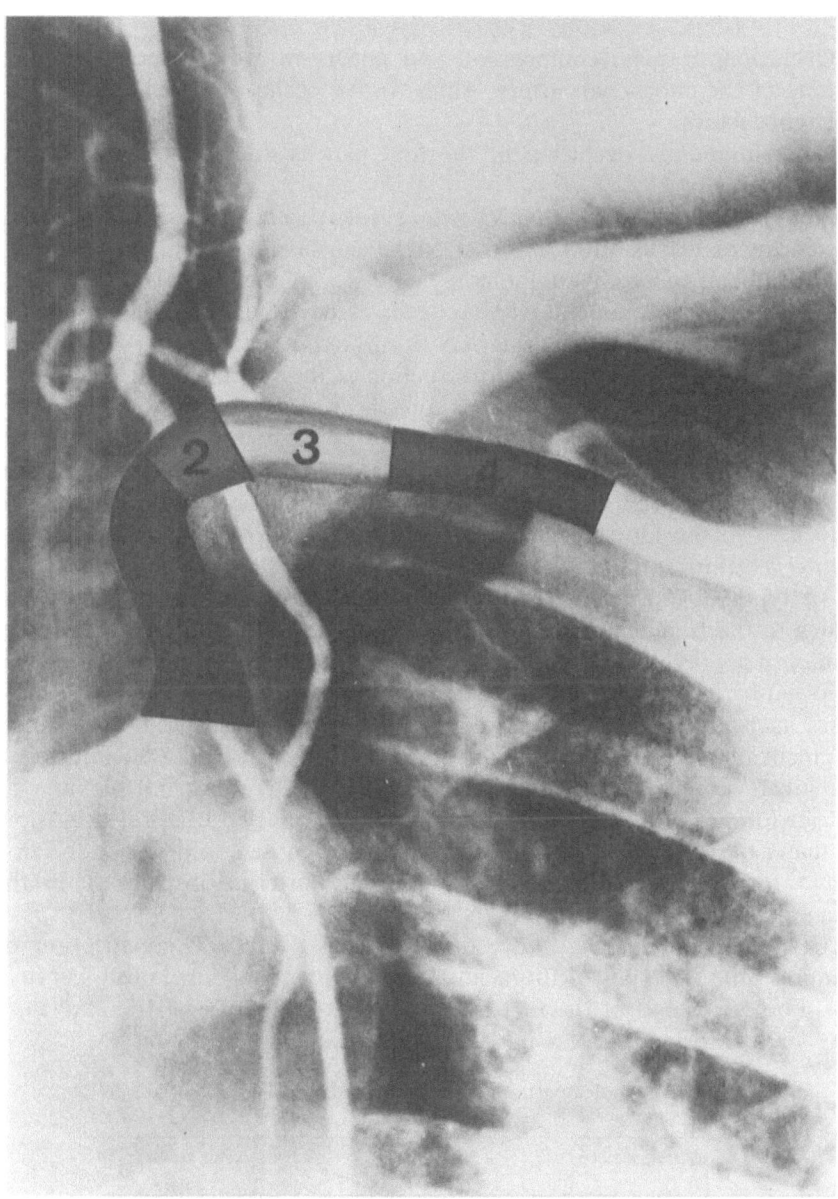

Figure 1. The subclavian artery can be divided into four segments (see text).

LESIONS OF THE SUBCLAVIAN ARTERY

Occlusion, trauma, compression and aneurysm are the most common lesions of the subclavian artery (Table 4). An occlusion can be caused by different factors.

– Most frequently occlusion of the first part is due to arterio sclerotic disease.
– Non-specific arteritis, better known as Takayashu's disease, may cause a stenosis or occlusion of any part of the subclavian artery.
– Thrombosis caused by radiotherapy for cancer of the breast is seldom seen. We observed four patients with occlusion of the distal part of the subclavian artery and the entire axillary artery due to radiotherapy.
– Ergot intoxication can cause obstruction of the subclavian artery, but in most cases the brachial artery and the arteries of the fore-arm are affected.
– Costoclavicular compression is seen at a point where the clavicle crosses the first rib. Occlusion due to this type of thoracic outlet syndrome is located in the fourth segment of the subclavian artery and may extend into the third part.

All types of blunt and penetrating trauma have the capacity to cause injury to the subclavian arteries. These injuries include laceration, transection, intimal avulsion, contusion and thrombosis. Less often trauma is followed by formation of a false aneurysm of the subclavian artery. In most cases such an aneurysm is secundary to a laceration, caused by a sharp fragment of the broken clavicle or first rib. Many patients with injuries of the subclavian artery have an associated lesion of the brachial plexus.

Clot formation in such an aneurysm may be followed by total occlusion. In many patients the aneurysm itself is not diagnosed before, but the first signs are the ischemic symptoms of an acute arterial obstruction in the arm.

Arterial aneurysms may arise distal to sites of arterial constriction or compression. All types of thoracic outlet compression – including cervical ribs, bony exostosis of the first rib, a mal-united fracture of the clavicle – may lead to formation of a post-stenotic subclavian aneurysm.

Table 4. Diagram demonstrating the causes and complications of lesions of the subclavian artery.

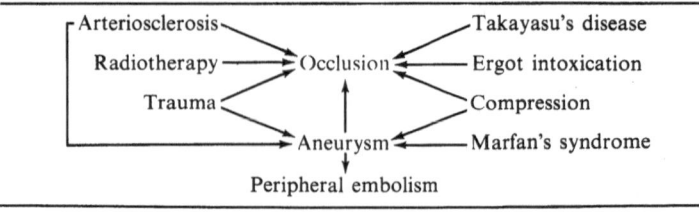

Occlusion by clot formation in the aneurysm may occur, and major gangrene of the arm has been reported, but more frequently the mural thrombus fragments and lodges in distal vessels causing peripheral embolic occlusion.

Formation of subclavian aneurysms may of course be due to arteriosclerotic disease, but this hardly happens.

Lastly aneurysms of the subclavian artery may occur in patients with other lesions of the vessel walls, for instance in Marfan's disease. All these aneurysms may also lead to occlusion or result in peripheral embolic complications.

APPROACH TO THE SUBCLAVIAN ARTERY; RECONSTRUCTIVE PROCEDURES

Many approaches have been suggested for exploring and reconstructing the subclavian artery. The clavicular part of the subclavian artery can be reached by a supraclavicular incision, but this incision is inadequate to perform a resection of an aneurysm or occluded arterial segment and to replace it by a graft. The most common approaches are median sternotomy, thoracotomy, combination of supraclavicular incision and thoracotomy and other extensive operative approaches.

In our experience such comprehensive approaches are seldom necessary. In most cases lesions of the subclavian artery can be treated in a more simple way.

In occlusions of the first portion of the left subclavian artery several different techniques can be used. It is possible to resect the occluded segment and to replace it by a prosthesis, or the occluded segment can be bypassed by a Dacron graft between the descending aorta and the subclavian artery beyond the occlusion. Endarterectomy and patch graft angioplasty is a third possibility for the correction of this kind of occlusion. In all these cases a left-sided thoracotomy is required and the descending aorta must be clamped off by means of a tangentially applied clamp.

More simple and less extensive is the extrathoracic procedure with insertion of a Dacron or venous graft between the left common carotid artery and the midportion of the subclavian artery. Only a simple supraclavicular incision is needed. The results are equally good and morbidity is less than after transthoracic procedures. There are no objections to this kind of reconstruction. There is no reason to be afraid of a new steal phenomenon, except in cases with associated stenosis of the origin of the left common carotid artery. Also in such cases both lesions can be corrected by extrathoracic approach. With the help of one prosthesis or venous transplant between the right common carotid artery and the left common carotid and subclavian arteries a complete correction is achieved in a simple manner (Figure 2).

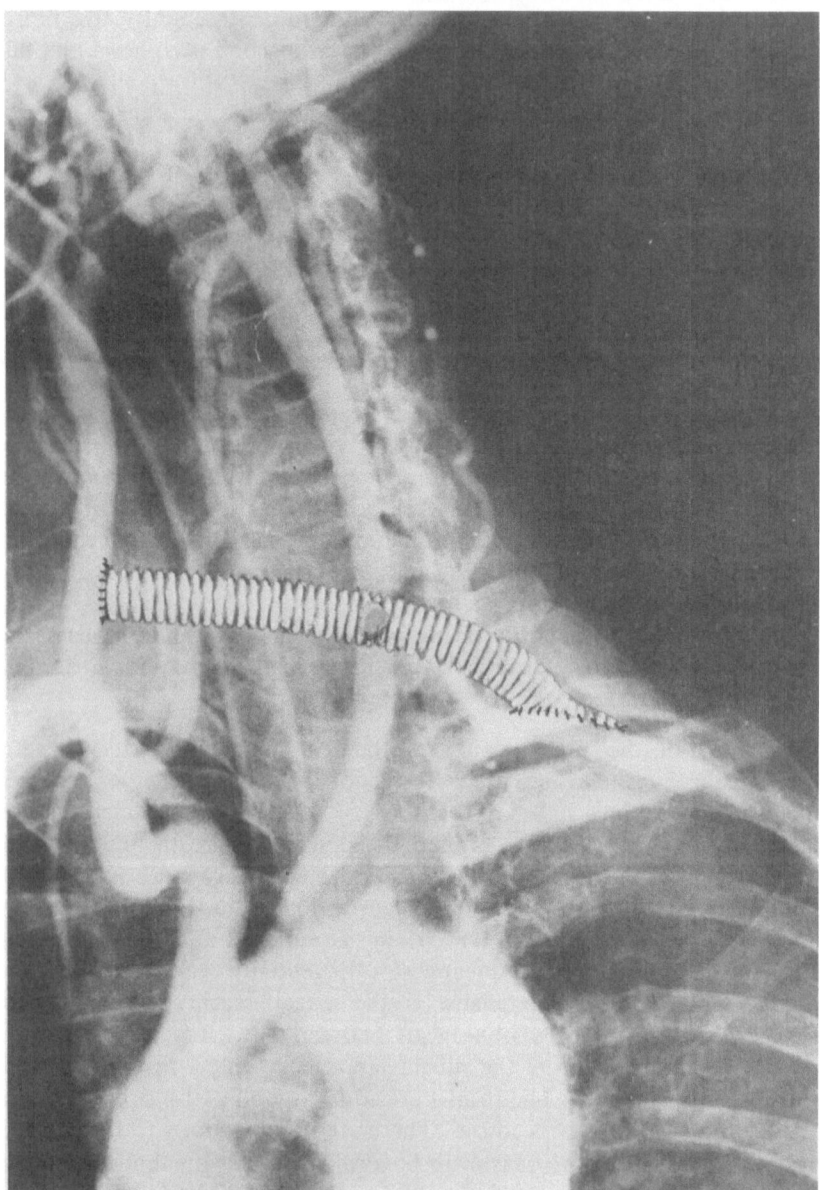

Figure 2. Total occlusion of the first part of the left subclavian artery and subtotal occlusion of the initial part of the left common carotid artery. Reconstruction with the help of one prosthesis between right common carotid artery and left common carotid and subclavian arteries.

Finally a subclavian-subclavian bypass graft can be inserted using an autogenous vein or a prosthetic graft. This also is an effective method for correction of the left-sided subclavian steal syndrome, especially in poor risk patients.

The proximal part of the right subclavian artery can be approached by a median plane sternotomy, after which the occlusion can be treated by endarterectomy and patch graft angioplasty. This technique requires clamping off the common carotid and innominate arteries because the arteriotomy must be continued into the wall of the innominate artery. For this reason an intraarterial shunt is used to be certain that the bloodflow to the brain will not be impaired.

There are two alternative techniques using an extrathoracic approach. In many cases it is possible to make an end-to-side anastomosis between the second part of the subclavian artery and the right common carotid artery, the first being transected just beyond the occlusion. On the other hand a bypass graft can be inserted between the second part of the subclavian artery and the common carotid artery. Either of these operations can be safely carried out using an extra-thoracic supraclavicular approach. From a haemodynamic point of view there are no problems to use the common carotid artery as a common trunk. Lord and Ehrenfeld have demonstrated that any of the brachiocephalic vessels can sustain a sixfold increase in blood flow. Therefore, the proximal portion of anyone of the four brachiocephalic vessels could serve as a common trunk for the distal segments of at least two of the four vessels.

The conventional procedures of approaching the second, third and fourth portion of the subclavian artery make use of supraclavicular or infraclavicular incisions in combination with clavicular resection and other comprehensive approaches. Moreover the first rib must be resected to prevent compression of the reconstructed vessel or the bypass graft.

All these are traumatic approaches. The procedures are risky because proximal control may be difficult, and the shoulder morbidity may be severe.

The transaxillary approach is much better and more convenient. We have used this technique in more than forty cases of stenoses, occlusions and aneurysms of the midportion and distal part of the subclavian artery and in all cases there were no technical problems. After resection of the first rib it was always possible to dissect free the subclavian artery up to the first segment. In all cases we were able to apply clamps on the proximal part of the subclavian artery and on the vertebral artery, and to pass loops of mersilene around the other branches of the subclavian artery for haemostatic control. This technique has been suggested by Roos in 1966 in his first publication dealing with the trans axillary approach for first rib resection

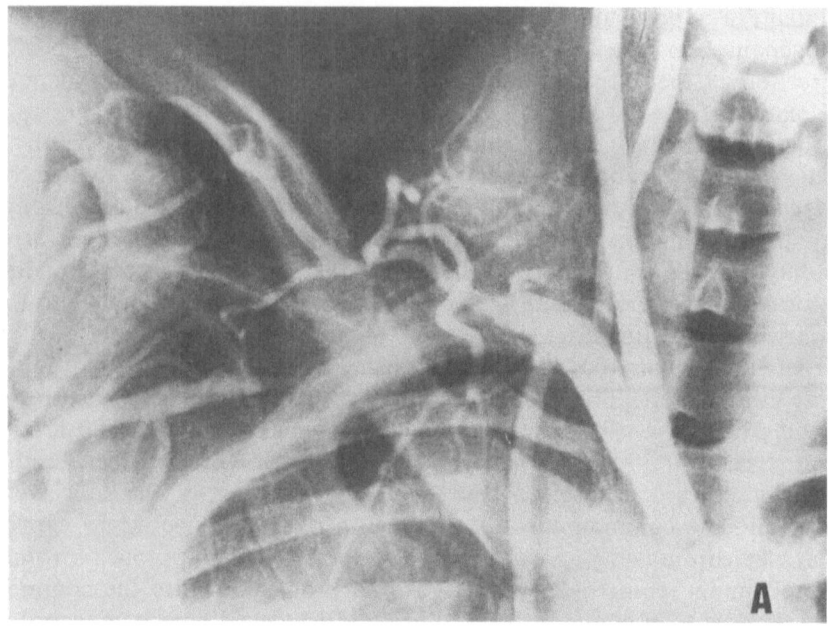

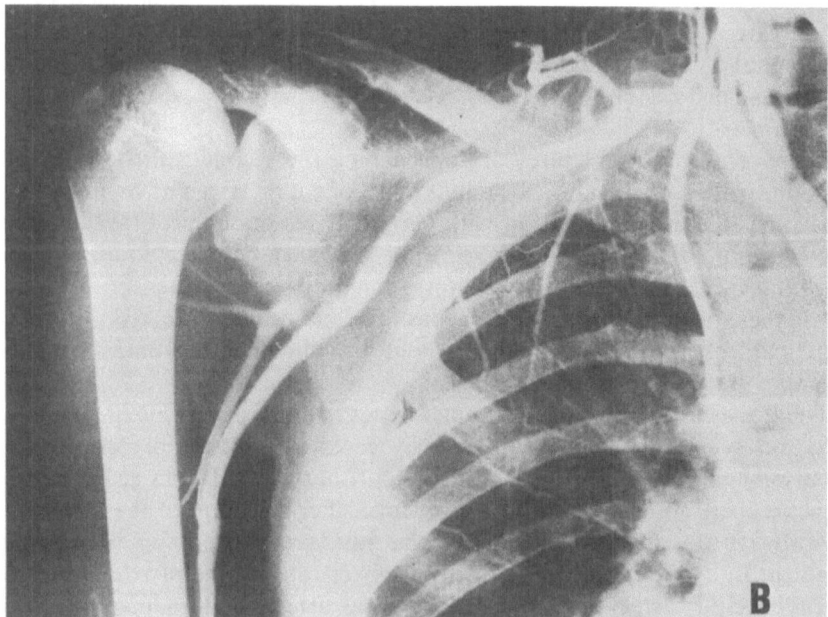

Figure 3A. Occlusion of the third and fourth segments of the right subclavian artery treated by venous bypass graft.
    B. Post-operative angiogram.

and in the same year he reported about one patient with an occluded aneurysm of the subclavian artery, treated by resection and Dacron prosthesis replacement, using this approach. It is amazing, that this technique in the reconstructive treatment of subclavian artery lesions is so rarely mentioned in literature.

In reconstructive surgery of the subclavian artery we prefer the use of autogenous veins (Figures 3a and b). A Dacron prosthesis is used only when it concerns an aneurysmatic formation of a large-sized artery. If the subclavian artery is of normal size and no suitable vein is available, we sometimes use a P.T.F.E. graft.

Most occlusions of the subclavian artery are caused by thoracic outlet compression, especially costoclavicular compression. Reconstructive surgery is necessary for two reasons. First to relieve the complaints caused by the arterial occlusion, and second to prevent proximal extension of the thrombosis. Such an extension may occlude the origins of the vertebral and even the right carotid artery and thereby interfering with cerebral blood flow. Distal spread of the thrombus may lead to severe ischaemic complaints and even to gangrene of the fingers.

There may be some problems in patients with Takayashu's disease. The artery proximal to the stenosed or occluded segment may be thick-walled and it may be difficult to reach a normal central part of the artery. In some patients with occlusion of the third and fourth portion of the subclavian artery due to Takayashu's disease it is not possible to reach a normal and suitable proximal subclavian artery. In such cases a bypass may be inserted between the aortic arch and the axillary artery, using a combination of sternotomy and distal infraclavicular incision. But there is in such cases a more simple method of reconstruction. Complete revascularisation of the arm can be achieved by means of a venous bypass between the common carotid artery and the axillary artery beyond the occlusion of the subclavian artery.

And now some examples of aneurysm of the subclavian artery. The first patient was admitted because of multiple peripheral embolic occlusions (Figure 4a). The source of the emboli was not known, but the X-ray picture showed a cervical rib. So we assumed the presence of a poststenotic aneurysm of the subclavian artery. This was confirmed by arteriography (Figure 4b). It was a small-sized aneurysm, just beyond the crossing first rib. Through a transaxillary approach the first rib was resected together with the cervical rib. The aneurysm has been removed and the artery restored by means of a Dacron graft. The opened aneurysm showed some small mural thrombus formation.

The same approach and technique is used in patients with arteriosclerotic aneurysms of the subclavian artery and aneurysms due to Marfan's disease. There are no technical problems with the proximal control in such

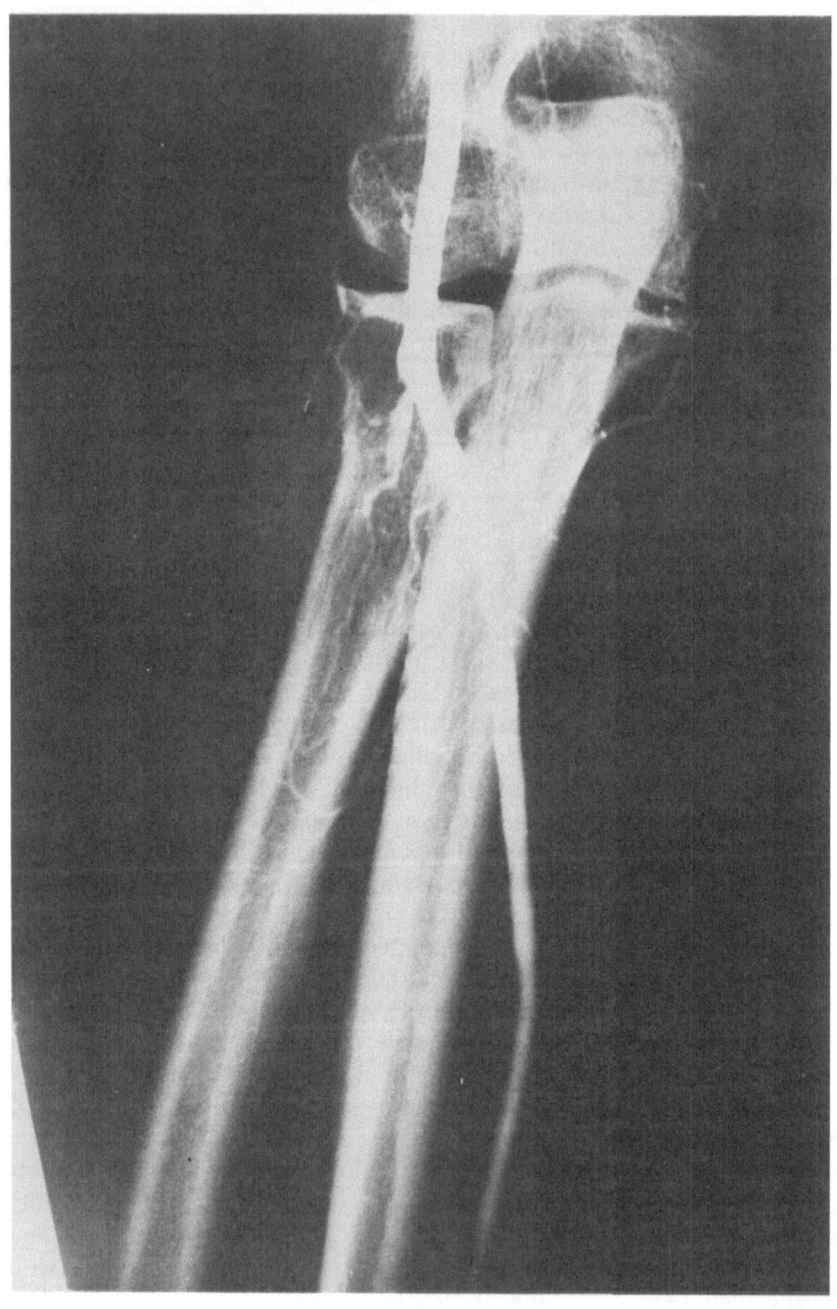

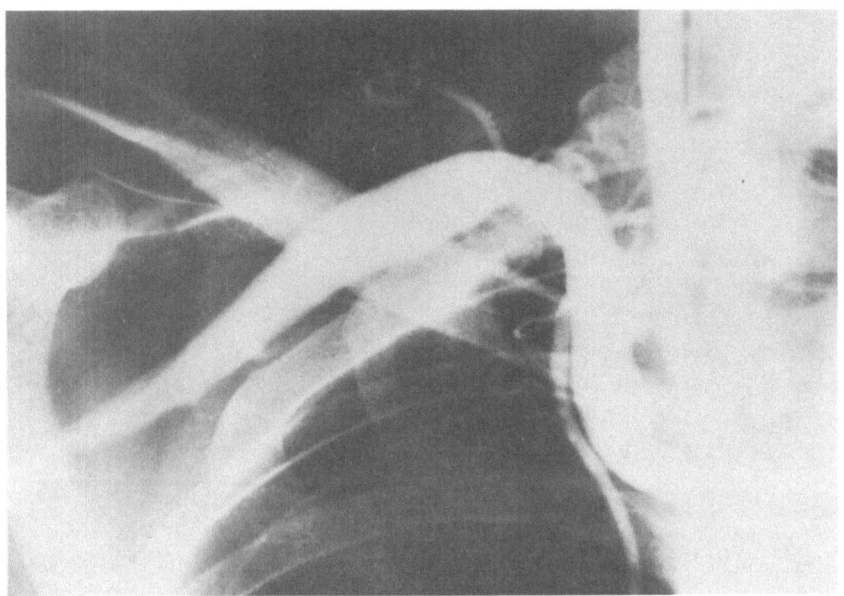

Figure 4*A*. Embolic occlusion of the radial artery.
  B. The emboli are coming from a post-stenotic aneurysm of the subclavian artery.

cases. In all patients resection and reconstruction could be performed safely by transaxillary approach.

REFERENCES

1. R.S.A. Lord, W.K. Ehrenfeld. Carotid-subclavian bypass: a hemodynamic study. Surgery 66: 521, 1969
2. D.B. Roos. Transaxillary approach for first rib resection to relieve thoracic outlet syndrome. Ann. Surg. 163: 354, 1966
3. D.B. Roos, J.C. Owens. Thoracic outlet syndrome. Arch. Surg. 93: 71, 1966

26. Operative management of vascular injuries of the thoracic outlet

J.M. GREEP M.D., Ph.D. AND
A.R. SMITH M.D., Ph.D.*

ABSTRACT

Vascular injuries of the thoracic outlet are rare. In the United States, injuries are mostly inflicted by gunshot or knife-wounds. In the Netherlands by falls from a bicycle or motorcycle. The experience with vascular injuries of the thoracic outlet will be presented. Plan of management emphasized an operative approach allows for rapid control after good exposure of the major vessels to the involved upper extremity. A median sternotomy was used for exposure and repair of a lesion of the right subclavian artery. A left anterior thoracotomy was used for control and exposure of the left sublcavian artery.

MATERIAL

Two patients were presented to the emergency-ward with hypotension after trauma to the thoracic outlet. In both cases uncontrollable intra-thoracic bleeding was the indication for exploration. In the patient with a lesion of the right subclavian artery there was no palpable pulse distal to the side of the injury. The patient with the left sided lesion had an entrance wound under the left clavicula. No arteriographies were made. Chest X-ray showed a hemothorax in both patients. Both patients were in rather unstable condition despite of volume replacement. The patient with the lesion of the right subclavian artery was managed with a median sternotomy extended into the soft tissue of the right side of the neck (Figure 1A, B, C, D.). A left thoracotomy was used in the patient with the left subclavian vessel injury (Figure 2A, B, C.). The patient with the right sided lesion had a considerable damage of the vessel due to fracture of the clavicula; resection of the vessel and end-to-end anastomosis was attempted but a synthetic graft was necessary for interposition (Figure 1D.). On the left side an end-to-end anastomosis could easily be established. The clavicula fracture on the right side was stabilized with an AO-compression plate with four screws. There was no associated neurologic injury. In the patient with the left sided lesion primary vein repair of the subclavian vein was also performed. There were no postoperative complications except for a delayed union of the clavicula.

*St. Annadal Hospital, Maastricht, The Netherlands.

J.M. Greep, H.A.J. Lemmens, D.B. Roos and H.C. Urschel (eds.).
Pain in shoulder and arm: an integrated view, 293–299. All rights reserved.
Copyright © 1979 by Martinus Nijhoff Publishers, The Hague/Boston/London.

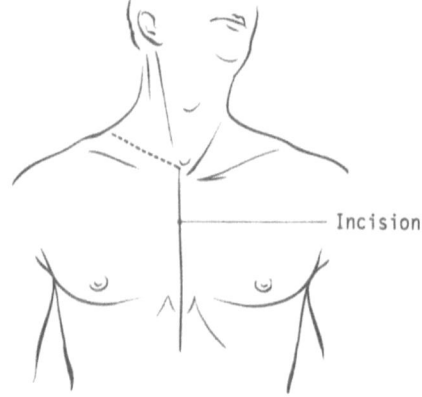

Figure 1*A*.

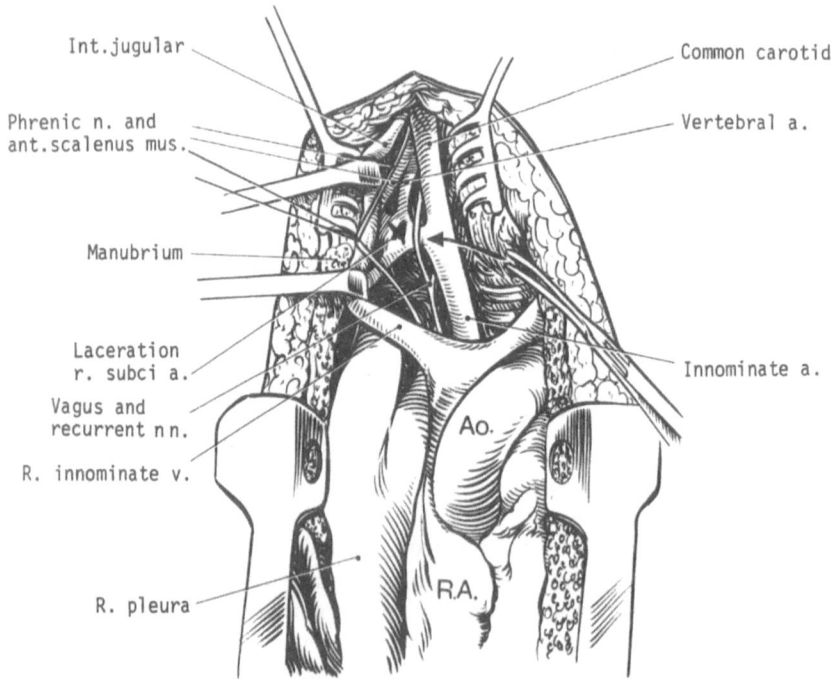

Figure 1*B*.

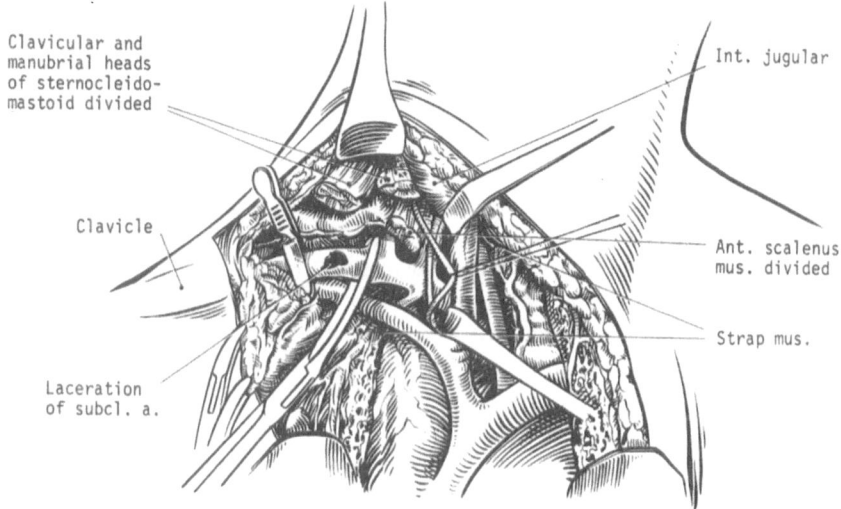

Figure 1*C*.

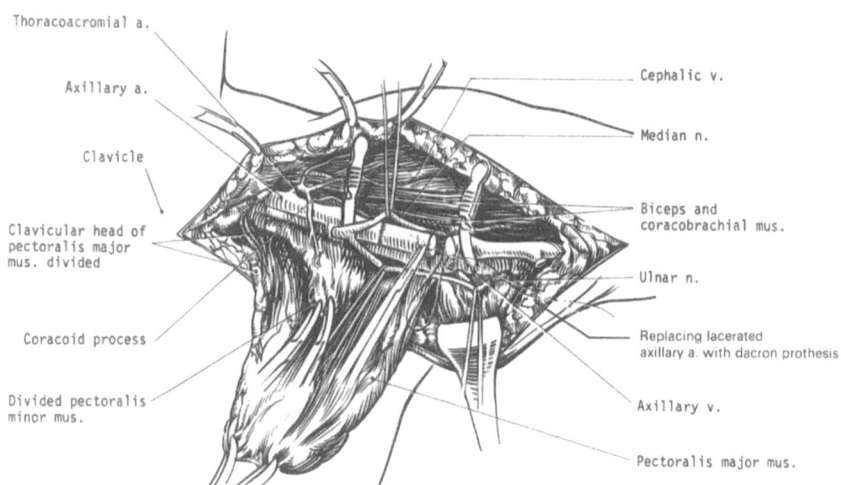

Figure 1*D*.

Both arteries were patent after re-examination in the out-patient clinic.

DETAILED CASE REPORTS

Case I (Figures 1A, B, C and D)

A 42-year old female was brought to the emergency-ward of the St. Luke's Hospital, Amsterdam, in October 1974, suffering from a fall from a bicycle on the right shoulder. Blood pressure was 90/40 mm Hg, heart rate of 140 beats/minute. Fracture of the right clavicula was easily noticed. Brachial and radial pulses in the right arm were faint. Despite volume replacement with hemacel and blood, patient remainded hypotensive. An X-ray showed a hematothorax and the patient was rushed to the operating-room where a median sternotomy was performed. The injury to the right subclavian artery was identified. First resection and primary anastomosis was tried, but the condition of the vessel did not allow primary anastomosis because of intimal tear. Not only the right subclavian artery, but also the pleura was punctured. A Dacron prosthesis of 6 cm, ($\emptyset$ 8 mm) was performed. The blood in the chest was evacuated and the chest drained. The patient did well. The fracture of the right clavicula was stabilized with an AO-compression plate.

Case II (Figures 2A, B and C)

The second patient, J.M., man of 42 years was brought to the emergency-ward of the St. Luke's Hospital, following a trauma to the left supra-clavicular area after collision with his motor cycle. A small wound over the left supraclavicular area was noticed. Vital signs were unstable. Chest X-ray showed a large hematothorax with suprapulmonic hematoma. The patient was taken to the operating room for subclavian artery exploration by an anterolateral thoracotomy. Lesions of the subclavian artery and vein were controlled. It was difficult to expose the distal left subclavian artery. The injured artery portion was excised. End-to-end reconstruction of the artery was performed, and pulses were restored. The vein lesion was easily repaired. The post-operative course was uneventful.

DISCUSSION

Injuries to the vascular structures of the thoracic outlet are uncommon. Recently Schaff and Brawley (1977) presented their 5-years experience with 20 patients who had penetrating vascular injuries of the thoracic outlet all presented to the emergency-ward of the Johns Hopkins Hospital. Drapanas

(1970) presented 226 cases of arterial wounds in civilian practice. Only in the 28 cases, lesions of the subclavian and axillary vessels were presented. All these wounds were accompanied by serious uncontrollable hemorrhage into the chest toward the clavicular area. In our 2 cases both required

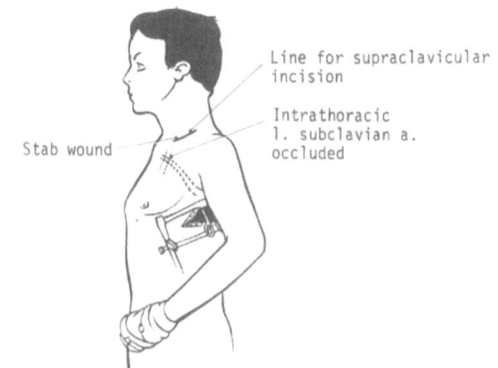

Figure 2*A*.

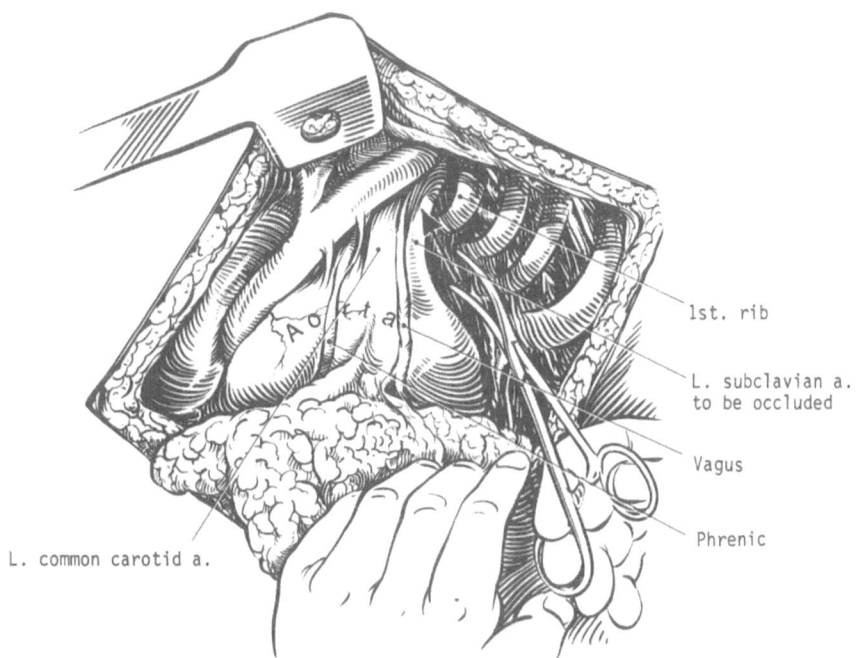

Figure 2*B*.

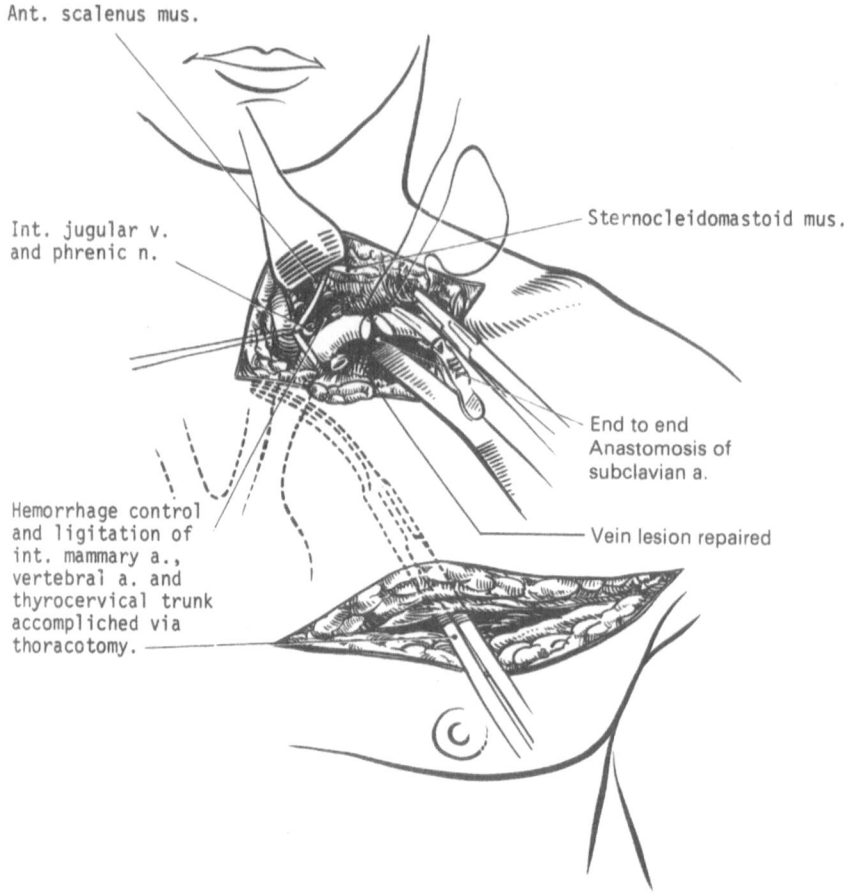

Ant. scalenus mus.

Int. jugular v.
and phrenic n.

Sternocleidomastoid mus.

End to end
Anastomosis of
subclavian a.

Hemorrhage control
and ligitation of
int. mammary a.,
vertebral a. and
thyrocervical trunk
accompliched via
thoracotomy.

Vein lesion repaired

Figure 2C.

prompt evaluation and surgical approach and rapid control of the bleeding. Both patients were transported quickly to the operating room, in order to get manual compression of the vessels within the chest. Emergency sternotomy and thoracotomy were performed. In both cases it was impossible to perform a pre-operative arteriography, which is normally used for the operative approach to vascular wounds. Hunt et al. amended already in 1969 median sternotomy for the exposures of the right subclavian artery. Brawley et al. recommended in 1970 anterolateral thoracotomy for exposure of the left subclavian artery and vein. This technique was used in the management of our second patient. There were no neurologic problems in both patients, but in the recent series of Schaff and Brawley (1977), inflicted by penetrating vascular injuries, at least 5 patients had brachial plexus injury with radial or ulnar nerve palsy.

SUMMARY

The operative management of 2 patients with vascular injuries of the thoracic outlet was presented. A median sternotomy with extension into the right neck was used to explore a patient with a right subclavian vascular injury caused by a fracture of the clavicula. The injury to the left subclavian vessel was explored through a left anterolateral thoracotomy. Both arteries were repaired and patent on follow-up examination. Associated venous injuries were dealt with on the left side. Both approaches gave an adequate exposure and good vessel control in our two patients.

REFERENCES

1. R.K. Brawley, G.F. Murray, C. Crisler et al. Management of wounds of the innominate, subclavian and axillary blood vessels. Surg. Gynecol. Obstet. 131: 1130, 1970
2. T. Drapanas, R.L. Hewitt, R.F. Weichut, et al. Civilian vascular injuries. A critical appraisal of three decades of management. Ann. surg. 172: 351, 1970
3. T.K. Hunt, F.W. Blaisdell, J. Okimoto. Vascular injuries of the base of the neck. Arch. surg. 98: 586, 1969
4. H.V. Schaff, R.K. Brawley. Operative management of penetrating vascular injuries of the thoracic outlet. Surgery 82: 182, 1977

Index of subjects